METHODS IN MOLECULAR BIOLOGY™

Series Editor
John M. Walker
School of Life Sciences
University of Hertfordshire
Hatfield, Hertfordshire, AL10 9AB, UK

For other titles published in this series, go to
www.springer.com/series/7651

Immunocytochemical Methods and Protocols

Third Edition

Edited by

Constance Oliver and Maria Célia Jamur

Department of Cell and Molecular Biology and Pathogenic Bioagents, Faculdade de Medicina de Ribeirão Preto, University of São Paulo, Ribeirão Preto, SP, Brazil

Humana Press

Editors
Constance Oliver
Department of Cell and Molecular Biology
and Pathogenic Bioagents
Faculdade de Medicina de Ribeirão Preto
University of São Paulo
Ribeirão Preto, SP
Brazil
coliver@fmrp.usp.br

Maria Célia Jamur
Department of Cell and Molecular Biology
and Pathogenic Bioagents
Faculdade de Medicina de Ribeirão Preto
University of São Paulo
Ribeirão Preto, SP
Brazil
mjamur1@aol.com

ISSN 1064-3745 e-ISSN 1940-6029
ISBN 978-1-58829-463-0 e-ISBN 978-1-59745-324-0
DOI 10.1007/978-1-59745-324-0
Springer New York Dordrecht Heidelberg London

Library of Congress Control Number: 2009942530

1st edition: Edited by Lorette C. Javois and is Volume 34 of the *Methods in Molecular Biology series*

Printed on acid-free paper

Human Press is part of Springer Science+Business Media (www.springer.com)

Preface

Antibodies tagged with fluorescent markers have been used in histochemistry for over 50 years. Although early applications were focused on the detection of microbial antigens in tissues, the use of immunocytochemical methods now has spread to include the detection of a wide array of antigens including proteins, carbohydrates, and lipids from virtually any organism. Today, immunohistochemistry is widely used to identify, in situ, various components of cells and tissues in both normal and pathological conditions. The method gains its strength from the extremely sensitive interaction of a specific antibody with its antigen. For some scientific areas, books have been published on applications of immunocytochemical techniques specific to that area.

What distinguished *Immunocytochemical Methods and Protocols* from earlier books when it was first published was its broad appeal to investigators across all disciplines, including those in both research and clinical settings. The methods and protocols presented in the first edition were designed to be general in their application; the accompanying "Notes" provided the reader with invaluable assistance in adapting or troubleshooting the protocols. These strengths continued to hold true for the second edition and again for the third edition. Since the publication of the first edition, the application of immunocytochemical techniques in the clinical laboratory has continued to rise and this third edition provides methods that are applicable to basic research as well as to the clinical laboratory. The third edition also provides sites for resources that are available on the Internet. As with the previous editions, chapters providing overviews of selected topics related to immunocytochemistry are interspersed throughout the book.

Immunocytochemical Methods and Protocols, Third Edition, begins with an overview of the use of antibodies in immunocytochemistry followed by methods for purifying and conjugating them for use in immunostaining protocols. The next set of protocols details the fixation and preparation, including antigen retrieval, of tissues and cells for light microscopic immunostaining. Various methods for the use and detection of fluorescently labeled antibodies are then given. The confocal microscope and laser-microbeam applications are discussed in detail. This section is followed by protocols used for immunodetection by bright field microscopy. The use of enzyme-conjugated antibodies and colloidal gold to localize antigens in a variety of preparations is considered at length. The following section concentrates on the preparation and staining of cells for flow cytometry using a fluorescence-activated cell sorter (FACS). This section is followed by protocols detailing the preparation and use of colloidal gold for immunostaining samples for transmission electron microscopy. The final section of the book focuses on the clinical laboratory, where regulations and troubleshooting guidelines are discussed. Many of the special applications discussed here are normally limited to applications within a specific area, and not given within the context of a broader work devoted to immunocytochemical methods and protocols. By bringing these methods together in a single volume, it enables both researchers and clinicians to be well informed about their options when considering an immunohistochemical approach.

We are deeply indebted to the authors of the various chapters in the first and second editions as well as to the additional authors who contributed to this edition, for their interest in this work. We appreciate all of the authors' hard work, dedication, and willingness to share their expertise. The authors are experts in their respective areas and routinely use these protocols in their own laboratories. With the "Notes" that the authors have provided, they share the details of each protocol that make the method work successfully in any laboratory. We would also like to thank Dr. John Walker, *Methods in Molecular Biology* series editor, for his help and encouragement throughout the process of compiling this third edition. Final thanks go to David Casey and the staff of Humana Press for making this book a reality.

Constance Oliver
Maria Célia Jamur

Contents

Part III Light Microscopic Detection Systems

Part IV Fluorescence-Activated Cell Sorter (FACS) Analyses

Part V Colloidal Gold Detection Systems for Electron Microscopic Analysis

Part VI The Clinical Laboratory

Contributors

ANDREA ABATI • *Laboratory of Pathology, Cytopathology Section, National Cancer Institute, National Institutes of Health, Bethesda, MD, USA*

DENIS BASKIN • *Division of Endocrinology/Metabolism, VA Puget Sound Health Care System, Seattle, WA, USA*

L. SCOT BASTIAN • *Division of Endocrinology/Metabolism, VA Puget Sound Health Care System, Seattle, WA, USA*

ELSA BERENSTEIN • *Receptors and Signal Transduction Section, Oral Infection and Immunity Branch, National Institute of Dental and Craniofacial Research, National Institutes of Health, Bethesda, MD, USA*

GARY L. BRATTHAUER • *Department of Gynecologic and Breast Pathology, Armed Forces Institute of Pathology, Washington, DC, USA*

ROBERT E. CUNNINGHAM • *Department of Biophysics, Armed Forces Institute of Pathology, Washington, DC, USA*

PATRICIA A. FETSCH • *Laboratory of Pathology, Cytopathology Section, National Cancer Institute, National Institutes of Health, Bethesda, MD, USA*

ANA CRISTINA GRODZKI • *Receptors and Signal Transduction Section, Oral Infection and Immunity Branch, National Institute of Dental and Craniofacial Research, National Institutes of Health, Bethesda, MD, USA*

ELAINE S. JAFFE • *Laboratory of Pathology, Hematopathology Section, National Cancer Institute, National Institutes of Health, Bethesda, MD, USA*

MARIA CÉLIA JAMUR • *Department of Cell and Molecular Biology and Pathogenic Bioagents, Faculdade de Medicina de Ribeirão Preto, University of São Paulo, Ribeirão Preto, SP, Brazil*

LASZLO KRENACS • *Laboratory of Tumor Pathology and Molecular Diagnostics, Bay Zoltan Foundation for Applied Research, Szeged, Hungary*

TIBOR KRENACS • *1st Department of Pathology and Experimental Cancer Research, Semmelweis University, Budapest, Hungary*

ELAINE VICENTE LOURENÇO • *Department of Cell and Molecular Biology, Faculdade de Medicina de Ribeirão Preto, University of São Paulo, Ribeirão Preto, SP, Brazil*

LUCIANA CLAUDIA HERCULANO MACHADO • *Department of Cell and Molecular Biology, Faculdade de Medicina de Ribeirão Preto, University of São Paulo, Ribeirão Preto, SP, Brazil*

LIVIA MARIA ROSATTO MODA • *Department of Cell and Molecular Biology, Faculdade de Medicina deRibeirão Preto, University of São Paulo, Ribeirão Preto, SP, Brazil*

SU-YAU MAO • *Gaithersburg, MD, USA*

J. MICHAEL MULLINS • *Department of Biology, The Catholic University of America, Washington, DC, USA*

CONSTANCE OLIVER • *Department of Cell and Molecular Biology and Pathogenic Bioagents, Faculdade de Medicina de Ribeirão Preto, University of São Paulo, Ribeirão Preto, SP, Brazil*

MARIA VERONICA DÁVILA PÁSTOR • *Universidade do Vale do Itajaí-UNIVALI, Centro de Ciências da Saúde, Itájaí, SC, Brazil*

P. SCOTT PINE • *Division of Applied Pharmacology and Research, Center for Drug Evaluation and Research, Food and Drug Administration, Silver Spring, MD, USA*

MARK RAFFELD • *Laboratory of Pathology, Hematopathology Section, National Cancer Institute, National Institutes of Health, Bethesda, MD, USA*

RICARDO GUELERMAN PINHEIRO RAMOS • *Department of Cell and Molecular Biology, Faculdade de Medicina de Ribeirão Preto, University of São Paulo, Ribeirão Preto, SP, Brazil*

MARIA-CRISTINA ROQUE-BARREIRA • *Department of Cell and Molecular Biology, Faculdade de Medicina de Ribeirão Preto, University of São Paulo, Ribeirão Preto, SP, Brazil*

EVA STELKOVICS • *Laboratory of Tumor Pathology and Molecular Diagnostics, Bay Zoltan Foundation for Applied Research, Szeged, Hungary*

WILLIAM D. SWAIM • *Molecular Physiology and Therapeutics Branch, National Institute of Dental and Craniofacial Research, National Institutes of Health, Bethesda, MD, USA*

MARK C. WILLINGHAM • *Department of Pathology, Wake Forest University School of Medicine, Winston-Salem, NC, USA*

Part I

Antibody Preparation

Chapter 1

Overview of Antibodies for Immunochemistry

Constance Oliver and Maria Célia Jamur

Abstract

Immunohistochemistry is widely used to identify, in situ, various components of cells and tissues in both normal and pathological conditions and is an exceptionally powerful method to demonstrate the localization of cellular components. Immunoglobulins (antibodies) are glycoproteins and are divided into five major classes. IgG, which composes approximately 75% of the immunoglobulins in human serum, is most commonly used for immunostaining. Two types of detection systems, fluorescent and enzyme based are used for immunostaining. The choice of detection system depends on the type of sample and the availability of fluorescent or bight field microscopes as well as the type of information the investigator would like to obtain. This chapter provides an overview of antibody characteristics, and their use in immunostaining.

Key words: Immunohistochemistry, Fluorescence microscopy, IgG, Primary antibody, Secondary antibody, Monoclonal antibody, Polyclonal antibody, Fluorochrome

1. Introduction

Immunohistochemistry is widely used to identify, in situ, various components of cells and tissues in both normal and pathological conditions (1–4). It is an exceptionally powerful method to demonstrate the localization of cellular components. Immunohistochemistry or immunocytochemistry derives its name from the root "immuno," in reference to antibodies used in the procedure, and "histo," meaning tissue or "cyto" meaning cell. Immunohistochemistry is based on the extremely sensitive interaction of a specific antibody (immunoglobulin) with its antigen. A given antibody binds specifically only to a small site on its antigen, called an epitope. An epitope usually consists of 1–6 monosaccarides or 5–8 amino acids. The epitope recognized by a specific antibody can be the linear primary sequence of a protein or it may consist of various sites on a molecule that are in

C. Oliver and M.C. Jamur (eds.), *Immunocytochemical Methods and Protocols*, Methods in Molecular Biology, Vol. 588, DOI 10.1007/978-1-59745-324-0_1, © Humana Press, a part of Springer Science+Business Media, LLC 1995, 1999, 2010

close proximity when the antigen is in its three-dimensional conformation. This is the reason that some antibodies work very well on living cells, but do not bind to fixed cells or do not function for Western blots. Although most commonly used antibodies are against proteins, antibodies can be raised against any cellular component including nucleic acids, lipids and carbohydrates. Today a wide variety of antibodies is commercially available. The supplier of an antibody against a particular antigen can be found by searching the scientific literature, searching the world wide web either by using a search engine such as Google or through a search engine linked to a commercial site such as Abcam's World's Antibody Gateway (http://www.abcam.com), by searching a site dedicated to immunohistochemisty such as ICH World (http://www.ichworld.com) or by searching Linscott's Directory of Immunological and Biological Reagents (http://www.linscotts-directory.com). Alternatively, antibodies can be obtained from a friend or a colleague or produced in the laboratory. Whatever the source, the antibodies used for immunocytochemistry should be of the highest purity available in order to avoid unwanted background and cross reactivity with other molecules.

2. Antibodies

Immunoglobulins are glycoproteins that may be divided into five major classes whose molecular weight and principle characteristics are given in Table 1. IgG, which composes approximately 75% of the immunoglobulins in human serum, is most commonly used for immunostaining. IgG can further be divided into subclasses and in humans there are four different subclasses (5) while five different subclasses have been reported in mouse. The best immunostaining results using monoclonal antibodies are obtained if the secondary antibody is directed against the subclass of the primary antibody. Subclass specific secondary antibodies can also be used to detect primary antibodies that were raised in the same species, but are of different subclasses. Although IgM may also be used for immunostaining, because of its high molecular weight, it does not readily penetrate cells and tissues. IgG (Fig. 1) is monomeric and is composed of two heavy chains and two light chains. Each molecule has two antigen binding sites. The whole IgG molecule can be used for immunostaining or it can be enzymatically digested into smaller fragments. Pepsin cleaves the IgG molecule behind the disulfide bridges, linking the Fc portions of the two heavy chains as well as in the middle of the Fc portion, producing one $F(ab)'_2$ fragment and one or more fragments from the Fc portion. In contrast, papain cleaves the IgG molecule before the disulfide bridges that link. The Fc portions of the two

Table 1
Molecular weight and characteristics of the major classes of human immunoglobulins

Immunoglobulin class	Subclass	Heavy chain	Light chain	Molecular weight	Characteristics
IgA	IgA_1 IgA_2	α1 α2	λ or κ	100,000 to 600,00	Primary immunoglobulin in mucosal secretions
IgD		δ	λ or κ	150,000	Present on surface of circulating B cells
IgE		ε	λ or κ	150,000	Bound to surface of basophils and mast cells
IgG	IgG_1 IgG_{2a} IgG_{2b} IgG_3 IgG_4	γ1 γ2 γ2 γ3 γ4	λ or κ	150,000	Major Immunoglobulin present in serum
IgM	μ		λ or κ	970,000	Pentameric, Largely confined to intravascular pool

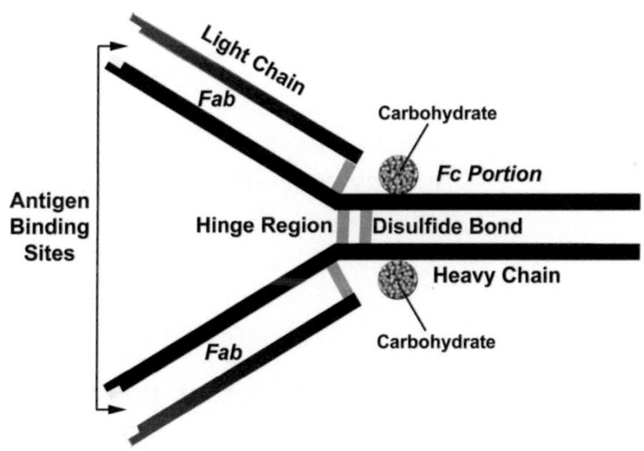

Fig. 1. A schematic diagram of an IgG molecule with carbohydrate bound to its Fc portion is shown.

heavy chains producing two Fab fragments, leaving the Fc portion relatively intact depending on the time of incubation with the enzyme. Kits that facilitate the production of IgG fragments are commercially available (http://www.thermo.com/pierce).

Antibodies are produced by B lymphocytes. Each B cell produces one type of antibody directed against a single epitope of a given antigen. When animals are immunized with an antigen, multiple clones of B cells are activated to produce antibodies to various epitopes of the antigen. This polyclonal mixture of antibodies in the serum may then recognize a variety of different epitopes on a given antigen. Polyclonal antibodies can be produced in virtually any species. However, polyclonal antibodies made in rabbit, goat and donkey are most frequently encountered. Monoclonal antibodies are produced by fusing a single B lymphocyte with an immortal cell, since B cells do not survive in culture. The usual method is to fuse the B cells from the spleen of an immunized animal with a myeloma cell line, thus producing hybridomas. The hybridomas are then cloned, with the result, that all antibodies produced by an individual clone recognize the same epitope on the antigen. Although theoretically B cells from any immunized animal can be used to produce hybridomas, in practice the spleens from small animals are most frequently used. The most common monoclonal antibodies are derived from mouse, although rat and hamster are also used. A wide array of monoclonal antibodies is available commercially. Hybridomas producing antibodies against many different antigens are also available commercially. Linscott's Directory of Immunological and Biological Reagents (http://www.linscottsdirectory.com) gives the sources of many hybridomas. Hybridomas may also be purchased from the American Type Culture Collection (http://www.atcc.org) and from the Development Studies Hybridoma Bank, University of Iowa (http://dshb.biology.uiowa.edu). Both polyclonal and monoclonal antibodies may be used for immunostaining. The advantages and disadvantages of each are given in Table 2. The choice of a monoclonal antibody over a polyclonal antibody depends on the availability of a good antibody and the application to be used.

Table 2
Comparison between the characteristics of polyclonal and monoclonal antibodies

	Polyclonal antibodies	**Monoclonal antibodies**
Signal Strength	Excellent	Antibody dependent (poor to excellent)
Specificity	Usually good, but may give some background	Excellent
Strengths	Stable, multi-valent interactions	Specificity Unlimited supply
Weaknesses	Non renewable background	Need high-affinity

In any application, the antibody chosen should be specific (i.e. react with only the desired antigen and not cross react with other cell or tissue components), have a high affinity (strength of non-covalent binding) and be produced at a high titre. An ideal antibody should also have a high avidity for its antigen. Antibody avidity is an indication of the functional affinity of a serum antibody to bind to its antigen. The avidity of an antibody is based on the rate at which the antigen–antibody complex is formed. Antibodies with these characteristics will give the best immunoreactions. Due to their specificity, they have minimal background. The high affinity will allow for numerous processing steps and sample washing with minimal loss of the specific antibody. If you are producing an antibody yourself or have immune serum, ascites fluid available, or culture medium available, it is important to screen these crude preparations before purifying the antibody for further use. This may be done by dot blotting (applying a drop of tissue or cell lysate onto nitrocellulose paper and immunostaining, using the same protocol used for Western Blots), Western Blotting, or by immunostaining, using various dilution of your crude antibody. Western blotting is the preferred method for assessing the specificity of an antibody. Ideally, only one specific band should be seen on a Western Blot. If the crude preparation shows that the antibody of interest is specific and present at a high titer, the antibody should then be purified (*see* Chapters 2–5) for use. Finally, the purified antibody should be characterized by the use of Western blots (http://www.westernblotting.org), binding curves, immunoprecipitation and/or immunostaining. Western Blotting should also be used to confirm the specificity of commercial antibodies.

3. Immunolabeling

Initial attempts at immunolabeling relied on the conjugation of a dye molecule to the antibody. However, because of the low signal generated in most instances, this approach was not very successful. In 1941, Coons (6) introduced the concept of fluorescently labeled antibodies using FITC as the fluorophore. At the time, this was considered an extremely laborious technique. Because of this impression, coupled with the lack of high quality fluorescent microscopes, fluorescent antibody methods did not come into wide-spread use for more than 40 years. In the 1960s Nakane and Pierce (7) introduced the use of enzymes, specifically horseradish peroxidase, linked to antibodies in order to increase the signal strength of the immune reaction. Today, both the detection systems, fluorescent (*see* Chapters 15–21) and enzyme based (*see* Chapters 24–28) are used extensively. The choice of one detection system over the other depends on the type of sample to be used and the availability of fluorescent or bight field microscopes as well as the type of information the investigator would like to obtain. For example, the development of various fluorophores along with highly sensitive instruments has seen FACS analysis become a routine technique for detecting cell associated antigens (*see* Chapters 31–36) and laser-capture microdissection (*see* Chapters 22 and 23) is being routinely applied to pathological samples. ELISA (*see* Chapter 29) has exploited the use of enzyme linked antibodies.

Other particulate labels are most commonly used for electron microscopy. These labels include ferritin, and colloidal gold (*see* Chapters 30, 37–42). More recently, the availability of Q-dot® nanocrystals (Invitrogen, Molecular Probes), small, intensely fluorescent, semiconductor crystals, has made it possible to use the same probe for electron microscopy as well as fluorescence microscopy.

The early immunolabeling methods concentrated on directly labeling the primary antibody with a fluorochrome or enzyme (*see* Chapters 6, 7, 16 and 24), later, indirect immunolabeling methods (*see* Chapters 17–19 and 25–28), where a secondary antibody is conjugated to a fluorochrome or enzyme, were introduced (8–10). The indirect method offers more versatility and often is more sensitive than the direct methods. However, tissue preparation may have a significant effect on the ability to detect a given antigen (*see* Chapters 8–14). A fixation method that is adequate for one antigen may completely denature another antigen (*see* Chapter 37). Unfortunately, there is no universal protocol for immunostaining that will apply to all samples in every situation. The exact conditions of immunostaining will have to be empirically developed by the user.

4. Controls

In any immunohistochemical procedure, proper controls are essential. Every new primary antibody should be characterized before beginning the immunostaining process. If the antibody is suitable for Western blotting, this will confirm the specificity of the antibody. A binding curve, using serial dilutions of the antibody should also be done in order to confirm that the staining is not due to non-specific binding to the cell surface, such as binding to Fc receptors (*see* Chapter 29, Note 7). The optimum working concentration of a particular primary antibody also needs to be determined. A negative control, where the primary antibody is omitted from the staining protocol should also be run. Another negative control is to substitute normal IgG from the same species as the primary antibody, in the place of the primary antibody during immunostaining. The antigen binding site of the antibody may also be blocked by adsorbing it with specific peptides or with the specific antigen, or tissue prior to use. In some cases, the antigen itself may be blocked with another primary antibody prior to staining.

References

1. Polak JM, VanNoorden S (2003) Introduction to Immunocytochemistry. BIOS Scientific Publishers, Oxford, UK 196 pp
2. Beesely J (1993) Immunocytochemistry: a practical approach. Oxford University Press, UK, p 276
3. Larson L-I (1988) Immunocytochemistry: theory and practice. CRC Press, Boca Raton, FL 298 pp
4. Sternberger LA (1979) Immunocytochemistry, 2nd edn. Wiley, New York
5. Hamilton RG (2001) The human IgG subclasses. Mohan C. (ed) Calbiochem-Novabiochem http://www.emdbiosciences.com/docs/docs/LIT/CB0051.pdf
6. Coons AH, Creech HJ, Jones RN (1941) Immunological properties of an antibody containing a fluorescent group. Proc Soc Exp Biol Med 47:200–202
7. Nakane P, Pierce G (1966) Enzyme-labeled antibodies: preparation and application for the localization of antigens. J Histochem Cytochem 14:929–931
8. Farr A, Nakane P (1981) Immunohistochemistry with enzyme labeled antibodies: a brief review. J Immunol Methods 47:129–144
9. Sternberger LA, Sternberger NH (1986) The unlabeled antibody method: comparison of peroxidase-antiperoxidase with avidin–biotin complex by a new method of quantification. J Histochem Cytochem 34: 599–605
10. Coons AH, Leduc EH, Connolly JM (1955) Studies on antibody production I. A method for the histochemical demonstration of specific antibody and its application to a study of the hyperimmune rabbit. J Exp Med 102: 49–60

Chapter 2

Introduction to the Purification of Antibodies

Ana Cristina Grodzki and Elsa Berenstein

Abstract

Antibodies are a powerful and essential tool in scientific laboratories being used in an array of applications such as immuno-histochemistry, immunobloting, immunoprecipitation and enzyme-linked immunosorbent assays (ELISA). The different sources for antibodies include polyclonal antisera from immunized animals and monoclonal antibodies from cells in culture or from ascites in animals. Both polyclonal and monoclonal antibodies have their advantages, and or disadvantages, but in general the production of monoclonal antibodies is more time consuming and requires tissue culture facilities and skills. The use of either monoclonal or polyclonal antibodies in some of the applications may require that the antibody is in a purified form. They can be purified by a variety of methods described in the next few chapters. The availability of commercially available kits primarily designed for the purification of IgG and IgM classes of antibodies derived from all common animal species should also be mentioned.

Key words: Monoclonal antibodies, Polyclonal antibodies, Antibody applications, IgG, Immunoglobulins, Serum, Ascitic fluid, Hybridoma

1. Purification of Antibodies

Antibodies have become useful, versatile reagents and essential tools in the scientific laboratory. The different sources of antibodies include polyclonal antisera from immunized animals and monoclonal antibodies from cells in culture or from ascites in animals.

Compared to monoclonal antibodies polyclonal antisera takes less time, effort and technical skill to produce. The serum from immunized animals contains antibodies with specificity to many different antigens or even to different antigenic groups (epitopes) in the antigen molecule. Even after hyperimmunization only a small fraction (usually a few percent) of the total IgG binds to the immunizing antigen. The variability in the response of the immunized animal accounts for differences in the binding

C. Oliver and M.C. Jamur (eds.), *Immunocytochemical Methods and Protocols*, Methods in Molecular Biology, Vol. 588, DOI 10.1007/978-1-59745-324-0_2, © Humana Press, a part of Springer Science+Business Media, LLC 1995, 1999, 2010

characteristics of different batches of polyclonal antibodies. Polyclonal antibodies can be produced in nearly any species.

In contrast, monoclonal antibodies require a fusion cell partner and they can only be made with cells of a few species. They also require tissue culture facilities and skills, but the outcome is an essentially limitless supply of uniform antibodies that recognize a single epitope. They can also be produced in large quantities with uniform characteristics. Among the advantages of the use of monoclonal antibodies, is the specificity of their binding: even impure antigens or whole cells can be used for immunization and the resulting monoclonal antibodies recognize one epitope and therefore one molecule. This is a very powerful tool for identifying unique populations of cells or molecules. Other rewards are that monoclonal antibodies are homogeneous in nature and can be produced in unlimited quantities.

Both polyclonal and monoclonal antibodies can be used in many of the same application such as immuno-histochemistry, immunoblotting, immunoprecipitation, and enzyme-linked immunosorbent assays (ELISAs).

Some assays or applications do not require a purified antibody. In this case the polyclonal antibodies can be used as antiserum and the monoclonals as either ascitic fluid or supernatants. Other assays require that the antibodies present in the serum, ascites or supernatants be in purified form; some examples include the following: (1) when the antibodies are used after chemical modifications such as labeling with fluorescent probes or isotopes; (2) for the preparation of IgG fragments such as $F(ab')_2$ or Fab; (3) when accurate concentrations of the antibody are required.

IgG can be purified, as described in the Chapters 3–5, by a variety of methods: Ammonium sulfate precipitation followed by size–exclusion (SE) chromatography are the least expensive option available for the purification of antibodies. Protein A- and protein G-affinity chromatography are the fastest methods for purifying antibodies, but they are not effective for all subclasses of antibodies. Ion-exchange (IEX) chromatography is indicated for purifying intact monoclonal and polyclonal antibodies and antibody fragments. A protocol for affinity chromatography purification of polyclonal antibodies with defined specificity or immunoglobulin class is also provided.

IgG purification from whole serum (such as by ammonium sulfate precipitation) effectively removes other contaminating proteins. However such IgG preparations will still contain both the specific (to the desired antigen) and non-specific IgG molecules. If necessary, this step can be followed by size-exclusion or ion exchange chromatography. Alternatively, Protein A, protein G or one of the newer commercial proprietary affinity chromatography columns can be used.

Table 1
Commonly used kits for antibody purification

Kit name	Manufacturer	Basis	Class
Econo-Pac^R Serum IgG Purification Kit	Bio-Rad	DEAE	Ion exchange
Montage^R Antibody Purification Kits	Millipore	Protein A, Protein G	Affinity
PURE1A	Sigma-Aldrich	Protein A	Affinity
Proteus A & G Kits	ProChem	Protein A, Protein G	Affinity
MAb Trap Kit	GE Healthcare	Protein G	Affinity
Protein A and Protein G	KPL	Protein A and G	Affinity
Immunopure (A) IgG purification kit	Pierce	Protein A	Affinity
N Ab™ Protein A,G,A/G, L Spin Kit	Pierce	Protein A,G,A/G, L	Affinity
IgM Purification Kit	Pierce	Mannan Binding Protein	Affinity
Immobilized Jacalin	Pierce	d-galactose binding lectin	Affinity

When antibodies are being purified, an assay for antibody activity and a method for determining the purity of the antibody are required. Contamination with other serum proteins can easily be checked by SDS–PAGE and staining the gels with Coomassie Blue. The activity of the antibodies can be determined by immunoassays such as any one of the methods that are described in this book.

There are commercially available kits primarily designed for the purification of IgG and IgM classes of antibodies derived from all common animal species. These kits are in general very reliable and work well, although they are more expensive than using the classical methods of purification described in these chapters. There are also kits for the fragmentation of antibodies (for example see Pierce Biotechnology, www.piercenet.com). Table 1 gives a list of some of the immunoglobulin purification kits that are available; it is by no means complete, but shows the diversity of products commercially available.

Acknowledgements

This work was supported by the Intramural Research Program of the NIH, NIDCR.

Chapter 3

Antibody Purification: Ammonium Sulfate Fractionation or Gel Filtration

Ana Cristina Grodzki and Elsa Berenstein

Abstract

Antibodies can be purified by a variety of methods based on their unique physical and chemical properties such as size, solubility, charge, hydrophobicity and binding affinity. This chapter focuses on ammonium sulfate precipitation as a convenient first step in antibody purification in that, it allows the concentration of the starting material and the precipitation of the desired protein. The principle of ammonium sulfate precipitation lies in "salting out" proteins from the solution. The proteins are prevented to form hydrogen bonds with water and the salt facilitates their interaction with each other forming aggregates that afterward precipitate out of solution. Gel filtration or size- exclusion chromatography is also discussed in this chapter. Gel filtration is based on the relative size of protein molecules and it is of great value to separate IgMs, exchange buffers and/or desalt solutions. The columns designed to separate the proteins are composed of porous beads and the proteins will flow through the packed column inside and around the beads, depending on its size.

Key words: Antibody purification, Ammonium sulfate precipitation, Fractional precipitation, Fractionation, Caprylic acid, Gel filtration, Size-exclusion chromatography, Fast Protein Liquid Chromatography, FPLC

1. Introduction

Antibodies, like other proteins, can be separated for analysis or characterization, on the basis of their unique physical and chemical properties such as size, solubility, charge, hydrophobicity and binding affinity. The strategy applied for their purification is mostly dependent on the source of the material. The advantage of serum or ascitic fluid is the high quantity of immunoglobulin produced, and the disadvantages are the numerous contaminating materials in the product. Hybridomas, on the other hand, can yield unlimited volume and amount of antibodies (1). Ammonium sulfate precipitation is frequently the first step in the purification

C. Oliver and M.C. Jamur (eds.), *Immunocytochemical Methods and Protocols*, Methods in Molecular Biology, Vol. 588, DOI 10.1007/978-1-59745-324-0_3, © Humana Press, a part of Springer Science+Business Media, LLC 1995, 1999, 2010

of antibodies from either serum or ascitic fluids. It also provides an inexpensive method for the concentration of large starting volumes of material (2,3). Table 1 indicates the source, type of antibody, the contaminants and the average yields from the different sources.

1.1. Ammonium Sulfate Precipitation or Fractional Precipitation

Sera or ascites contain large aggregates and lipids and lipoproteins. The aggregates are removed by centrifugation at 10,000 × *g* for 30 min at 4° C, while the lipids and lipoproteins are removed by delipidation (*see* Note 1). Ammonium sulfate is the salt of choice to precipitate antibodies from solutions since it yields precipitated proteins that are not denatured, and concentrates the antibodies into a small volume. Phenol red, a pH indicator often present in the culture supernatants of hybridomas, may bind to some chromatographic media and must be removed from the sample before purification. It can be removed by ammonium sulfate precipitation (*see* Subheadings 1.1 and 1.2) or by a buffer exchange column (*see* Subheading 2.1, Note 3). Alternatively, culture supernatants can be collected from cells grown in the absence of phenol red.

Ammonium sulfate precipitation (*see* Note 2) or fractional precipitation is based on the solubility of the particular immunoglobulin. Solubility is illustrated by salt precipitation. It is a convenient first step that allows the reduction of the large volume of the starting material and the precipitation of the desired protein. Contaminant proteins can be trapped or co-precipitated with the target protein, so other methods must follow the ammonium

Table 1
Characteristics of antibodies from different sources

Source	Type	Contaminants	Amount
Serum	Polyclonal	Albumin, transferrin, α2-macroglobulin, other serum proteins	IgG: 8–16 mg/mL IgM:0.5–2.0 mg/mL IgD: <0.4 mg/mL IgA : 1–4 mg/mL IgE: 10–400 ng/mL
Hybridoma culture medium with 10% fetal calf serum	Monoclonal	Albumin, transferrin, α2-macroglobulin, bovine IgG, Phenol red, other serum proteins, viruses	Usually ~10 μg/mL; but with special conditions up to 1 mg/mL
Ascites fluid	Monoclonal	Lipids, albumin, transferrin, lipoproteins, endogenous IgG, other host proteins	1–15 mg/mL

sulfate precipitation step if very pure preparations are needed. Immunoglobulins precipitate at different ammonium sulfate saturations depending somewhat on the immunoglobulin subclass and the species in which they were produced, e.g., rat and mouse IgG precipitates in the range of 40–50% ammonium sulfate saturation, while rabbit immunoglobulins precipitate at 33% (*see* Note 2).

The principle of fractionation lies in "salting-out" proteins from the solution. In solution, the proteins form hydrogen bonds with water through their charged and polar side chain groups. The interaction of the antibody molecules with the solvent can be prevented if the antibody molecules interact with each other and form aggregates that then precipitate out of solution. Therefore, as the concentration of salt is increased in a solution, the amount of solvent available to interact with antibody molecules is reduced because of the competition of the ions for the solvent, leading to interaction between hydrophobic groups and the formation of a precipitate. The molecular weight of the antibody, the amount of polar groups, pH of the solution and temperature can affect the concentration at which a particular antibody will precipitate out of solution (4).

The concentration of ammonium sulfate used can be adjusted depending on the purpose of that step in purification. Instead of purifying the target molecule, a small amount of ammonium sulfate can be added first to precipitate the less soluble impurities, which are then removed by centrifugation. The target protein and other, more soluble proteins remain in the liquid phase. More ammonium sulfate is then added to the supernatant fraction, until the desired immunoglobulins are precipitated. Approximately half to two-thirds of contaminating proteins are removed from the sample by this salting out step.

Ammonium sulfate precipitation can be achieved by two approaches: the addition of solid ammonium sulfate salt or by adding saturated ammonium sulfate solution. The addition of solid ammonium sulfate to the sample is not recommended for most applications because it results in localized high salt concentrations in the sample that might precipitate more contaminants. The addition of saturated ammonium sulfate solution (100% solution) (*see* Note 2) is highly recommended since the solution is quickly mixed with the sample. Precipitate formation is a time dependent process and can be tracked by measuring the turbidity of the solution. Complete precipitation occurs between 3 and 8 h at 4° C. The precipitate once formed, is collected by centrifugation and solubilized in an appropriate volume of buffer and stored at –80° C or dialyzed in the buffer of choice for further purification.

Other water miscible solvents (ethanol, methanol, and acetone), and other salts can also be used to differentially precipitate out proteins. Caprylic acid can precipitate proteins as effectively as ammonium sulfate, however, unlike ammonium sulfate, it does not aggregate the IgG molecules but they stay in solution and the contaminants are aggregated and precipitated. The combination of both ammonium sulfate and caprylic acid precipitations can be used to improve the yield and purification of some particular proteins.

Immunoglobulins can also be precipitated out of solution with polymers. The most frequently used polymer is polyethylene glycol (PEG or antifreeze). PEG tends to stabilize proteins and the antibody solution can be stored in the cold for long periods with PEG.

Ammonium sulfate can easily be removed from the precipitated antibody preparations by dialysis of the solution against large volumes of the desired buffer. Gel filtration or size-exclusion chromatography is another method used for salt removal and buffer exchange.

1.2. Gel Filtration/Size-Exclusion Chromatography

Size-exclusion chromatography or gel filtration (*see* Note 3) is based on the relative size of protein molecules. This procedure is of great value to separate IgMs (which are larger molecules compared to other immunoglobulins), exchange buffers and/or desalt solutions. The column designed to separate the proteins by size is composed of porous beads and the proteins will flow through the packed column inside the beads and around beads. The key to this procedure is to determine the dimensions of the bead pores and the hydrodynamic diameter of the proteins. In solution, the proteins acquire a three dimensional shape, which with their molecular size determines their hydrodynamic flow through the column. Both molecular weight and three dimensional shape contribute to the degree of retention on the column. The larger a molecule, the faster it will be eluted from the column as these molecules just flow around the beads. The smaller molecules, compared to the pore size of the beads, enter and penetrate the matrix being retarded as they move through the column. This procedure gives a relatively low resolution of target proteins that are not retained by the column, but it is still a valuable method to use in combination with other types of purification. For proteins that are retained in the beads, the resolution can be increased when the volume of the sample is no more than 1–2% of the volume of the column. The parameters for optimal resolution by gel filtration are the inclusion and exclusion range of the matrix, the column dimensions and the volume of the sample. The matrix should also be compatible with the buffers of choice, exhibit good flow characteristics and not interact significantly with the proteins in the sample. The eluting buffer should therefore contain a certain concentration of salt (between 50 and 150 mM) to minimize nonspecific protein-matrix interactions. Some examples of gel filtration matrices are: Sephadex G series, Sephacryl, Superose and Superdex (5,6). These gel filtration matrices come in a variety of different pore sizes and/or packings (GE Healthcare Bio-Sciences Corp. 800 Centennial Avenue. P.O. Box 1327. Piscataway, NJ 08855-1327. USA).

2. Materials

1. Serum or ascites (100 mL).
2. BBS (borate buffered saline): 0.2 M borate buffer, 0.16 M NaCl, pH 8. Dissolve 8.75 g of boric acid, 5.61 g of sodium borate and 9.35 g of NaCl in a total of 1 L of distilled H_2O. Check the pH of the solution and adjust to 8.0 with 1 N NaOH. Filter through a 0.45 μm filter. Store at room temperature.
3. Saturated ammonium sulfate (*see* Note 4).
4. Dialysis tubing (*see* Note 5).
5. Steriflip filter units with 0.22 and 0.45 μm pore size and 50 mL volume. Also Stericup units with volumes between 150 mL and 1,000 mL. They have fast flow, low protein binding membranes with a 0.22 μm pore size (Millipore Corporation, 290 Concord Rd. Billarica, MA 01821.).
6. Graduated cylinders, beakers and pipettes.
7. Centrifuge.
8. Spectrophotometer and UV-light cuvette (*see* Note 6). FPLC system (P-500 pumps, Frac-100 fraction collector, Flow cell, Uvicord SII monitor, V-7 valve and Recorder 101) (GE HealthCare, Amersham Biosciences, 800 Centennial Avenue, Piscataway, NJ 08855). Alternatively, use a syringe column filled with the gel of your choice, a peristaltic pump, an UV-monitor and a recorder or a compact purification system e.g., AKTAprime (GE HealthCare – Amersham Biosciences, 800 Centennial Avenue, Piscataway, NJ 08855) that offers the convenience of being compact and flexible (*see* Note 7).
9. Concentrators (Millipore Microcon, Centricon or similar ones, depending on protein to be concentrated.
10. Sephadex G-25, (coarse, medium, fine, superfine) is recommended for buffer exchange with minimal dilution of the sample. For most applications, medium or fine grade should be used. Packed columns of different grades and sizes are also available commercially (GE HealthCare, Amersham Biosciences, 800 Centennial Avenue, Pidcataway, NJ 08855).
11. Commercially available column or a syringe of at least 10 cm height.

12. Glass wool, Stoppers (preferably rubber).
13. Sephacryl S-300 prepacked column. It has the range to purify antibodies, serum proteins and midsize proteins. (GE Health-Care, Amersham Biosciences, 800 Centennial Avenue, Piscataway, NJ 08855).

3. Methods

3.1. Ammonium Sulfate Precipitation and Dialysis

3.1.1. Fractional Ammonium Sulfate Precipitation

1. Filter (through a 0.45 μm filter) or centrifuge the sample for 30 min at 10,000 ×*g* at 4° C to remove large aggregates.
2. Transfer the supernatant to a beaker with a stirring bar and measure its volume. The volume of the beaker should be at least four times the volume of the sample.
3. With continuous stirring, at 4° C, slowly add the volume of saturated ammonium sulfate required to achieve a final concentration of 25%. A 50–60 mL syringe barrel with an attached 19 GA 1 ½ TWA hypodermic needle is an easy way of adding the saturated ammonium sulfate solution so that it will drip slowly (*see* Note 2).
4. Incubate for 6 h to overnight at 4° C with continuous stirring.
5. Centrifuge 30 min at 10,000 ×*g* at 4° C. The antibody should be in the supernatant.
6. Transfer to a new beaker and measure the volume of the new supernatant.
7. Again with continuous stirring, slowly add the volume of saturated ammonium sulfate necessary to achieve a final concentration of 50%.
8. Incubate for 6 h or overnight at 4° C with continuous stirring.
9. Centrifuge 30 min at 10,000 ×*g* at 4° C.
10. Remove and save the supernatant. The antibody should be in the pellet.
11. Resuspend the pellet in PBS (1/5 of the starting volume) avoiding foaming and bubbles.
12. Prepare and fill dialysis tubing approximately half way with the resuspended ammonium sulfate precipitate. Leave a small pocket of air (this will prevent the bag from sinking to the bottom of the beaker or cylinder) before closing the tube with a knot followed by another knot 1 cm apart or use a dialysis tubing clip.
13. Place the tubing in a cylinder or beaker where it should be able to move freely when stirred.

14. Dialyze with stirring at 4° C against four to five changes of PBS or 10 mM Tris–HCl for a minimum of 4 h each. Alternatively use a Sephadex G-25 column to desalt and change the buffer of the sample (*see* Subheading 2.1 and Note 7).
15. Determine the protein concentration by absorbance measurement at 280 nm (aromatic amino acids) and store at 4° C (*see* Note 6).

3.1.2. Direct Ammonium Sulfate Precipitation

1. Filter sample (through a 0.45 µm filter) or centrifuge the sample for 30 min at 10,000 × *g* at 4° C to remove large aggregates.
2. Add 1 part 1 M Tris–HCl, pH 8.0 to 10 parts sample volume to maintain pH.
3. With continuous stirring, add saturated ammonium sulfate solution slowly, drop by drop, to achieve a final concentration of 50%. The solution becomes turbid at about 20% saturation. Incubate at 4° C for at least 6 h with continuous stirring.
4. Centrifuge for 30 min at 10,000 × *g*.
5. Discard supernatant and wash pellet twice by resuspension in a 50% ammonium sulfate solution.
6. Dissolve pellet in a small volume of buffer (PBS, BBS or 10 mM Tris–HCl pH 7.4) which is about 5–10% of the original volume.
7. Dialysis and subsequent steps are the same as in Subheading 3.1.1.

3.2. Gel Filtration/ FPLC

3.2.1. Desalting and Buffer Exchange

This method is a description of the use of gel filtration for desalting or buffer exchange, while Subheading 3.2.2 describes the use of gel filtration for purification of some classes of antibodies. Desalting and buffer exchange of protein samples are particular examples of gel filtration in which the size difference of the molecules to be separated is large (at least a factor of 10).

1. Prepare the dry Sephadex according to the manufacturer's instructions (*see* Note 8).
2. Pack the column (*see* Note 9).
3. Pour the set volume of degassed slurry in a single operation down the wall of the syringe using a glass rod or similar device. Avoid introducing bubbles.
4. Connect the pump to the top of the syringe using a stopper or another adapter and pack the column for 10 min or longer, using water. When the column is packed pass 2–3 column volumes of buffer through it until the bed is equilibrated. You can use a flow rate of at least 10 mL/min.

5. Add the sample ready for buffer exchange, desalting or other group separation (the volume of the sample should not exceed 30% of the column volume and the protein concentration of the sample should not be greater than 25 mg/mL). Maintain or increase the flow rate of the buffer (*see* Note 10).
6. The concentration of the protein eluted in or just after the void volume is measured with the spectrophotometer at $\lambda = 280$ in the UV region (*see* Note 6).

3.2.2. Separation of Biomolecules using Fast Protein Liquid Chromatography or FPLC

Gel filtration is used in high resolution fractionation to separate the components of a sample according to the differences in their molecular weights. It is usually the polishing or last step in protein purification. It is most successful when the sample originally consists of few components or when the protein has been previously purified by another method. It can be used to separate aggregates from monomers, to isolate one or more components and to determine the molecular weight of the different components present in the sample.

While desalting columns can separate sample volumes of up to 30% of the total volume of the column, high resolution columns can only handle samples with volumes equivalent to 0.5–4% of the total column volume.

1. Degas and filter (0.22 or 0.45 μm filtration membrane) BBS or any other buffer that will be used.
2. Unpack the Sephacryl S-300 or any other sizing column. Connect the column to the FPLC system. If the column is new or it has been in storage for a long time, equilibrate the column with distilled water. Use at least 0.5 column volumes at the flow rate indicated by manufacturer.
3. Equilibrate the column with at least two column volumes of buffer, in this case BBS, at the flow rates suggested by the manufacturer.
4. Inject the filtered sample. Use a lower flow rate to optimize the resolution. The sample should be approximately 2% of the total column volume. Sample volumes should be around 0.5–4 % of the total column volume. Smaller sample volumes will increase the separation of the proteins in the mixture.
5. Elute with buffer at the lower flow rate and monitor the eluate at $\lambda = 280$ nm (*see* Note 11).
6. Collect the IgG containing fractions, and determine the concentration using the spectrophotometer at $\lambda = 280$.
7. Before running another sample run at least a whole column volume of BBS.
8. To store the column, clean with at least a 0.5 column volumes of 0.2 M NaOH and then with 2 column volumes of BBS at the flow rates recommended by the manufacturer.

9. For long term storage, wash with at least 4 column volumes of H_2O and then with 4 column volumes of 20% ethanol. Close the ends of the column and store between 4° C and 25° C.

4. Notes

1. Delipidation (removal of the lipids and lipoproteins from plasma, serum and ascites) is a necessary first step prior to the use of chromatographic methods for the purification of immunoglobulins. One of the simplest ways to selectively remove the lipids and lipoproteins is to use commercially available reagents (e.g., PHM-L LIPOSORB absorbent from Calbiochem). It is fast, simple and easy to use and it has a high lipoprotein binding capacity. Additional methods are described below: *Dextran sulfate method:* Dextran sulfate precipitates lipoproteins in the presence of divalent cations such as Ca^{2+}. (1) Mix 40 μL of 10% dextran sulfate solution and 1 mL of 1 M $CaCl_2$ with 1 mL of sample; (2) Gently mix for 15 min (3)Centrifuge at 10,000 × *g* for 10 min; (4) Discard the precipitate (5) Add buffer suitable for purification. *Polyvinylpyrrolidine(PVP):* PVP produces a pH dependent precipitation effect. PVP precipitates lipoproteins at pH 7. The lipoproteins remain in solution if the pH is below 4.0. (1) Add solid PVP to the sample solution to a final concentration of 3% (w/v). The pH should be 7.0; (2) Stir for 4 h at 4 °C; (3) Centrifuge at 17,000 × *g* for 30 min; (4) Discard precipitate; (5) Exchange buffer by dialysis or by using a desalting column.
2. Ammonium sulfate precipitation. Mixing of the ammonium sulfate with the antibody solution is not instantaneous and takes time, which depends on the properties of the components as well as on the processing conditions, i.e., mixing intensity, the volume, density and viscosity of the medium as well as on the power input for mixing. The volume of saturated ammonium sulfate solution in mL that has to be added to a sample to salt out proteins at any concentration is given by the equation: V (mL) = 100 mL X (S2–S1)/(1–S2) where S1 and S2 are expressed as fractions of the saturated solution, 100 is the volume of the sample and V(mL) is the volume of saturated ammonium sulfate that has to be added to the sample to obtain the desired concentration. For example: A 100 mL sample is precipitated sequentially first to an initial saturation of 25% and then to a final 50% ammonium sulfate saturation. V(mL) = 100 × (0.25–0)/(1–0.25). V(mL) = 33.3 mL. The volume of 33.3 mL of saturated ammonium sulfate is added

to the 100 mL sample, with stirring for at least 6 h to obtain a 25% saturated solution. After centrifugation the volume of the supernatant is going to be approximately 133 mL and the initial ammonium sulfate concentration will be 25%. The volume of saturated ammonium sulfate solution to precipitate the protein at 50% is calculated as follows: V(mL) = 133 × (0.5–0.25)/1–0.5. V(mL) = 66.5 mL. The volume of 66.6 mL is the volume of saturated ammonium sulfate that is added to the 25% sample, in order to raise the concentration to 50%. In this case the desired proteins, immunoglobulins, are going to be in the precipitate. The extent of supersaturation determines the nature of the precipitates: high supersaturation gives gelatinous precipitate. The saturation of ammonium sulfate can be adjusted to precipitate the target antibody or the contaminants. This step removes proteins aggregates and less soluble proteins. If DEAE chromatography is used for subsequent purification, dialyze the antibody against 10 mM Tris–HCl, pH 8.5. Ammonium sulfate can be removed by desalting columns, buffer exchange columns or dialysis. IgGs are readily precipitated with ammonium sulfate since they are highly hydrophobic when compared to many other proteins (7,8).

3. Gel filtration: To increase the capacity of the columns, the samples can be concentrated up to 70 mg/mL. Above this concentration, the viscosity of the sample starts to interfere with the separation. If the sample is a complex mix, start with a load equivalent to 0.5% of the total column volume to optimize resolution. To minimize sample dilutions, use the maximum volume load that will give you the desired separation between two peaks. The height of the bed pack affects the resolution and also the time of elution. Doubling the bed height will increase the resolution by approximately 40%. Most columns give satisfactory results with heights of 30–60 cm. If a bed height larger than this is required it is better to use 2 or 3 columns in tandem. A gel filtration step is frequently used to separate dimeric and monomeric forms of the antibodies. The large proteins will rapidly flow through the column and the small proteins will enter and migrate through many of the beads, and their flow through the column then will be slow. The smaller the protein, the later it elutes from the column.
4. The solubility of ammonium sulfate [$(NH4)_2$ SO_4] changes with temperature. The amount of $(NH4)_2$ SO_4 needed to saturate 1,000 mL of H_2O at 4° C is about 707 g. The saturated ammonium sulfate solution is prepared at room temperature by adding the solid salt to the desired volume of H_2O with continuous stirring until some does not dissolve. Continue the stirring overnight. Adjust the pH to 7.4 with

1 M Tris or solid Tris base powder and store at 4° C. Always stir before use to insure that the solution is homogenous.

5. Cut dry tubing in reasonable lengths (Spectra/por, mol wt cut off 1–8,000 daltons. Serva Electrophoresis.GmbH, Carl-Benz-Str 7, D-69115 Heidelberg; other tubing from Serva includes, Membra-cel, Servapor and Visking). Boil for 10 min in a large volume of 2% sodium bicarbonate, 1 mM EDTA stirring the tubing with a polished glass rod. Then rinse in deionized distilled water and boil for 10 min in distilled water. Let cool and store in 20% ethanol at 4° C until needed. Remove the desired amount of tubing and rinse well with water to remove all traces of ethanol. Tie a knot at one end of the tubing and then another 1 cm away. Fill the tubing with water and check for leaks. Alternatively, one can use prepared dialysis cassettes. One such source is Pierce Biotechnology, Slide-A-Lyzer (Pierce Biotechnology. 3747 N. Meridian Rd. P.O.Box 117. Rockford, IL 61105 USA). They come with different molecular weight cut offs and sizes for different volumes.
6. The purified and concentrated protein can be stored in BBS or PBS. The concentration is determined by measuring the absorbance at 280 nm in the UV range. It is preferable to use minicuvettes with a maximum volume of 100 μL. Use the storage buffer (either PBS or BBS) as a blank and read the absorbance of a tenfold (10 μL of protein solution + 90 μL of PBS or BBS) diluted solution. A 1 mg/mL solution of immunoglobulin will have an absorbance of ~1.4 using a 1 cm path length cuvette. To obtain the concentration divide the absorbance by 1.4 and multiply by the dilution factor, in this case 10. Purified samples can be analyzed by SDS–PAGE under both non-reducing and reducing conditions in 10% gels and the gels stained with Coomasie blue. This would indicate the removal of impurities such as albumin or transferrin (2).
7. For smaller separations including the removal of small molecular weight labels, the use of prepacked PD-10 columns is easy, fast and there is no equipment requirement since the separations are made using gravity flow. For other prepacked Sephadex-25 desalting columns, you should have at least a rudimentary system to do the separation. It is convenient, in this case, to follow the manufacturer's instructions.
8. The dry Sephadex must be allowed to swell in excess buffer for at least 3 h. Heating in a boiling water bath can accelerate the process. After swelling, decant the fines (smaller particles than the average bead size floating in the buffer) and resuspend

the slurry so that when settled it is 75% of the total volume in medium. Dry Sephadex G-25 powder of all grades will give an approximate bed volume of 4–6 mL/g.

9. If using a syringe, plug the end with glass wool. Attach the syringe vertically to a stand and fill the syringe with distilled water to approximately 2 cm above the glass wool.
10. The elution profile of the separation shows that large molecules elute in or just after the void volume and the small molecules such as salts, low molecular weight labels, cofactors or inhibitors are eluted just before one total column volume.
11. In this column the monomeric form of IgG will elute at approximately the midpoint of the total column volume.

Acknowledgement

This work was supported by the Intramural Research Program of the NIH, NIDCR

References

1. Bonifacino JS, Dasso M, Harford JB, Lippincott-Schwartz J, Yamada KM (eds) (2007) Current protocols in cell biology. Wiley, Hoboken, NJ
2. Halow E, Lane D (1988) Storing and purifying antibodies. In: Harlow E, Lane D (eds) Antibodies: a laboratory manual. Cold Spring Harbor Laboratory, Cold Spring Harbor, NY
3. Antibody purification handbook. Amersham Pharmacia Biotech, Piscataway, NJ. http://www6.gelifesciences.com/APTRIX/upp00919.nsf/content/handbooks
4. Ausubel FM, Brent R, Kingston RE, Moore DD, Seidman JG, Smith JA, Struhl K (eds) (2007) Current protocols in molecular biology. Wiley, Hoboken, NJ
5. Stellwagen E (1990) Gel filtration. Methods Enzymol 182:317–328
6. Gel filtration chromatography: principles and methods. Amersham Pharmacia Biotech, Piscataway, NJ. http://www6.gelifesciences.com/APTRIX/upp00919.nsf/content/handbooks
7. Protein purification handbook. Amersham Pharmacia Biotech, Piscataway, NJ. http://www6.gelifesciences.com/APTRIX/upp00919.nsf/content/handbooks
8. Jason JC, Ryden L (eds) (1998) Protein purification: principles, high resolution methods, and applications. Wiley, Hoboken, NJ

Chapter 4

Antibody Purification: Ion-Exchange Chromatography

Ana Cristina Grodzki and Elsa Berenstein

Abstract

Ion exchange chromatography techniques are the focus of this chapter and they showcase the power of this method for the purification of proteins and monoclonal antibodies. The technique is powerful and can separate biomolecules that have minor differences in their net charge, e.g., two protein molecules differing by a single charged amino acid. Given the amphoteric character of proteins the pH of the solution is important in the determination of the type of ion exchanger used. Immunoglobulins, although they can be purified by either cation or anion exchange chromatography, are most frequently purified by anion exchange with DEAE resins. The purification of the rabbit IgG fraction from serum using a DEAE column is detailed as well as the purification of IgG from ascitic fluid using FPLC, from loading to elution of the purified and concentrated protein.

Key words: Ion-exchange chromatography, Net surface charge, Isoelectric point, Cation exchanger, Anion exchanger, Ionic strength, DEAE column, Chromatographic matrix

1. Introduction

A detailed discussion of the principles and theory that are the fundamentals of Ion Exchange Chromatography can be found in Himmelhoch (1) and on the GE Health Care web site (2). While this is a powerful method for the purification of proteins, it should be preceded by ammonium sulfate fractionation (*see* Chapter 3) or followed by affinity chromatography (*see* Chapter 5) or gel filtration (*see* Chapter 3) when used to purify immunoglobulins from crude materials. This section only intends to be a short introduction to the theoretical basis of this technique.

Ion exchange chromatography relies on the separation of biomolecules according to their net surface charge. Molecules vary considerably in their charge properties and will exhibit

C. Oliver and M.C. Jamur (eds.), *Immunocytochemical Methods and Protocols*, Methods in Molecular Biology, Vol. 588,
DOI 10.1007/978-1-59745-324-0_4, © Humana Press, a part of Springer Science+Business Media, LLC 1995, 1999, 2010

different degrees of interaction with charged chromatography media, depending on differences in their overall charge, charge density and surface charge distribution. The charged groups within a molecule that contribute to the net surface charge, possess different p*K*a values (the pH at which an acid is 50% dissociated) depending on their structure and chemical microenvironment. In brief, ion-exchange chromatography is based on the binding of charged sample molecules to oppositely charged groups attached to an insoluble matrix. The immunoglobulins or other proteins will bind to the ion exchangers when they carry a net charge opposite to that of the ion exchanger. Such binding is electrostatic and reversible (3).

All molecules with ionizable groups have a net surface charge that is highly pH dependent. Proteins, which are made up of many different amino acids containing weak acidic and basic groups, are amphotheric: i.e., their net surface charge will change gradually as the pH of the solution changes. The pH value at which a biomolecule carries no net charge is called the isoelectric point (p*I*). When exposed to a pH below its p*I*, the biomolecule will carry a positive net charge and will bind to a cation exchanger (SP and CM). At a pH above its p*I*, the biomolecule will carry a negative net charge and will bind to an anion exchanger (Q, DEAE and ANX). If the sample components are most stable below their p*I*, a cation exchanger should be used; if they are more stable above their p*I* then an anion exchanger is used. If, on the other hand, the sample stability is high over a wide pH range on both sides of the p*I*, either type of ion exchanger can be used. The technique is powerful and can separate biomolecules that have minor differences in their net charge, e.g., two protein molecules differing by a single charged amino acid.

Immunoglobulins, although they can be purified by either cation or anion exchange chromatography (*see* Note 1), are most frequently purified by anion-exchange chromatography with DEAE resins (4–7). Since the p*I* of immunoglobulins is near neutrality, a DEAE column and a low ionic strength (low salt concentration) buffer with a pKa around 8 and pH 8–8.5 will provide almost optimal conditions when the column and the sample are equilibrated with buffer approximately 1 pH unit above the sample p*I*. The immunoglobulins in the sample that binds to the ion exchange matrix are effectively concentrated under these conditions.

After binding of the target proteins to the exchanger, the same equilibration buffer is used to wash the column and remove all the molecules that do not bind under the conditions chosen for the target protein. The elution of the immunoglobulins bound to the column is done by increasing the ionic strength of the buffer and only occasionally by changing the pH. As the salt concentration increases, the salt ions, usually Na^+ and Cl^-, compete with the proteins that are bound to the matrix and one or more of the bound proteins starts to elute and moves down the column. At the selected pH, the proteins with the lowest net charge will be the first to elute. In a similar manner the proteins with the highest net charge will be the last to elute. By changing the ionic strength, either using a linear gradient or step increases, the proteins bound to the matrix are eluted differentially in a purified and concentrated form.

2. Materials

1. Serum or ascites (10–100 mL). Hybridoma cell culture supernatant (100–1,000 mL) (*see* Notes 2 and 3).
2. PD-10 columns or other prepacked desalting columns (GE HealthCare 800 Centennial Avenue, Piscataway, NJ 08855).
3. 0.0175 M phosphate buffer, pH 6.3 (*see* Note 4).
4. 20 mM Tris buffer, pH 8.0.
5. 20 mM Tris buffer, 0.5 M NaCl, pH 8.0.
6. 20 mM Tris buffer, 1 M NaCl, pH 8.0.
7. 0.2 M Borate buffer, 0.16 M NaCl, pH 8.0 (*see* Chapter 3, Subheading 3.2).
8. Saturated ammonium sulfate (*see* Chapter 3, Subheading 3.2).
9. Dialysis tubing or prepared dialysis cassettes (*see* Chapter 3, Subheading 3.2).
10. Steriflip and Stericup filter units (*see* Chapter 3, Subheading 3.2).
11. Graduated cylinders, beakers and pipettes.
12. Centrifuge.
13. Spectrophotometer and cuvettes that can be used at UV wavelengths.
14. The column can be prepared with the exchanger of choice, anion or cation, weak or strong according to the characteristics of the protein to be purified. If packing your own column, use a syringe or a commercial column. If using a prepacked column follow the manufacturer's instructions. A variety of ion exchange media either dry or as prepacked (*see* Note 5) columns are available from GE HealthCare (GE HealthCare, 800 Centennial Avenue, Piscataway, NJ 08855).
15. DEAE Sephadex A50 or other exchanger with similar characteristics. It is a mixed weak and strong anion exchanger.

It comes as a dry powder and it should be swollen following the manufacturer's protocol (GE HealthCare, 800 Centennial Avenue, Piscataway, NJ 08855).

16. HiTrap DEAE FF prepacked in 1 mL or 5 mL column size (GE HealthCare, 800 Centennial Avenue, Piscataway, NJ 08855) (*see* Note 6).
17. FPLC system (P-920 Pumps, UPC-900 Monitor; sensitive in the UV range, conductivity and pH monitor, FRAC-900 or FRAC-950 Fraction Collector INV-907 Injection valve, sample loops and a Unicorn Control System). Alternatively, use a syringe column filled with the matrix of your choice, a peristaltic pump, a UV-monitor and a recorder or a compact purification system e.g., AKTAprime (GE HealthCare, 800 Centennial Avenue, Piscataway, NJ 08855) that offers the convenience of being compact and flexible.
18. Concentrators (Millipore Microcon, Centricon or similar depending on protein to be concentrated).
19. Commercially available column or a syringe of at least 10 cm height.
20. Glass wool, Stoppers (preferably rubber).

3. Methods

3.1. Purification of Rabbit IgG Fraction from Rabbit Serum on DEAE Ion Exchange Column

1. The serum is centrifuged at 10,000 × *g* for 30 min at 4° C to remove large aggregates.
2. The immunoglobulins and other proteins present in the rabbit serum sample are precipitated with saturated ammonium sulfate at a final concentration of 33% (*see* Chapter 3, Subheading 3.3.1.1, and Note 2).
3. Centrifuge at 10,000 *g* for 30 min at 4° C and resuspend the precipitated proteins in 0.0175 M phosphate buffer pH 6.3 using 1/10 to 1/5 of the original volume.
4. Dialyze the sample against 0.0175 M buffer pH 6.3 or conversely, the buffer may be exchanged using a Sepadex PD-10 column or another prepacked buffer exchange column.
5. Prepare (DEAE Sephadex A50) or use a prepacked DEAE column (HiTrap DEAE FF, 1 mL) and equilibrate with 0.0175 M phosphate buffer until the conductivity of the sample and the column flow through are the same.
6. Load the sample onto the column and elute with the same buffer. Rabbit IgG will not bind to the matrix and it will elute with the flow through.

7. Collect the peak and dialyze or exchange this buffer against PBS. The peak is the rabbit IgG fraction.

3.2. DEAE Ion-Exchange Chromatography using FPLC

1. The FPLC system should be set up and assembled according to the manufacturer's instructions. A 5 mL HiTrap DEAE FF prepacked column is used. The start buffer is 20 mM Tris, pH 8 and the elution buffer 20 mM Tris, 0.5 M NaCl, pH 8.0.
2. The sample, either serum, ascites, or hybridoma culture medium is prepared for loading into the column (*see* Notes 1–3 and 6).
3. The column is equilibrated with 5–10 column volumes of start buffer at a flow rate of 5 mL/min.
4. The sample is applied to the column via the injection loop at a flow rate of 5 mL/min.
5. Wash the column with at least 25 mL (5 column volumes) of start buffer or until no material appears in the effluent as determined by monitoring the absorbance at $\lambda = 280$ nm.
6. Elute with 5–10 column volumes of a continuous salt gradient of start buffer to start buffer +0.5 M NaCl at a flow rate of 5 mL/min.
7. Collect 1 mL fractions and monitor the effluent at $\lambda = 280$ nm.
8. The IgG should be the major peak and should elute between 0.2 and 0.3 M NaCl.
9. The pooled fractions containing the mouse IgG can be desalted by dialysis or by using a desalting column.
10. The column can be reused. It can be regenerated by washing with 5 column volumes 20 mM Tris, 1 M NaCl followed by 5–10 column volumes of start buffer.
11. After this treatment the column can be used again for another purification or it can be prepared for storage.
12. To store, wash the column with water and then with 5 column volumes of 20% ethanol to prevent microbial growth. Close both ends and store between 4° C and 30° C.

4. Notes

1. The starting pH for anion exchangers should be around 1 pH unit above the p*I* of the protein that is to be bound to the matrix and the sample should be stable at this pH. For cation exchangers the starting pH should be around 1 pH unit below the protein p*I*.

2. If the source of the sample is ascitic fluid or serum, then ammonium sulfate fractionation should be the first step. It should be followed by extensive dialysis or gel filtration with the starting buffer. It is very important that the conductivity of the sample and the column be the same.
3. The amount of protein loaded in the columns should not exceed 30 mg.
4. All buffers should be prepared with high quality water, filtered and degassed.
5. Strong and weak ion exchanger do not refer to the binding strength between the ionized groups in the matrix and the proteins but to the fact that strong exchangers do not take up or lose protons with changes in pH. Strong exchangers remain fully charged over a broad pH range, and they do not show a variation in ion exchange capacity. Weak exchangers can take or lose protons with changing pH and their ion exchange capacity also changes with it.
6. For some samples, the buffer pH or gradient conditions will require modification in order to optimize the results. GE Healthcare offers a HiTrap IEX Selection Kit, which consists of 7 HiTrap 1 mL columns prepacked with different ion exchangers, i.e., strong and weak cation and anion exchangers. It provides a convenient way to find the best exchanger and buffer system for a given protein.

Acknowledgement

This work was supported by the Intramural Research Program of the NIH, NIDCR.

References

1. Himmelhoch SR (1971) Chromatography of proteins on ion-exchange adsorbents. Methods Enzymol 22:273–286
2. Ion-exchange chromatography: principles and methods. GE Health Care, http://www6.gelifesciences.com/APTRIX/upp00919.nsf/content/handbooks.
3. Karlsson E, Ryden L, Brewer J (1998) Ion exchange chromatography. In: Janson JC, Ryden L (eds) Protein purification: principles, high resolution methods and applications. Wiley, New York, NY, pp 145–205
4. Halow E, Lane D (1988) Storing and purifying antibodies. In: Halow E, Lane D (eds) Antibodies: a laboratory manual. Cold Spring Harbor Laboratory, Cold Spring Harbor, NY
5. Hardy RR (1986) Purification and characterization of monoclonal antibodies. In: Weir DM (ed) Handbook of experimental immunology, vol 1, Immunochemistry. Blackwell Scientific, Oxford, UK, pp 13.1–13.13
6. Antibody. production, purification, fragmentation, labeling. Pierce Biotechnology. P.O. Box 117, Rockford, IL61105. Part 1: http://www.piercenet.com/files/1601323%20Antibodies_1.pdf; Part 2: www.piercenet.com/files/1601323%20Antibodies_2.pdf; Part 3: http://www.piercenet.com/files/1601323%20Antibodies_3.pdf
7. Antibody purification handbook. GE Health Care, http://www6.gelifesciences.com/APTRIX/upp00919.nsf/content/handbooks. Excellent handbook on the theory and practice of antibody purification

Chapter 5

Antibody Purification: Affinity Chromatography – Protein A and Protein G Sepharose

Ana Cristina Grodzki and Elsa Berenstein

Abstract

Affinity chromatography relies on the reversible interaction between a protein and a specific ligand immobilized in a chromatographic matrix. The sample is applied under conditions that favor specific binding to the ligand as the result of electrostatic and hydrophobic interactions, van der Waals' forces and/or hydrogen bonding. After washing away the unbound material the bound protein is recovered by changing the buffer conditions to those that favor desorption. The technique has been used not only to isolate antigen-specific antibodies but also to remove specific contaminants from biological samples. Methods are described for the purification of immunoglobulins, namely IgG, IgG fragments and subclasses, using the high affinity of protein A and protein G coupled to agarose. In the Subheading 3 there are also protocols for affinity purification using a specific ligand coupled to commercial matrices like CNBr- Sepharose 4-B and Affigel.

Key words: Affinity chromatography, Affinity matrices, Antigen-specific antibodies, Hapten-specific antibodies, Specie-specific antibodies, Cross-reacting immunoglobulin, Sepharose, Affigel, IgM, IgA, Mannan binding protein, Jacalin, Protein A, Protein G, Protein L

1. Introduction

Affinity chromatography relies on the separation of protein (s) on the basis of their reversible interaction with a specific ligand immobilized in a chromatographic matrix, e.g., the protein to be purified is specifically and reversibly bound to the ligand coupled to the matrix. The sample is applied under conditions that favor specific binding to the ligand and the resulting interactions are the result of electrostatic and hydrophobic interactions, van der Waals' forces and/or hydrogen bonding. The unbound material is washed away and the bound protein is recovered by changing the buffer conditions to those that favor desorption. In general, the bound protein can be eluted from the matrix specifically by

C. Oliver and M.C. Jamur (eds.), *Immunocytochemical Methods and Protocols*, Methods in Molecular Biology, Vol. 588, DOI 10.1007/978-1-59745-324-0_5, © Humana Press, a part of Springer Science+Business Media, LLC 1995, 1999, 2010

using a competitive ligand or nonspecifically by changing the pH, ionic strength or polarity of the eluting buffer.

Affinity chromatography has been used to isolate antigen-specific antibodies, hapten-specific antibodies, species-specific antibodies or to separate cross-reacting immunoglobulins from the antibody of interest. It has also been used to remove specific contaminants, e.g., serine proteases such as trypsin, thrombin, factor Xa or other contaminating proteins such as albumin.

Some typical biological interactions, frequently used in affinity chromatography are; enzyme to: substrate analogue, inhibitor, or cofactor; antibody to: antigen, virus, or cell; lectin to: polysaccharide, glycoprotein, cell surface receptor, or cell; nucleic acid to: complementary base sequence, histones, or nucleic acid polymerase; hormone or vitamin to: receptor, or carrier protein; glutathione to: glutathione-S-transferase (GST) or GST fusion proteins; and metal ions to: poly (His) fusion proteins, or native proteins with histidine, cysteine and/or tryptophan residues on their surfaces.

Several types of affinity matrices are commercially available. The most convenient coupling chemistries are directed to the –NH2 and –SH groups because they are reactive at physiological pH and their presence in a sequence is either unique or they are present in limited number. If there is no primary amine available in the ligand (or the amine group is involved in specific interactions at the binding site) then, other affinity matrices for ligand attachment via hydroxyl, carboxyl or thiol groups should be considered. Some of the most popular affinity matrices for coupling molecules are commercially available already activated and ready for use (*see* Note 1). They are manufactured with or without spacer arms. These are well suited for affinity chromatography in that agarose has low nonspecific protein adsorption, the matrix is stable over a wide pH range, it can be used with denaturants and reagents, and it has a high capacity. The chemical group in the ligand involved in covalent coupling at pH 8.0 to 9.0 is an –NH2 or -SH group (*see* Note 2) (1–3).

On the other hand, the purification of immunoglobulins, namely IgG, IgG fragments and subclasses, use the high affinity of protein A and protein G for the Fc region of polyclonal and monoclonal IgG-type antibodies from a number of species (*see* Note 3)(4, 5). When coupled to a Sepharose matrix, they are very useful in many routine applications such as the purification of IgG monoclonal antibodies from ascites or culture supernatants, the purification of polyclonal IgG subclasses from serum and also the adsorption of immune complexes involving IgG.

Protein L is another protein that can be used for antibody purification as it binds *kappa* light chains (*see* Note 4). Mannan Binding Protein (MBP) and jacalin (extracted from Jackfruit) bind fairly specifically to mouse or human IgM and human IgA respectively and have also been used in the affinity purification of antibodies. The following sections will describe three different protocols as examples of affinity purification of antibodies.

2. Materials

1. CNBr-activated Sepharose 4B (GE Health Care) coupled to rat, mouse or any other species immunoglobulins. The coupling is done following the manufacturer‘s instructions. For short instructions *see* Note 1.
2. Empty, disposable columns (GE Health Care, 800 Centennial Avenue, Piscataway, NJ08855) to pour the resin. A regular syringe can also be used.
3. A peristaltic pump, tubes to collect the elution, UV cuvettes, spectrophotometer.
4. 0.2 M carbonate buffer, 0.5 M NaCl.
5. BBS: 0.2 M borate buffer, 0.16 M NaCl, pH 8.0. To prepare 1 L of BBS: 8.75 g of boric acid, 5.61 g of sodium borate and 9.35 g of NaCl. Check the pH and if not pH 8.0 adjust with either 0.2 M boric acid or 0.2 M sodium borate as necessary.
6. 0.2 M glycine: dissolve 15.01 g of glycine in carbonate buffer (0.2 M carbonate buffer, 0.1 M NaCl, pH 8.3).
7. 1 M ethanolamine: 30 mL of ethanolamine in 470 mL of carbonate buffer (0.2 M carbonate buffer, 0.1 M NaCl, pH 8.3).
8. Elution buffer: 0.1 M glycine, pH 3: To 900 mL of deionized water, add 7.51 g of glycine. Adjust pH to 3 with 5 N HCl. Add water to a final volume of 1,000 mL.
9. 0.5 M acetic acid, pH 3: To 900 mL of water, carefully add 29 mL of glacial acetic acid. Adjust pH to 3 with 5 *N* ammonium hydroxide. Add water to a final volume of 1,000 mL.
10. 1 M Tris: To 900 mL of water, add 121 g of Tris-base. Mix until dissolved. Add water to 1,000 mL. The pH should be between 10 and 11.
11. Mouse anti-rat IgG serum. 5–15 mL.
12. Affigel 10 (Bio-Rad Laboratories Inc., 2000 Alfred Nobel Dr, Hercules, CA 94547). Use sufficient slurry to give a 3–5 mL packed gel.
13. Concentrators (Millipore, Microcon, Centricon among others; Millipore Corporation, 290 Concord Road, Billerica, MA 01821) depending on protein to be concentrated.

14. Slide-A-Lyzer (Pierce Biotechnologies, PO Box 117, Rockford, Ill 61105). Dialysis tubing (*see* Chapter 3)
15. Sephadex G-25, (coarse, medium, fine, superfine) for buffer exchange (GE HealthCare, 800 Centennial Avenue, Piscataway, NJ08855).
16. 150 mM phosphotyramine in PBS
17. 10 mM *p*-nitrophenyl phosphate in PBS.
18. PBS, pH 7.4
19. Chromatography cartridges protein A/G (Pierce Biotechnology, PO Box 117, Rockford, Ill 61105). rProtein G Agarose, Protein A Agarose (Invitrogen, 1600 Faraday Avenue. P.O. Box 6482, Carlsbad, California 92008). Protein G Sepharose 4 Fast Flow, rmpProtein A Sepharose (GE HealthCare, 800 Centennial Avenue, Piscataway, NJ08855).
20. Binding Buffer: 0.01 M sodium phosphate buffer pH 7, 0.15 M NaCl. To 900 mL of deionized water, add 0.53 g of monobasic sodium phosphate monohydrate ($NaH_2PO_4 \cdot H_2O$) and 0.87 g of dibasic sodium phosphate anhydrous (Na_2HPO_4). Add 8.77 g of sodium chloride (NaCl) and dilute to a final volume of 1,000 mL with deionized water.
21. Stripping Buffer: 1.0 M acetic acid, pH 2.4. For 1 L: To 943 mL of deionized water carefully add 57 mL of glacial acetic acid.
22. Storage Buffer: Binding Buffer + 0.05% thimerosal. To 1 L of binding buffer, add 0.5 g of thimerosal.

3. Methods

3.1. Affinity Purification of Mouse Anti-rat IgG Using Previously Coupled Rat IgG: CNBr-Sepharose 4-B

This protocol describes the purification of anti-rat antibodies using rat IgG coupled to Sepharose beads (*see* Note 1).

1. Pack the rat IgG-Sepharose resin in the syringe or commercially available column. If using a syringe put some glass wool at the bottom of the syringe before adding the resin.
2. The packed volume will depend on the size of the sample that you want to purify.
3. Attach to a peristaltic pump and wash the column with 2–3 column volumes of BBS at 0.5–1 mL/min or until the absorbance of the eluted buffer is approximately the same as that of the buffer itself.
4. Load the volume of serum or ascites that will not exceed the capacity of the column (*see* Note 5). Recirculate the sample for at least 1 h at 0.2–0.5 mL/min.

5. At the end of the recirulation period, run the whole sample through the column and collect it in a tube.
6. Wash the column with at least 10 column volumes of BBS. The absorbance of the wash should be less than 0.02 AU at 280 nm and comparable to the absorbance of the column buffer before you start the elution from the column. Collect the fractions.
7. Elute the bound antibody with 0.1 M glycine, pH 3 at 0.5–1 mL /min.
8. Collect 1 mL fractions into tubes containing 0.5 mL of 1 M Tris, pH 8
9. Pool the immunoglobulin containing samples, dialyze against several changes of BBS or PBS and concentrate if necessary.
10. Wash the column with 2–3 column volumes of 0.2 M glycine, pH 3 and regenerate by washing with 5 column volumes of BBS to neutralize the acid. Store in BBS at 4° C.
11. If the column is going to be stored for a long period of time, store it in 20% ethanol.

3.2. Affinity Purification of Rabbit Polyclonal or Mouse Monoclonal Antiphosphotyrosine Antibodies on Phosphotyramine Coupled to Affigel 10

This protocol describes the purification of mouse monoclonal anti-phosphotyrosine antibodies using a hapten coupled to Affigel 10.

1. In this case, the hapten (phosphotyramine) is coupled to Affigel 10 (Bio-Rad Laboratories Inc., 2000 Alfred Nobel Dr, Hercules, CA 94547) following the manufacturer instructions.
2. Pour the matrix into a commercially available column or a syringe and wash with PBS.
3. Centrifuge the sample at 10,000×*g* for 30 min at 4° C to remove any precipitates from the polyclonal or monoclonal antiphosphotyrosine immunoglobulins. Delipidate (*see* Chapter 3, Delipidation) and dialyze or mix 1:1 with PBS, pH 7.4 loading buffer.
4. Connect the column to the pump and wash with PBS, pH 7.4 loading buffer. Wash with 3–5 column volumes at 0 0.5 -1 mL/min.
5. Load the antiphosphotyrosine immunoglobulins in a volume of 5–20 mL and circulate the sample through the column for at least 3 h at 0.2–0.5 mL/min.
6. Drain the column and save the eluent.
7. Start washing with the loading buffer. Wash with at least 10 column volumes and save the wash eluent. Before ending the wash, step check that the absorbance of the eluent is <0.02 AU at 280 nm.

8. Elute the antiphosphotyrosine antibodies with 10 mM *p*-nitrophenol phosphate in PBS, pH 7.4. Use a step wise approach. Add a column volume of the elution buffer and wait for 30 min. Apply a second column volume, save the first volume and again incubate for 30 min. Repeat once more, if necessary. The last column volume of eluate is collected by using PBS as the buffer.
9. The elution sample is pooled and extensively dialyzed to remove the hapten (the hapten will give it a yellow coloration). The hapten can also be removed by using a sizing column (*see* Chapter 3).
10. Concentrate the sample.
11. The column can be regenerated and stored for future use. Wash the column with PBS, pH 7.4 (at least 10 column volumes).
12. Wash the column with 0.1 M glycine, pH 3.0 or 0.1 M acetic acid to remove any residual bound material. Use at least 3 column volumes.
13. Wash the column again with PBS, pH 7.4 until all the acid has been removed. Test the pH of the effluent with pH paper.
14. Store in PBS, pH 7.4 containing 0.02% sodium azide at 4° C.

3.3. Purification of Mouse Monoclonal Antibodies with Protein G Coupled to Agarose

Protein A, Protein G and Protein A/G are ready to use affinity chromatography matrices for the purification of IgG antibodies. They can also be prepared in the laboratory by coupling either one of the proteins or both to agarose. They can be used to purify IgG from most mammalian species including mouse, human, rabbit, rat, goat, cow and horse. If you purchase the ready to use columns or cartridges follow the indications of the manufacturer. As an example, this protocol describes the use of Invitrogen rProtein G Agarose for the purification of mouse monoclonal antibodies from ascites.

1. Ascites should be clear and without particulates. Centrifuge or filter ascites before loading onto column.
2. Delipidate the ascites (*see* Chapter 3, Note 1).
3. Pack a column or a syringe (remember to put glass wool or similar at the bottom) with 2 mL of rProtein G Agarose (*see* Note 6). Connect column to the pump.
4. Wash the column with at least 10 volumes of binding buffer. Use a flow rate of 0.5–1 mL/min.
5. Load sample into column. Sample pH should be between 6 and 7.5. If necessary, dialyze the sample against binding buffer or dilute the sample with binding buffer.

6. Wash the column with 6–12 bed volumes of binding buffer or until the absorbance at 280 nm of the column eluate reaches that of the buffer.
7. Elute bound IgG with 6 bed volumes of elution buffer.
8. Immediately adjust pH of eluted IgG to 7.0 with 1.0 M Tris Base.
9. Reequilibrate column with 4 volumes of binding buffer.
10. The column may be reused beginning at step 5 or may be prepared for storage.
11. After the last sample has been processed, the gel should be cleaned by washing with 5 bed volumes of stripping buffer.
12. Equilibrate the column with 5 volumes of storage buffer and store at 2–8° C.

5. Notes

1. It has become fairly easy to couple peptides, proteins and haptens to Sepharose or agarose beads to form an affinity matrix. The most convenient coupling chemistries are directed at –NH2 and –SH groups because these groups are reactive at physiological pH and their presence in a sequence is either unique or they are in limited number. Some activated affinity matrixes such as CNBr-activated Sepharose (GE HealthCare, 800 Centennial Avenue, Piscataway, NJ 08855) and Affigel (Bio-Rad Laboratories Inc., 2000 Alfred Nobel Dr, Hercules, CA 94547) for amido group chemistry and SulfoLink (Pierce, PO Box 117, Rockford, Ill 61105) for thiol group chemistry are commercially available. The procedures for the coupling reactions are described by the manufacturers. The following is a short description for coupling a protein to CNBr-Sepharose 4B: the resin is hydrated with 10 mM HCl. The hydration step serves to wash the resin of additives as well as to swell the matrix and prepare it for coupling. One gram of dry gel will yield approximately 3.5 mL of coupled resin. Before addition of the protein, the resin is resuspended in coupling buffer. The protein to be coupled (5–10 mg) at 1 mg/mL in coupling buffer (0.1 M NaHCO3, pH 8.3 containing 0.5 M NaCl) is added to the gel and mixed end over end, overnight at 4° C. After overnight coupling the supernatant is saved to determine the concentration of the unbound protein, the resin is washed with coupling buffer to remove unbound ligand and blocked for at least two hours at room temperature or overnight at 4° C with 1 M ethanolamine pH 8.0, 0.2 M glycine, pH 8,

or any other buffer containing amines. The gel is finally washed with alternating cycles (3–6 times) of high and low pH. Buffers such as 0.1 M Tris–HCl, pH 8–9 containing 0.5 M NaCl followed by 0.1 M acetate buffer pH 3–4 containing 0.5 M NaCl can be used. The coupled gel is suspended in a storage buffer such as BBS (0.2 M borate buffer, 0.16 M NaCl, pH 8.0) at 4° C or 20% ethanol. For a detailed protocol see GE Health Care web site at http://www6.gelifesciences.com/aptrix/upp00919.nsf/Content/3DC5E0509E2624FEC1256EB400418007/$file/71500015AD.pdf.

2. Matrix should be chemically and physically inert. Preactivated matrices have been chemically modified to facilitate the coupling of a specific type of ligand. When the affinity medium is not available for a particular purification, one can be designed by coupling a specific ligand to a preactivated chromatography matrix. Antibodies, antigens, enzymes, receptors, peptides as well as small nucleic acids can be used as affinity ligands to enable the purification of their binding partners. Sepharose provides a macroporous matrix with high chemical and physical stability. It also has low non-specific adsorption to facilitate a high binding capacity and sample recovery. The ligand must selectively and reversibly interact with the target molecule and must be compatible with the binding and elution conditions. It must carry chemically modifiable functional groups through which it can be attached to the matrix. Too low affinity will result in poor yields since the protein may leak or wash from the column. Too high affinity will result in poor yields since it will not dissociate during the elution. The ligands should be of the highest purity. When using a small ligand (Mr <5,000) there is a risk of steric hindrance between the ligand and the matrix that restricts the binding of the target molecule, in which case one should select a preactivated matrix with a spacer arm (it is used to improve the binding between ligand and target molecule by overcoming the effects of steric hindrance). In general for ligands Mr >5,000 no spacer arm is necessary.

3. Both proteins are of bacterial origin; protein A is a 42,000 Da polypeptide isolated from the cell walls of *Staphylococcus aureus* and protein G from a cell surface protein from Group G streptococci. Recombinant protein A and G are also available. Both have specificity for the Fc region of IgG. Protein A is used more in the purification of rabbit, pig, dog and cat IgGs while protein G has a better range for human and mouse IgG subclasses. Since protein A and G bind to the Fc region of IgGs they have been useful in the separation of Fc and Fab fragments after proteolytic digestion. Protein A/G is a

recombinant fusion protein that includes the IgG-binding domains of both Protein A and Protein G. It contains the four binding domains from Protein A and the two from Protein G and it has a molecular weight of 50,450 Da. Protein A/G binds to the broadest range of IgG subclasses from rabbit, mouse, human and other mammalian samples. It binds to all human IgG subclasses and also to IgA, IgE, IgM and also slightly to IgD. It also binds well to all mouse IgG subclasses but does not bind to mouse IgA, IgM and murine serum albumin, this makes it a tool of choice for the purification of mouse monoclonal antibodies.

4. Protein L is an immunoglobulin-binding protein obtained from the bacteria *Peptostreptococcus magnus.* It binds Igs through interactions with kappa light chains. Kappa light chains occur in members of all classes of immunoglobulin (i.e., IgG, IgM, IgA, IgE and IgD) and Protein L can purify these different classes of antibody. However, only those antibodies within each class that possess the appropriate kappa light chains will bind.
5. The serum should have been previously centrifuged, delipidated and either dialyzed against the loading buffer or mixed with at least 1:1 volume of loading buffer (*see* Chapter 3, Delipidation).
6. The commercial slurry is at 50% so add 4 mL of the slurry to the column.

Acknowledgement

This work was supported by the Intramural Research Program of the NIH, NIDCR.

References

1. Protein purification handbook. GE Health Care 800 Centennial Avenue, Piscataway, NJ08855. (http://www1.gelifesciences.com/aptrix/upp00919.nsf/Content/9C7BA3 DA 6539F07AC1256EB40044A8B2/$file/1811 3229AC.pdf)
2. Affinity chromatography handbook. Principles and methods. Amersham Biosciences. (http://www1.gelifesciences.com/aptrix/upp00919.nsf/Content/91D3DF5DE303E8B6C1256 EB400417F34/$file/18102229AD.pdf)
3. Antibody. production, purification, fragmentation, labeling. Pierce Biotechnology. P.O. Box 117, Rockford, IL61105. Part 1: http://www.piercenet.com/files/1601323%20 Antibodies_1.pdf; Part 2: http://www.piercenet.com/files/1601323%20Antibodies_2.pdf; Part 3: http://www.piercenet.com/files/1601323%20 Antibodies_3.pdf
4. Bauer K, Bayer PM, Deutsch E, Gabl F (1980) Binding of enzyme-IgG complexes in human serum to Protein-A Sepharose CL-4B. Clin Chem 26:297–300
5. Protein A agarose. Invitrogen. Carlsbad, CA. (https://www.invitrogen.com/content/sfs/manuals/15918014.pdf)

Chapter 6

Conjugation of Fluorochromes to Antibodies

Su-Yau Mao and J. Michael Mullins

Abstract

Immunolocalization of antigen via fluorescence requires that fluorochromes be linked either to the primary antibody (direct method) or to a second antibody (indirect method) to provide a fluorescent signal to mark the site of antibody-antigen binding. Of these two methods, the indirect technique is generally more useful and practical. Fluorochromes can be covalently conjugated to antibodies through reactions with thiol or amine groups. Typically, fluorochromes containing isothiocyanate, succinimidyl ester, or sulfonyl chloride reactive groups are conjugated to amines on the antibody molecules. Provided are step-by-step instructions for conjugating isothiocyanate derivates of fluorescein and sulfonyl chloride derivatives of rhodamine to the amine groups of antibodies.

Key words: Antibody, Immunolocalization, Fluorochrome, Conjugation,Thiol, Amine

1. Introduction

Fluorescence-based immunolocalization of biomolecules within cells and tissues requires that fluorochromes, or fluorescent markers such as quantum dots, be covalently conjugated to antibodies. Techniques for antibody-fluorochrome conjugation were first devised by A. H. Coons and his associates, who pioneered the use of immunofluorescence microscopy in the 1940s and 1950s. Initially, the conjugation of fluorochrome to antibody was done directly to the antibody with the desired antigenic specificity (1). Subsequently, an indirect method (2) of immunolocalization was introduced that proved advantageous for most routine work.

For indirect immunolabeling, the antibody of desired specificity, referred to as the primary antibody, is applied first, without fluorochrome conjugation. After excess primary antibody is washed away, a fluorochrome-conjugated, second antibody is introduced. Antigenic specificity of the second antibody is to immunoglobulin

C. Oliver and M.C. Jamur (eds.), *Immunocytochemical Methods and Protocols*, Methods in Molecular Biology, Vol. 588, DOI 10.1007/978-1-59745-324-0_6, © Humana Press, a part of Springer Science+Business Media, LLC 1995, 1999, 2010

isotypes from the same animal species that produce the primary antibody. Thus, if the primary antibody was produced in a mouse, the second antibody could consist of anti-mouse immunoglobulins produced by immunizing a goat with mouse antibodies. Secondary antibodies bind to the primary antibody, and so deliver fluorochromes to the antigenic site of primary antibody binding. Unless fluorochrome labeling of the primary antibody is demanded by the specific requirements of a project, the indirect method of immunofluorescence labeling provides distinct advantages: (1) The antigenic specificity of the primary antibody is not altered by the process of fluorochrome conjugation. (2) Since secondary antibodies are usually polyclonal, more than one secondary antibody can bind to each primary antibody molecule, delivering additional fluorochromes and thus providing increased fluorescence intensity. (3) A single preparation of fluorochrome-conjugated secondary antibody can be used to localize many different primary antibodies that were all obtained from the same animal species, greatly minimizing the number of conjugations that must be done.

The choice of a fluorochrome to conjugate to the second antibody preparation depends upon the particular application to be undertaken. Chapter 15 (3) reviews the relevant properties of commonly employed fluorochromes. Fluorescein, rhodamine, Texas Red® (4), and phycoerythrin (5, 6) have been common choices, but the more recently introduced fluorochrome families, such as the Alexa series, offer advantages in photostability and other optical properties (7).

Of the chemical groups common to biomolecules, thiol and amine groups are the only ones that can be reliably modified in an aqueous solution. Of these, the thiol group is easier to modify with high selectivity. Nonetheless, amines are common targets for conjugating fluorochromes to antibodies or other proteins, given their availability. In addition to the amine group displayed at the free, amino terminus of a protein, virtually all proteins contain lysine residues as part of their primary structure. The ε-amino group of lysine is moderately basic, and reactive with acylating reagents. At pH values lower than 8.0, the concentration of the freebase form of aliphatic amines is quite low, making the kinetics of acylation reactions of amines by isothiocyanates, succinimidyl esters, and other reagents strongly pH-dependent. Amine acylation reactions are typically carried out above pH 8.5. However, since acylation reagents degrade in the presence of water, with the rate increasing directly with an increase in pH value, a pH in the range of 8.5–9.5 is considered optimal for modifying lysines.

Where possible, the antibodies used for labeling should be pure (*see* Chapters 2–5). Fluorochrome-labeled, affinity-purified antibodies produce less background and lower non-specific fluorescence than are obtained with fluorescent antiserum or immunoglobulin fractions. The instructions provided below give the procedures for labeling antibodies with the isothiocyanate derivatives of fluorescein and sulfonyl chloride derivatives of rhodamine (8). The major problem encountered in these procedures is either over- or under-coupling (*i.e.*, too high or too low a ratio of fluorochrome to antibody), but the level of conjugation can be determined by simple absorbance readings.

For many researchers, the wide range of fluorochrome-conjugated secondary antibodies that are commercially available will likely obviate the need to undertake conjugation in the laboratory. Where it is necessary to do so, the researcher should give consideration to the commercially available kits (*see* Note 6). Such kits provide a convenient way to obtain reliable and reproducible conjugation of fluorochromes antibodies or other proteins.

For some purposes, it may be desirable to conjugate antibodies to quantum dots (3) rather than to organic fluorochrome molecules. Reliable conjugation of quantum dots to proteins has been undertaken through two basic approaches (reviewed in (9, 10)). Either antibodies are covalently conjugated directly to the surface cap of the quantum dots (11), or a linker molecule, such as avidin or genetically modified protein G, is electrostatically assembled onto the quantum dot surface and used to bind the antibody (12). Conjugation methodologies are still being explored (13, 14). For researchers looking to try quantum dot-based immunofluorescence, manufacturers such as Invitrogen, Molecular Probes (www.invitrogen.com/site/us/en/home/brands/Molecular-Probes.html) now provide a variety of secondary antibodies already conjugated to quantum dots, as well as kits to allow conjugation of quantum dots to antibodies or other proteins.

2. Materials

1. Purified IgG.
2. Borate-buffered saline (BBS): 0.2 M boric acid, 160 mM NaCl, pH 8.0.
3. Fluorescein isothiocyanate (FITC) or Lissamine rhodamine B sulfonyl chloride (RBSC).
4. Sodium carbonate buffer: 1.0 M $NaHCO_3$–Na_2CO_3 buffer, pH 9.5, prepared by titrating 1.0 M $NaHCO_3$ with 1.0 M Na_2CO_3 until the pH reaches 9.5.
5. Absolute ethanol (200 proof) or anhydrous dimethylformamide (DMF).
6. Sephadex G-25 column.
7. Whatman DE-52 column.
8. 10 mM sodium phosphate buffer, pH 8.0.

9. 0.02% (w:v) sodium azide.
10. UV spectrophotometer.

3. Methods

3.1. Coupling of Fluorochrome to IgG

1. Prior to coupling, prepare a gel-filtration column to separate the labeled antibody from the free fluorochrome after the completion of the reaction. The size of the column should be 10 bed volumes/sample volume (*see* Note 1).
2. Equilibrate the column in phosphate buffer. Allow the column to run until the buffer level drops just below the top of bed resin. Stop the flow of the column by using a valve at the bottom of the column.
3. Prepare an IgG solution of at least 3 mg/mL in BBS, and add 0.2 volume of sodium carbonate buffer to IgG solution to bring the pH to 9.0. If antibodies have been stored in sodium azide, the azide must be removed prior to conjugation by extensive dialysis (*see* Note 2).
4. Prepare a fresh solution of fluorescein isothiocyanate at 5 mg/mL in ethanol or RBSC at 10 mg/mL in DMF immediately before use (*see* Note 3).
5. Add FITC at a 10-fold molar excess over IgG (about 25 μg of FITC/mg IgG). Mix well and incubate at room temperature for 30 min with gentle shaking. Add RBSC at a fivefold molar excess over IgG (about 20 μg of RBSC/mg IgG), and incubate at 4°C for 1 h.
6. Carefully layer the reaction mixture on the top of the column. Open the valve to the column, and allow the antibody solution to flow into the column until it just enters the bed resin. Carefully add phosphate buffer to the top of the column. The conjugated antibody elutes in the excluded volume (about one-third of the total bed volume).
7. Store the conjugate at 4°C in the presence of 0.02% sodium azide (final concentration) in a light-proof container. The conjugate can also be stored in aliquots at –20°C after it has been snap-frozen on dry ice. Do not refreeze the conjugate once thawed.

3.2. Calculation of Protein Concentration and Fluorochrome-to-Protein Ratio

1. Read the absorbance at 280 and 493 nm. The protein concentration is given by Eq. 1, where 1.4 is the optical density for 1 mg/mL of IgG (corrected to l-cm path length)

$$\text{Fluorescein - conjugated IgG conc.}\left(\text{Fl IgG conc.}\right)$$
$$\left(\text{mg/mL}\right) = (A_{280\text{ nm}} - 0.35 \times A_{493\text{ nm}}) / 1.4$$

2. The molar ratio (F/P) can then be calculated, based on a molar extinction coefficient of 73,000 for the fluorescein group, by Eq. 2 (*see* Notes 4 and 5).

$$F/P = (A_{493\text{ nm}}/73{,}000) \times (150{,}000/\text{Fl IgG conc})$$

3. For rhodamine-labeled antibody, read the absorbance at 280 and 575 nm. The protein concentration is given by Eq. 3.

$$\text{Rhodamine - conjugated IgG conc.}(\text{Rho IgG conc.})\ (\text{mg/mL}) = (A_{280\text{ nm}} - 0.32 \times A_{575\text{ nm}})/1.4$$

4. The molar ratio (F/P) is calculated by Eq. 4.

$$F/P = (A_{575\text{ nm}}/73{,}000) \times (150{,}000/\text{Rho IgG conc.})$$

4. Notes

1. Sephadex G-25 resin is the recommended gel for the majority of desalting applications. It combines good rigidity, for easy handling and good flow characteristics, with adequate resolving power for desalting molecules down to about 5,000 Da mol wt. If the volume of the reaction mixture is <1 mL, a prepacked disposable Sephadex G-25 column (PD-10 column from Pharmacia, Piscataway, NJ) can be used conveniently.
2. When choosing a buffer for conjugation of fluorochromes, avoid those containing amines (e.g., Tris, azide, glycine, and ammonia), which can compete with the ligand.
3. Both sulfonyl chloride and isothiocyanate will hydrolyze in aqueous conditions; therefore, the solutions should be made freshly for each labeling reaction. Absolute ethanol or dimethyl formamide (best grade available, stored in the presence of molecular sieve to remove water) should be used to dissolve the reagent. The hydrolysis reaction is more pronounced in dilute protein solution and can be minimized by using a more concentrated protein solution. Caution: DMSO should not be used with sulfonyl chlorides, because it reacts with them.
4. An F/P ratio of two to five is optimal, since ratios below this yield low signals, whereas higher ratios show high background. If the F/P ratios are too low, repeat the coupling reaction using fresh fluorochrome solution. The IgG solution needs to be concentrated prior to reconjugation (e.g., Centricon-30 microconcentrator from Amicon Co., Beverly, MA, can be used to concentrate the IgG solution).

5. If the F/P ratios are too high, either repeat the labeling with appropriate changes or purify the labeled antibodies further on a Whatman DE-52 column (diethylaminoethyl microgranular preswollen cellulose, l-mL packed column/ l-2 mg of IgG). DE-52 chromatography removes denatured IgG aggregates and allows the selection of the fraction of the conjugate with optimal modification. Equilibrate and load the column with 10 mM phosphate buffer, pH 8.0. Wash the column with equilibrating buffer and elute with the same buffer containing 100 mM NaCl (first) and 250 mM NaCl (last). Measure the F/P ratios of each fraction, and select the appropriate fractions.
6. Alexa fluorochromes are available only as a protein labeling kit from Invitrogen, Molecular Probes, Inc. (Carlsbad, CA, USA; www.probes.com). The reactive dye has a succinimidyl ester moiety that reacts with primary amines of proteins. The conjugation steps are similar to those for fluorescein isothiocyanate.

References

1. Coons AH, Creech HJ, Jones RN (1941) Immunological properties of an antibody containing a fluorescent group. Proc Soc Exp Biol Med 47:200–202
2. Coons AH, Leduc EH, Connolly JM (1955) Studies on antibody production I. A method for the histochemical demonstration of specific antibody and its application to a study of the hyperimmune rabbit. J Exp Med 102:49–60
3. Mullins JM (1999) Fluorochromes: Properties and characteristics. Methods Mol Biol
4. Titus JA, Haugland R, Sharrow SO, Segal DM (1982) Texas Red, a hydrophilic, red-emitting fluorophore for use with fluorescein in dual parameter flow microfluorometric and fluorescence microscopic studies. J Immunol Methods 50:193–204
5. Oi VT, Glazer AN, Stryer L (1982) Fluorescent phycobiliprotein conjugates for analyses of cells and molecules. J Cell Biol 93:981–986
6. Bochner BS, McKelvey AA, Schleimer RP, Hildreth JE, MacGlashan DW Jr (1989) Flow cytometric methods for the analysis of human basophil surface antigens and viability. J Immunol Methods 125:265–271
7. Panchuk-Voloshina N, Haugland RP, Bishop-Stewart J, Bhalgat MK, Millard PJ, Mao F, Leung WY, Haugland RP (1999) Alexa dyes, a series of new fluorescent dyes that yield exceptionally bright, photostable conjugates. J Histochem Cytochem 47:1179–1188
8. Schreiber AB, Haimovich J (1983) Quantitative fluorometric assay for detection and characterization of Fc receptors. Methods Enzymol 93:147–155
9. Jaiswal JK, Simon SM (2004) Potentials and pitfalls of fluorescent quantum dots for biological imaging. Trends Cell Biol 14:497–504
10. Jovin TM (2003) Quantum dots finally come of age. Nat Biotechnol 21:32–33
11. Wu X, Liu H, Liu J, Haley KN, Treadway JA, Larson JP, Ge N, Peale F, Bruchez MP (2003) Immunofluorescent labeling of cancer marker Her2 and other cellular targets with semiconductor quantum dots. Nat Biotechnol 21:41–46
12. Jaiswal JK, Mattousi H, Mauro JM, Simon SM (2003) Long-term multiple color imaging of live cells using quantum dot bioconjugates. Nat Biotechnol 21:47–21
13. Hua X-F, Liu T-C, Cao Y-C, Liu B, Wang H-Q, Wang J-H, Huang Z-L, Zhao Y-D (2006) Characterization of the coupling of quantum dots and immunoglobulin antibodies. Anal Bioanal Chem 386:1665–1671
14. Susumu K, Uyeda HT, Medintz I, Pons T, Delehanty JB, Mattoussi H (2007) Enhancing the stability and biological functionalities of quantum dots via compact multifunctional ligands. J Am Chem Soc 129:13987–13996

Chapter 7

Biotinylation of Antibodies

Su-Yau Mao

Abstract

Using the characteristic of a high-affinity complex between avidin and biotin, biotinylated antibodies have wide applications in various immunochemical assays, especially where signal amplification is required. A method is described here for the biotinylation of immunoglobulins. The procedure utilizes water-soluble succinimidyl ester of biotin that reacts with primary amines of the lysine residues or the amino terminus on the antibody to form amide bonds. The method is simple and specific and results in stable conjugates retaining full immunologic activity.

Key words: Biotinylation, Antibody, Immunoglobulin, IgG, Biotin, Avidin, Streptavidin, NHS–biotin, sulfo-NHS–biotin

1. Introduction

The high affinity and specificity of the avidin–biotin interaction permit diverse applications in immunology, histochemistry, in situ hybridizations, affinity chromatography, and many other areas (1) (*see* Chapters 26 and 27). This reaction was first exploited in immunocytochemical applications in the mid-1970s (2, 3), and has since been commonly used to localize antigens in cells and tissues. In this technique, a biotinylated primary or secondary antibody is first applied to the sample, and the detection is accomplished by using labeled avidin. Avidin with a variety of labels is available commercially, including fluorescent, enzyme, iodine, ferritin, or gold conjugates.

Both avidin and its bacterial counterpart, streptavidin, are standard reagents for histochemical procedures. Avidin is a 66-kDa, positively charged glycoprotein with an isoelectric point of about 10.5 (4). The positively charged residues and the oligosaccharide component of avidin can interact nonspecifically with

C. Oliver and M.C. Jamur (eds.), *Immunocytochemical Methods and Protocols*, Methods in Molecular Biology, Vol. 588, DOI 10.1007/978-1-59745-324-0_7, © Humana Press, a part of Springer Science+Business Media, LLC 1995, 1999, 2010

negatively charged cell surfaces and nucleic acids, sometimes causing background problems in histochemical and cytometric applications. Avidin is inexpensive, however, and remains one of the most commonly used reagents for these applications. On the other hand, streptavidin, a 60-kDa nonglycosylated protein with a near-neutral isoelectric point, exhibits less nonspecific binding than avidin. Both avidin and streptavidin bind four biotin equivalents per molecule with high affinity (K_a is about 10^{14} M^{-1}) and low reversibility, thus permitting numerous combinations of avidin, biotin, and antibody. It is possible to create a widely branching complex and build up high amounts of label over the original antigenic site to increase the sensitivity. One such technique was developed by Hsu et al. (5).

Labeling antibodies by covalent coupling of a biotinyl group is simple and, usually, does not have any adverse effect on the antibody (6). Most biotinylations are performed using a succinimidyl ester of biotin. The reagent reacts with primary amines of the lysine residues or the amino terminus on the antibody to form amide bonds. The protocol described below (7, 8) uses a water-soluble analog of *N*-hydroxylsuccinimide biotin (available from Pierce (Thermo Fisher Scientific), Rockford, IL, or Molecular Probes (Invitrogen), Eugene, OR), which can be dissolved directly in the reaction buffer. Biotin-coupled antibodies are stable under normal storage conditions.

2. Materials

1. Purified IgG.
2. Sulfosuccinimidobiotin: 2 mg/mL in sodium borate buffer (*see* Note 1).
3. Sodium borate buffer: 0.2 M boric acid, 160 mM NaCl, pH 8.5.
4. Dialysis tubing.
5. Phosphate-buffered saline (PBS): 10 mM sodium phosphate, 150 mM NaCI, pH 7.4.
6. UV spectrophotometer.
7. 0.02% (w:v) sodium azide.

3. Methods

1. Prepare an IgG solution of at least 3 mg/mL in sodium borate buffer. If the antibodies have been stored in sodium azide, the azide must be removed prior to conjugation. Dialyze extensively against the borate buffer (*see* Note 2).

2. Add the sulfosuccinimidobiotin at a 30-fold molar excess over IgG (about 90 μg/mg IgG). Mix well, and incubate at room temperature for 30 min with gentle shaking (*see* Note 3).
3. Dialyze extensively against several changes (>10^6-fold dilution) of phosphate-buffered saline or other desired buffer to remove uncoupled biotin.
4. Centrifuge dialysate (8,000 × *g*, 10 min, 4 °C) to remove any precipitate formed during dialysis.
5. Determine the IgG concentration by measuring the absorbance at 280 nm (absorbance of 1 mg/mL = 1.4, measured using cuvette with l-cm path length).
6. Store the conjugate at 4 °C in the presence of 0.02% sodium azide (final concentration). The conjugate can be stored in aliquots at –20 °C for very long periods if previously snap-frozen on dry ice (*see* Notes 4 and 5).

4. Notes

1. The sulfonated esters will hydrolyze in aqueous conditions. Therefore, the solutions should be made freshly before each use. The hydrolysis reaction is more pronounced in dilute protein solutions and can be minimized by increasing protein concentration.
2. When choosing a buffer for biotinylations, avoid those containing amines (e.g., Tris, azide, glycine, and ammonia), which can compete with the ligand. Phosphate buffers may result in the "salting out" of the biotin reagents containing sulfo-N-hydroxysuccinimide moieties.
3. Alternatively, the water-insoluble biotinylated succinimidyl ester can be first dissolved in fresh distilled dimethylsulfoxide (10 mg/mL), and then added to the IgG solution.
4. Many biotinylated succinimidyl esters are now available. Most of these variations alter the size of the spacer arm between the succinimide coupling group and the biotin. The additional spacers could facilitate avidin binding and, thus, may be critical for some applications (9).
5. If a free amino group forms a portion of the protein that is essential for activity (e.g., the antigen-combining site for antibody), biotinylation with the succinimidyl ester will lower or destroy the activity of the protein, and other methods of labeling should be tried. Biotin hydrazide has been used to modify the carbohydrate moieties of antibodies (10, 11). Other alternatives are the thiol-reactive biotin maleimide (12) or biotin iodoacetamide (13).

References

1. Roffman E, Meromsky L, Ben-Hur H, Bayer EA, Wilchek M (1986) Selective labeling of functional groups on membrane proteins or glycoproteins using reactive biotin derivatives and ^{125}I-streptavidin. Biochem Biophys Res Commun 136:80–85
2. Becker JM, Wilchek M (1972) Inactivation by avidin of biotin-modified bacteriophage. Biochim Biophys Acta 264:165–170
3. Heitzmann H, Richards FM (1974) Use of the avidin-biotin complex for specific staining of biological membranes in electron microscopy. Proc Natl Acad Sci U S A 71:3537–3541
4. Green NM (1975) Avidin. Adv Protein Chem 29:85–133
5. Hsu SM, Raine L, Fanger H (1981) Use of avidin–biotin–peroxidase complex (ABC) in immunoperoxidase techniques: a comparison between ABC and unlabeled antibody (PAP) procedures. J Histochem Cytochem 29: 577–580
6. Guesdon JL, Ternynck T, Avrameas S (1979) The use of avidin–biotin interaction in immunoenzymatic techniques. J Histochem Cytochem 27:1131–1139
7. Lee WT, Conrad DH (1984) The murine lymphocyte receptor for IgE II. Characterization of the multivalent nature of the B lymphocyte receptor for IgE. J Exp Med 159:1790–1795
8. LaRochelle WJ, Froehner SC (1986) Determination of the tissue distributions and relative concentrations of the postsynaptic 43-kDa protein and the acetylcholine receptor in Torpedo. J Biol Chem 261:5270–5274
9. Suter M, Butler JE (1986) The immunochemistry of sandwich ELISAs II. A novel system prevents the denaturation of capture antibodies. Immunol Lett 13:313–316
10. O'Shannessy DJ, Dobersen MJ, Quarles RH (1984) A novel procedure for labeling immunoglobulins by conjugation to oligosaccharide moieties. Immunol Lett 8: 273–277
11. O'Shannessy DJ, Quarles RH (1987) Labeling of the oligosaccharide moieties of immunoglobulins. J Immunol Methods 99:153–161
12. Bayer EA, Zalis MG, Wilchek M (1985) 3-(N-Maleimido-propionyl)biocytin: a versatile thiol-specific biotinylating reagent. Anal Biochem 149:529–536
13. Sutoh K, Yamamoto K, Wakabayashi T (1984) Electron microscopic visualization of the SH1 thiol of myosin by the use of an avidin–biotin system. J Mol Biol 178:323–339

Part II

Tissue Preparation for Light Microscopic Analysis

Chapter 8

Cell Fixatives for Immunostaining

Maria Célia Jamur and Constance Oliver

Abstract

Fixation is one of the most critical steps in immunostaining. The object of fixation is to achieve good morphological preservation, while at the same time preserving antigenicity. Tissue blocks, sections, cell cultures or smears are usually immersed in a fixative solution, while in other situations, whole body perfusion of experimental animals is preferable. Fixation can be accomplished by either chemical or physical methods. The chemical methods include cross-linking agents such as formaldehyde, glutaraldehyde and succinimide esters as well as solvents such as acetone and methanol, which precipitate proteins. Of the physical methods, freezing tissue and air drying are most widely used. This chapter deals with the chemical fixation methods most commonly used for light microscopy.

Key words: Fixation, Formaldehyde, Glutaraldehyde, Methanol, Acetone, PLP, Methacarn, Carnoy's, Bouin's

1. Introduction

Fixation is one of the most critical steps in immunostaining. The object is to achieve good morphological preservation while at the same time preserving antigenicity (1, 2). This becomes more problematic when one is dealing with intracellular antigens and the sample must be permeabilized to allow access to the antigen. The goal of fixation is to preserve cells and tissues in a life-like manner. Tissue blocks, sections, cell cultures or smears are usually immersed in a fixative solution (3). In some cases, perfusion of the whole animal via its circulatory system with fixative solutions is preferred. Fixation is also necessary to stabilize the sample and protect it from the deleterious effects of the immunostaining process. Fixation also helps to prevent artifactual diffusion of cell components, arrests enzymatic activity,

C. Oliver and M.C. Jamur (eds.), *Immunocytochemical Methods and Protocols*, Methods in Molecular Biology, Vol. 588,
DOI 10.1007/978-1-59745-324-0_8, © Humana Press, a part of Springer Science+Business Media, LLC 1995, 1999, 2010

and avoids decomposition of the tissue. Furthermore, the process of fixation helps to preserve the sample by inhibiting bacterial and fungal growth and by inhibiting lysosomal enzymes whose activity could lead to autolysis. Tissues vary in their composition, having different protein and lipid content. They also differ in the structural arrangement of these components. The fixatives, formaldehyde and glutaraldehyde, which are best for the preservation of tissue and protein structure (4) do so by cross-linking proteins making access of reagents difficult and possibly masking some epitopes. There is no universal fixative and with some antigens it may be necessary to try multiple fixatives. Any given fixative may preserve the immunoreactivity of one epitope, but it may destroy other epitopes on the same antigen (1). Fixation can be accomplished by either chemical or physical methods. The chemical methods include cross-linking agents such as formaldehyde, glutaraldehyde and succinimide esters as well as solvents such as acetone and methanol, which precipitate proteins (5). A new proprietary fixative, HOPE (Hepes-glutamic acid buffer-mediated Organic solvent Protection Effect), that uses no cross-linking agents has recently been developed (6). The physical methods most commonly used are freezing (*see* Chapter 10) and air drying. The most widely used fixative for immunostaining is formaldehyde (*see* Note 1), either alone or in combination with a solvent such as methanol or another substance such as picric acid (trinitrophenol) that coagulates proteins. Formaldehyde is a pungent, colorless, toxic, water-soluble gas that rapidly polymerizes into paraformaldehyde. Methanol is often added to commercial preparations to stabilize the formaldehyde (*see* Note 2). Most of the formaldehyde in a freshly prepared aqueous solution is in the form of methylene glycol, a small molecule that penetrates the tissue rapidly. Formaldehyde-based fixatives stabilize tissues by reacting primarily with basic amino acids to form methylene cross-links. The number of methylene bridges formed depends on the concentration of formaldehyde, temperature, pH and time of exposure (7). These fixatives are relatively gentle and are partially reversible. Formaldehyde is usually used as a 2–10% solution in buffer, such as phosphate-buffered saline, or in cold methanol. It is also a component of Bouin's fixative. This chapter deals primarily with fixatives most commonly used for light microscopy. However, for electron microscopy, formaldehyde is frequently used in combination with low concentrations of glutaraldehyde (*see* Note 3 and Chapter 37). Of the physical methods, freezing tissue is most widely used (*see* Chapter 10). Tissue blocks may be fixed before freezing or unfixed frozen sections may be fixed in situ.

2. Materials

1. 8% Paraformaldehyde Stock (*see* Note 4): Heat 800 mL of distilled H_2O to 55° C. Add 80 g of paraformaldehyde prill type and stir continuously on heat/stir plate. Do not allow powder to settle. Do not allow temp to exceed 60° C (*see* Note 5). Stir solution for 15 min at 55° C. Add a few drops of 1 *N* NaOH until the solution just clears. A small amount of flocculent material may remain. Filter through Whatman No. 1 filter paper. Bring volume to 1 L and store at 4° C for up to 1 month.
2. Lysine Stock: Dissolve 16.4 g of l-Lysine in 300 mL distilled H_2O. Adjust pH to 7.4 with 0.1 M Na_2HPO_4. Bring volume to 450 mL with distilled H_2O. Bring volume to 900 mL with 0.1 M Sorenson's Phosphate buffer. This may be stored at 4° C for up to 3 weeks.
3. 0.4 M Sorenson's phosphate buffer Stock: Dissolve 7.176 g sodium phosphate monobasic monohydrate ($NaH_2PO_4{\cdot}H_2O$) in 100 mL distilled H_2O. Dissolve 49.4 g of sodium phosphate ($NaPO_4$) in 750 mL distilled H_2O. Mix the sodium phosphate monobasic monohydrate and sodium phosphate solutions in a 1 L cylinder. Bring volume to 1 L with distilled water. The pH should be 7.6. Do not adjust pH. This may be stored at room temp for up to 6 months. For use dilute with distilled water to 0.1 M.
4. Paraformaldehyde/Lysine/Periodate Fixative (PLP) (2) (*see* Note 6): Place 30 mL of lysine stock in a 50 mL screw cap tube. Add 10 mL 8% paraformaldehyde. Add 0.085 g of Sodium *m*-periodate powder. Shake until powder dissolves.
5. Phosphate Buffered Saline (PBS): 8.0 g NaCl, 0.2 g KCl, 0.2 g KH_2PO_4, 2.16 g Na_2HPO_4 bring to 1 L with distilled water. pH should be 7.4.
6. Methacarn Methanol Carnoy's fixative: Freshly prepare, by volume, a solution of 60% methanol, 30% chloroform and 10% glacial acetic acid.
7. Glutaraldehyde should be purchased as a 70% solution of purified glutaraldehyde packaged in glass ampules under nitrogen.
8. Bouin's Fixative (*see* Note 7): Mix together 300 mL saturated picric acid (*see* Note 8), 100 mL commercial formalin (*see* Note 9) and 20 mL glacial acetic acid.

3. Methods

3.1. Paraformaldehyde/ Lysine/Periodate

1. Place sample in PLP fixative for a maximum of 24 h.
2. Rinse sample with 0.1 M Sorrensons phosphate buffer.
3. Process for immunomicroscopy.

3.2. Formaldehyde in PBS

1. Dilute formaldehyde (*see* Note 10) to 1–4% in PBS.
2. Immerse sample in formaldehyde solution for 15 min to 12 h at room temperature depending on the specimen.
3. Rinse well, a minimum of three times, in PBS.
4. Process as desired.

3.3. 2% Formaldehyde in Methanol (see Note 11)

1. Dilute freshly prepared formaldehyde stock or commercial formaldehyde to 2% in absolute methanol at –20° C (*see* Note 12).
2. Place sample on ice (*see* Note 13).
3. Add fixative and fix for 2–5 min on ice.
4. After 2–5 min, dilute the methanol-formaldehyde with cold PBS (*see* Note 14).
5. Remove half the solution.
6. Replace with cold PBS.
7. Repeat two more times.
8. Rinse in cold PBS.
9. Process as usual.

3.4. Cold Methanol or Acetone (see Note 11)

1. Place sample on ice (*see* Note 13).
2. Add absolute methanol or acetone at –20° C (*see* Note 12) and fix for 2–5 min on ice.
3. After 2–5 min, dilute the methanol or acetone with cold PBS (*see* Note 14).
4. Remove half the solution.
5. Replace with cold PBS.
6. Repeat two more times.
7. Rinse in cold PBS.
8. Process as usual.

3.5. Methacarn (Methanol Carnoy's fixative) (see Note 15)

1. Fix thin slices or small blocks of tissue for 6–8 h at room temperature in Methacarn.
2. Rinse in two changes of methanol, 1 h each.
3. Rinse in several changes of methyl benzoate.
4. Clear, infiltrate and embed as usual.

3.6. Glutaraldehyde–Formaldehyde (see Note 16)

1. Dilute stock glutaraldehyde solution to 0.5% in PBS containing 2% formaldehyde (*see* Note 17).
2. Fix samples for 20 min to 1 h in fixative.
3. Rinse three times in PBS.
4. Process as usual.

3.7. Bouin's Fixative (see Note 18)

1. Fix tissue by immersion for 1–12 h depending on sample size (*see* Notes 19 and 20).
2. Wash in 70% alcohol to precipitate soluble picrates.
3. Wash in water.
4. Dehydrate and embed tissue in paraffin.
5. Cut sections may be treated with 5% aqueous sodium thiosulfate followed by washing in water to remove any residual picric acid.

4. Notes

1. Commercial formalin preparations should not be used. Formalin is an aqueous solution of formaldehyde that typically contains 37–40% formaldehyde, 10–15% methanol and <0.05% formic acid and usually contains impurities. It has a high background fluorescence.
2. For immunostaining formaldehyde should be freshly prepared from paraformaldehyde powder or purchased as an EM grade aqueous paraformaldehyde solution sealed in ampoules under nitrogen.
3. Since glutaraldehyde is autofluorescent, it should not be used as a fixative for immunofluorescence.
4. *Paraformaldehyde is toxic. Prepare in fume hood.*
5. If the temperature exceeds 60° C, formic acid will form.
6. PLP fixative should be made just before use.
7. Bouin's fixative is *carcinogenic, irritant and toxic*. If you do not use it routinely, it is better to buy small amounts of the fixative ready-made than to make it.
8. To make a saturated solution of picric acid, add distilled water to the manufacturer's container and let it stand in a dark place. Do not let the picric acid dry out as it can become explosive.
9. Commercially available formalin is 37–40% formaldehyde (*see* Note 1) and may destroy many epitopes.

10. Formaldehyde should either be freshly prepared from paraformaldehyde or purchased as a purified solution (*see* Note 2).
11. This method is better suited to cultured cells grown on coverslips or to frozen section on glass slides. It is not well suited to blocks of tissue.
12. Absolute methanol or acetone may be stored in the freezer at –20° C until just before use.
13. Sample should be transferred to glass containers before fixation.
14. PBS should be added to the solvent to prevent evaporation of methanol or acetone and drying of the sample.
15. Methacarn is a fixative used on tissues to be paraffin-embedded and immunochemically stained in which methanol has been substituted for the ethanol in Carnoy's fluid. This methanol–Carnoy mixture is referred to as methacarn solution. It preserves certain tissue and cell components such as collagen and cytoskeletal elements exceptionally well for immunoperoxidase and other immunochemical staining (8).
16. Glutaraldehyde crosslinks proteins and may alter protein configuration and mask epitopes. Because of its cross-linking properties, penetration of reagents may be impaired. For immunocytochemistry, it is usually used in low concentration in combination with formaldehyde.
17. The concentration of glutaraldehyde may vary between 0.25 and 1% and the concentration of formaldehyde may vary between 2 and 4%.
18. Work in a well-ventilated area, wear gloves, lab coat and goggles. Avoid contact and inhalation. Toxic through skin exposure.
19. Tissues fixed for longer than 12–24 h become very brittle.
20. Lipids may be extracted or altered, so lipid-containing antigens may be affected.

References

1. Larsson L-I (2000) Immunocytochemistry: theory and practice. CRC Press, Boca Raton, FL
2. McLean IW, Nakane PK (1974) Periodate-lysine-paraformaldehyde fixative A new fixative for immunoelectron microscopy. J Histochem Cytochem 22:1077–1083
3. Presnell JK, Schreibman MP (1997) Humanson's animal tissue techniques. The Johns Hopkins University Press, Baltimore and London
4. Mason JT, O'Leary TJ (1991) Effects of formaldehyde fixation on protein secondary structure: a calorimetric and infrared spectroscopic investigation. J Histochem Cytochem 39:225–229
5. Kiernan JA (1981) Histological and histochemical methods: theory and practice. Pergamon, Oxford, UK
6. Olert J, Wiedorn KH, Goldmann T, Kuhl H, Mehraein Y, Scherthan H, Niketeghad F,

Vollmer E, Muller AM, Muller-Navia J (2001) HOPE fixation: a novel fixing method and paraffin-embedding technique for human soft tissues. Pathol Res Pract 197:823–826
7. Werner M, Chott A, Fabiano A, Battifora H (2000) Effect of formalin tissue fixation and processing on immunohistochemistry. Am J Surg Path 24:1016–1019
8. Holde P, Waldrop FS, Meloan SN, Terry MS, Conner HM (1970) Methacarn (methanol–Carnoy) fixation. Histochem Cell Biol 21:97–116

Chapter 9

Permeabilization of Cell Membranes

Maria Célia Jamur and Constance Oliver

Abstract

In order to detect intracellular antigens, cells must first be permeabilized especially after fixation with cross-linking agents such as formaldehyde and glutaraldehyde. Permeabilization provides access to intracellular or intraorganellar antigens. Two general types of reagents are commonly used: organic solvents, such as methanol and acetone, and detergents such as saponin, Triton X-100 and Tween-20. The organic solvents dissolve lipids from cell membranes making them permeable to antibodies. Because the organic solvents also coagulate proteins, they can be used to fix and permeabilize cells at the same time. Saponin interacts with membrane cholesterol, selectively removing it and leaving holes in the membrane. The disadvantage of detergents such as Triton X-100 and Tween-20 is that they are non-selective in nature and may extract proteins along with the lipids. This chapter provides methods for the use of organic solvents and detergents to permeabilize cell membranes.

Key words: Permeabilization, Organic solvents, Detergents, Saponin, Triton X-100, Tween 20

1. Introduction

In order to detect intracellular antigens, cells first must be permeabilized especially after fixation with cross-linking agents such as formaldehyde and glutaraldehyde (1). Permeabilization provides access to intracellular or intraorganellar antigens (*see* Fig. 1). Two general types of reagents are commonly used: organic solvents, such as methanol and acetone, and detergents. The organic solvents dissolve lipids from cell membranes making them permeable to antibodies. Because the organic solvents also coagulate proteins, they can be used to fix and permeabilize cells at the same time (*see* Chapter 8). However, these solvents may also extract lipidic antigens or lipid associated

C. Oliver and M.C. Jamur (eds.), *Immunocytochemical Methods and Protocols*, Methods in Molecular Biology, Vol. 588, DOI 10.1007/978-1-59745-324-0_9, © Humana Press, a part of Springer Science+Business Media, LLC 1995, 1999, 2010

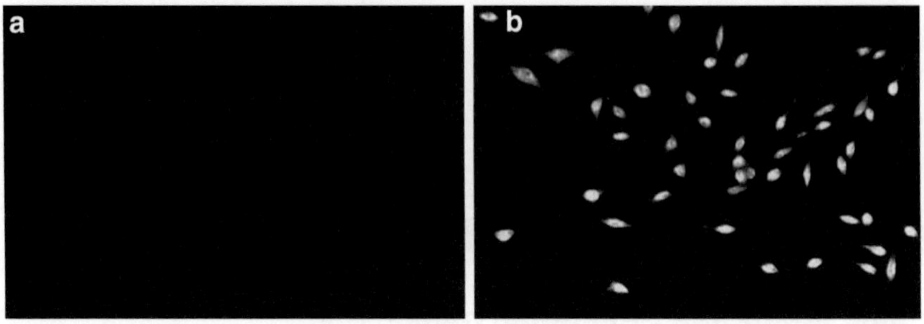

Fig. 1. Cultured RBL-2H3 cells unpermeabilized (**a**) and permeabilized with acetone (**b**) for 5 min at –20°C. Without permeabilization, there is no immunostaining. However, after permeabilization, the antibody has access to the antigen and the cells immunolabel.

antigens from cells. Paraffin embedded tissues often do not need further permeabilization since they are exposed to organic solvents during embedding and preparation of sections for immunostaining. The other large class of permeabilization agents is detergents. Saponin, a plant glycoside, interacts with membrane cholesterol, selectively removing cholesterol and making ~100Å holes in the membrane (2). In addition to forming membrane holes, antibodies may be incorporated into saponin/cholesterol micelles facilitating their entry into the cells. Saponin permeabilization is not effective on cholesterol-poor membranes such as mitochondrial membranes and the nuclear envelope (3). Non-ionic detergents such as Triton X-100 and Tween 20 are also widely used to permeabilize cells and tissues. These detergents contain uncharged, hydrophilic head groups that consist of polyoxyethylene moieties (4). The disadvantage of these detergents is that they are non-selective in nature and may extract proteins along with the lipids, resulting in a false negative during immunostaining. Depending on the antigen, a combination of permeabilizing agents may be preferable (3).

2. Materials

1. Absolute methanol or acetone, –20°C.
2. 0.01% saponin in PBS.
3. Phosphate Buffered Saline (PBS): 8.0 g NaCl, 0.2 g KCl, 0.2 g KH_2PO_4, 2.16 g Na_2HPO_4 bring to 1 L with distilled water. pH 7.4.

3. Methods

3.1. Methanol or Acetone

1. Place sample on ice (*see* Note 1).
2. Add absolute methanol or acetone at –20°C (*see* Note 2) and permeabilize for 1–2 min on ice.
3. After permeabilization, dilute the methanol or acetone with cold PBS (*see* Note 3).
4. Remove half the solution.
5. Replace with cold PBS.
6. Repeat two more times.
7. Rinse in cold PBS.
8. Process as usual.

3.1.1. Saponin

1. After fixation, rinse, quench and block tissue or cells (*see* Note 4).
2. Immunostain tissue using primary antibody diluted in buffer containing 0.01% saponin (*see* Note 5).
3. Rinse five times in PBS with or without saponin.
4. Incubate in secondary antibody diluted in PBS with or without saponin.
5. Rinse ten times in PBS.
6. Mount for immunofluorescence or process for enzyme-linked secondary antibodies (*see* Note 6).

3.2. Triton X-100

1. After fixation, rinse, quench and block tissue or cells (*see* Note 4).
2. Samples should be permeabilized by immersion in 0.1–1% Triton X-100 in PBS for 10–15 min (*see* Note 7).
3. Rinse five times in PBS.
4. Immunostain as usual.

4. Notes

1. Samples should be placed in glass containers.
2. Methanol and acetone may be stored in a –20°C freezer until just before use.
3. PBS should be added to solvent to prevent evaporation of methanol or acetone and drying of the sample.

4. If the sample is fixed with aldehyde fixatives it should be quenched with a solution of 0.1 M glycine that binds to free aldehyde groups. Non-specific binding of antibodies should be blocked using 1–2% BSA (Bovine Serum Albumin) in PBS with or without 5 μgm/mL of normal IgG from the same species as the secondary antibody.
5. Saponin may also be added to the blocking solution.
6. Depending on the sample saponin may be omitted after staining with the primary antibody.
7. The concentration and time of incubation in Triton X-100 has to be determined for each sample. Care should be taken that antigen is not being extracted by detergent exposure.

References

1. Larsson L-I (2000) Immunocytochemistry: theory and practice. CRC Press, Boca Raton, FL
2. Seeman P, Iles SD, Iles GH (1973) Structure of membrane holes in osmotic and saponin hemolysis. J Cell Biol 56:519–527
3. Goldenthal KL, Hedman K, Chen JW, August JT, Willingham MC (1983) Postfixation detergent treatment for immunofluorescence suppresses localization of some integral membrane proteins. J Histochem Cytochem 33:813–820
4. Bhairi SM (2001) Detergents: a guide to the properties and uses of detergents in biological systems. Calbiochem-Novabiochem Corporation, San Diego, CA

Chapter 10

Preparation of Frozen Sections for Analysis

Gary L. Bratthauer

Abstract

The analysis of frozen tissue by antibodies can be accomplished by the quick freezing of a small tissue sample in liquid nitrogen. Super-cooled isopentane can also be used to further the preservation process. Freezing preserves the available proteins in a near-native state for their identification by antibodies raised against naturally folded proteins. The tissues are sectioned onto charged glass slides where they can be optimally fixed in weakly or non-denaturing solutions such as acetone or those that are alcohol-based. Following mild pretreatment steps to allow for antibody use with low background, (the endogenous peroxidase enzyme or oxidative compounds quenched in a hydrogen peroxide solution and available charged sites blocked by incubation in a normal serum solution) the sections are ready for antigen detection.

Key words: Cryostat, Liquid nitrogen, Fixation, Frozen tissue, Isopentane, Charged slides

1. Introduction

Fresh tissue must be preserved in some manner before analysis because the substances to be tested in the tissue are often labile and cannot withstand analytical procedures without first being preserved. The best method for antigen preservation in immunocytochemical analysis is freezing. Freezing is a very suitable means for preserving antigens that lose their immunoreactivity (1). Fresh tissue, after being obtained, is quick frozen in a flask of liquid nitrogen for a few seconds depending on the size of the sample. The rapid introduction of ultra cold temperatures prevents soluble materials from degrading and reinforces the structural components steadfastly holding them in place. This method of preservation does not specifically alter the tissue in any way other than to cause some labile or low concentration solutes to degrade slightly or lyophilize. In performing assays

C. Oliver and M.C. Jamur (eds.), *Immunocytochemical Methods and Protocols*, Methods in Molecular Biology, Vol. 588,
DOI 10.1007/978-1-59745-324-0_10, © Humana Press, a part of Springer Science+Business Media, LLC 1995, 1999, 2010

on frozen specimens, there is always a bit of denaturation as the sections are placed on glass slides. There is also the risk of lyophilization of important components as well as the threat of freeze/thaw conditions occurring in the freezer after the specimens are preserved. However, this method of producing frozen specimens for analysis by antibody labeling is the closest one can come to in vivo conditions since no chemical changes have been forced upon the tissue. Instead, the tissue is bathed in the cold liquid form of nitrogen gas until frozen. The quickness with which this occurs is the reason this process is so good for preservation. Sometimes it is desirable to speed up the process even further, and an organic medium directly bathes the specimen. In this case, penetration occurs more quickly than with liquid nitrogen alone.

2. Materials

2.1. Cutting Sections

1. Gloves.
2. Goggles.
3. Liquid nitrogen, in tank (–196°C).
4. Dewar flask, styrofoam, or some such insulated thermos.
5. Mounting block.
6. Medium such as Tissue-Tek OCT media (Sakura Finetek USA, Inc., Torrance, CA) or Gum Tragacanth (Fisher Scientific, Pittsburgh, PA) 7% in H_2O.
7. Large forceps.
8. Cryostat microtome.
9. Clean glass slides or positively charged glass slides.
10. Freezer, –70°C.
11. Staining racks and dishes.
12. Stirring block with stir bars.
13. Zip-lock bags and slide boxes.
14. Tin foil.
15. Isopentane.
16. 60–80°C Oven.

2.2. Immunostaining of Frozen Sections

1. 0.1% Poly-L-lysine solution (Sigma Aldrich, St. Louis, MO).
2. Fixative solution of 95% ethanol, 5% glacial acetic acid, which should be prepared in advance and kept in the cold (4°C).
3. Phosphate-buffered saline (PBS): 0.01 M sodium phosphate, 0.89% sodium chloride, pH 7.40 ± 0.05.

4. Endogenous enzyme-blocking solution, 1.5% hydrogen peroxide (H_2O_2) in PBS prepared from a dilution of 30% H_2O_2.
5. Serum-blocking solution, 10% animal serum in PBS (the species of serum should match the detecting system antibody, *see* Note 8).

3. Methods

3.1. Preserving Tissue in Liquid Nitrogen

1. Fill a dewar flask half full with liquid nitrogen (*see* Note 1).
2. Apply some OCT embedding medium or 7% suspension of Gum Tragacanth compound in tap water to the end of a mounting block. Attach long forceps to the other end.
3. Immerse in liquid nitrogen for two seconds to adhere compound to the block.
4. Obtain the fresh specimen and set it into the compound on the end of the mounting block. Make sure the tissue is in the desired orientation (*see* Note 2).
5. Plunge the sample directly into the liquid nitrogen immediately after securing it to the block (*see* Note 3).
6. Time to freeze is dependent on the size of the specimen, but for most applications it should only be 10–15 s (*see* Note 3).
7. Remove frozen sample and place in ultra low freezer in zip lock bag to prevent lyophilization (*see* Note 4).

3.2. Sectioning Frozen Tissue

3.2.1. Preparing Coated Slides (If Uncharged)

1. Place Clean glass slides in a staining rack.
2. Immerse the slides for 30 min in a large staining dish containing a 1:10 dilution of 0.1% Poly-l-lysine solution in deionized water (*see* Note 5).
3. Remove the slides and oven dry for 1 h at 60°C.

3.2.2. Preparing the Sections

1. Fasten the mounting block to the block holder in the cryostat.
2. Align the knife to touch the surface of the tissue.
3. Set the thickness to 4 μm.
4. Begin cutting slowly until a nice section clings to the knife.
5. Touch a commercially prepared charged slide or Poly-l-lysine coated slide to the section so that it binds to the surface of the glass. Allow it to air dry (*see* Notes 5 and 6).
6. Store cut sections at –70°C in slide boxes.

3.3. Preparation of Section for Immunostaining

1. Sections in slide rack should be rapidly removed from the freezer and placed in a staining dish with the ethanol/acetic acid fixative solution for 2–10 min depending on tissue and antigen assayed (*see* Note 6).

2. Rinse the fixed sections with three changes of tap water, for 5 min each to remove the fixative solution.
3. Block endogenous peroxidase and peroxidase-like activity by incubation in 1.5% H_2O_2 in PBS endogenous enzyme-blocking solution for 15 min with constant stirring (*see* Note 7).
4. Rinse in water with three changes for 5 min each to remove all of the Hydrogen peroxide.
5. Block charged sites on tissue surface with incubation in the 10% serum in PBS serum blocking solution overnight at 4°C (*see* Note 8).

4. Notes

1. Be extra careful around the liquid nitrogen as it can cause serious injury. Wear goggles and gloves when handling the liquid nitrogen.
2. It is important to work quickly because the tissue will start to deteriorate the moment it is obtained. As always, when handling fresh tissue, it is imperative to wear gloves and protective clothing. If desired, specimens may be wrapped in tin foil and immersed into the liquid nitrogen directly. This way, the sample may be refrozen at a later date with proper orientation on an embedding medium-coated mounting block.
3. It is more detrimental to stop the freezing too soon than to let it continue too long, so add a few seconds to the actual freezing time. It may be necessary to quick freeze with a minimum of artifact. This may be accomplished by the use of isopentane cooled by immersion into liquid nitrogen, and used as the freezing medium. This liquid nitrogen super-cooled isopentane will preserve the tissue more rapidly and thus more efficiently. Isopentane will penetrate the tissue and allow the cold temperatures to freeze the tissue more quickly; however, it will freeze with too much liquid nitrogen exposure. (a) Place the isopentane in a pyrex beaker or large test tube which is small enough to be put in the dewar flask. Add the isopentane and surround the beaker with liquid nitrogen. (b) After 2 min the temperature should be –140°C. Plunge the specimen in the isopentane for 10 s. Rapid freezing is the best preservation tool. Liquid nitrogen and cooled isopentane serve the purpose of cooling quickly. The tissue should be relatively small in size to allow for rapid and thorough penetration of the cold temperature chemicals.
4. To store a block for later cutting, place in an air-tight container preferably one that is not too much bigger than the

block. Small zip lock bags are good for this. Place into an ultra low freezer (–70°C) as soon as possible. Avoid freezers with automatic freeze/thaw cycles such as "frost-free" types.

5. The sections should be cut as thin as possible on glass slides that are coated to prevent the tissue from coming off later in the process. Immunocytochemical procedures require the sections to be in buffers and solutions for hours or days, and they can float off of the slides during that time if not affixed properly. Many manufacturers sell positively charged slides that are ideal for these applications. Sometimes, though, extra coating is desired and it is quite simple to create your own charged slides in the laboratory. Some charged slides and some slide coatings like Poly-l-lysine can create background staining with certain techniques. Experimentation can determine the slide or slide coating, which provides clean backgrounds with the technique of choice. In addition to the use of Poly-l-lysine-coated glass slides, slides may also be coated with gelatin as follows: (a) Prepare a solution of 0.5% gelatin in deionized H_2O (heat to dissolve). (b) Immerse the slides for 15 min. (c) Allow to air dry 24 h. Also, slides may be coated with silane in the same manner as Poly-l-lysine, to control the loss of tissue sections common with these techniques.

6. Optimum time of fixation can be experimentally determined. The use of alternate fixatives may also be employed to identify specific compounds. One of the reasons for using a frozen preparation is to examine the tissue or cells in as close to the in vivo state as possible. Also, there are many antigens which cannot be evaluated in fixed tissues (2). Therefore when analyzing these sections, it is unwise to fix them in an efficiently cross-linking fixative such as glutaraldehyde or formalin. However, alcohol, while a relatively mild fixative, can still cause enough distortion to warrant the use of even milder agents. The classic is acetone, which is also frequently recommended. (a) The sections are fixed for 10 min in cold acetone. (b) The sections are allowed to air dry. A large number of antibodies are being generated against acid-precipitated proteins, and the presence of acid denaturation in the tissue preparations is often required for antibody recognition. This is the reason the ethanol/acetic acid fixation protocol is featured in this chapter. It should be stated though, that for sections to be the closest to in vivo conditions, simple acetone fixation is preferred. Other possible fixatives to try may include methanol, Bouin's fluid, or formalin - for the best morphologic preservation and only if the antigen is known to survive aldehyde cross-linking (3). Formalin fixation, if attempted, should be brief, 30 s to 1 min. The fixative used is important because frozen sections inherently sacrifice some morphology for the improved protein

viability and one doesn't want to negate that advantage with the choice of the wrong fixative. If a particularly labile antigen is to be detected, the sections can be immediately fixed after adhering to the glass slide. Sections fixed immediately can be stored in PBS at 4°C for up to 5 days (4) (*see* Chapter 8).

7. The enzyme or the chromogen detection system determines whether any endogenous material must first be destroyed. If a peroxidase marker molecule is to be used, endogenous peroxidase or peroxidase-like activity should be blocked. As these preparations are more fragile than a fixed, embedded, sample, endogenous enzyme is inactivated with a weaker blocking solution than would otherwise be used. The standard endogenous oxidation blocking solution, when using peroxidase enzymes, is a solution of 3% hydrogen peroxide in methanol. For frozen sections though, PBS is substituted for the same reason formalin is avoided. The compound of interest should not be subjected to any more denaturing agents than is necessary (5). Also the amount of H_2O_2 can be reduced; a 1.5% solution is usually sufficient. Sometimes even 1.5% H_2O_2 will cause visible bubbles of gas to develop, and if this is too intense it may succeed in lifting the section off of the slide. Careful monitoring and gentle tapping of the container will help to prevent this from happening. Wear gloves and exercise caution when handling the 30% H_2O_2, since it is caustic and can cause burns.

8. The tissue cells exist in an electrically charged environment. To prevent antibodies from binding due to excess charges on the tissue surface, a proteinaceous solution is used to bind to these sites in advance of the antibody incubations. A 10% normal animal serum in PBS is used, from the same species as that providing the secondary or detecting system antibody. The charged protein molecules of the serum will bind to the charged areas on the section, preventing the antibody reagents from binding to these areas non-specifically. The use of other species' sera may cause the antibodies to adhere non-specifically or cross-react. A problem that sometimes occurs when dealing with frozen or fresh material is that the tissue, being less denatured, is often more prone to protein binding to functionally preserved receptors (6). In this instance, the use of serum may cause difficulties by functionally reacting with the tissue and creating "exogenous antigen." This is especially true when assaying for a substance present in high concentrations in the serum. When applying serum to a section, the desired antigen is also applied and it may bind to areas which would be unavailable in a formalin-fixed, paraffin-embedded section. If the antibody to be used has a broad spectrum of reactivity and can detect antigen in various species, the antigen could be

identified where it has bound inadvertently. Also, sometimes an overly charged slide will bind sticky serum proteins and result in slight background staining. If these are potential concerns, charged sites on frozen sections may be blocked with the use of 2% bovine serum albumin. An overnight incubation at 4°C is best for the complete removal of available charged sites for non-specific binding, but a 2 h room temperature incubation will suffice.

The opinions or assertions contained herein are the private views of the author and are not to be construed as official or as reflecting the views of the Department of the Army or the Department of Defense.

References

1. Cuello AC (1993) Immunocytochemistry II. Wiley, New York, NY
2. Nadji M, Morales A (1984) Immunoperoxidase: part II. Practical applications. Lab Med 15:33–37
3. Tse J, Goldfarb S (1988) Immunohistochemical demonstration of estrophilin in mouse tissues using a biotinylated monoclonal antibody. J Histochem Cytochem 36:1527–1531
4. Miller R (1991) Immunohistochemistry in the community practice of pathology: part I. Lab Med 22:457–464
5. Van Bogart L (1985) Present status of estrogen-receptor immunohistochemistry. Acta Histochem 76:29–35
6. Ditzel H, Erb K, Nielsen B, Borup-Christensen P, Jensenius J (1990) A method for blocking antigen-independent binding of human IgM to frozen tissue sections when screening human hybridoma antibodies. J Immunol Methods 133:245–251

Chapter 11

Processing of Cytological Specimens

Gary L. Bratthauer

Abstract

Individual cells often need to be examined with antibodies apart from the surrounding tissue. They may be cells in fluid, cells encased in mucus from a swab, or cells directly extracted from a piece of tissue. Cells can be viewed on a glass slide as cell smears produced from a cell enriched source, introduced as a touch preparation from a piece of wet tissue, concentrated on a slide by the use of a cytocentrifuge, or applied directly to a slide from a solid medium such as a cotton swab. These cell preparations can then be optimally fixed in weakly or nondenaturing solutions such as acetone or those that are alcohol based. They can also be postfixed in formalin if desired. Incubation in buffers containing 0.25% Triton X-100 and 5% dimethylsulfoxide (DMSO) allow for easier antibody penetration. The endogenous peroxidase enzyme or oxidative compounds can be quenched in a mild hydrogen peroxide solution. The sections are then ready to test with antibody after an incubation in a normal serum solution blocks any available charged sites.

Key words: Cytocentrifuge, Cells, Smears, Touch preparations/imprints, DMSO, Fixation, Antibody penetration, Charged slides

1. Introduction

Immunocytochemistry can be a valuable tool for the determination of cellular contents from individual cell suspensions. Samples which can be analyzed include blood smears, aspirates, and swabs from any cellular site. Each sample is treated differently and yet all the methods are interchangeable. There is no one way to prepare these types of cell samples for immunocytochemical analysis. This chapter will deal with the most common forms of cell sample: the swab, aspirate, smear, and touch preps. Blood can be analyzed as a smear but it presents more of a problem owing to the concentration of red blood cells. These cells have an oxidative type function and when using a peroxidase based detection system it can greatly interfere with the test. Concentrated cellular suspensions

C. Oliver and M.C. Jamur (eds.), *Immunocytochemical Methods and Protocols*, Methods in Molecular Biology, Vol. 588,
DOI 10.1007/978-1-59745-324-0_11, © Humana Press, a part of Springer Science+Business Media, LLC 1995, 1999, 2010

which exist in a low viscosity medium make good candidates for smear preparations. Dilute cell suspensions existing in a dilute medium are best suited for the preparation of cytospins through cytocentrifugation. Cell suspensions which exist in a high viscosity medium are best suited to be tested as swab preparations (1). One consistent feature among these preparations is that the whole cell is present on the slide surface. For any intracellular reaction to take place, immunoglobulin must first traverse the cell membrane which is intact in these preparations. Reactions taking place in the nucleus can be more difficult and the extracellular fluids can create unique obstacles in the performance of immunocytochemistry. If the smears or aspirates cannot be adequately produced, or the sample is too small for extra studies, touch preparations can provide a means of quick cell identification or examination (2). Touch preparations, or imprints, enable the examination of the whole cell apart from the tissue aspect. The cells are obtained by touching a wet tissue with a glass slide. Cells adhere to the glass in roughly the same orientation as they exist on the surface of the tissue touched. Fixing them in place enables one to examine the cells for a rapid investigation without having to freeze and cut through a tissue block. If cytological information is needed, touch preparations can be obtained easily from the surface of otherwise large tissue fragments. Cells which are acquired in this manner can provide information about such things as membrane receptors and some cell adhesion molecules in the absence of the tissue's structural components. Sometimes tissue structural elements can interfere with the ability to identify a substance associated with a particular cell. Cell touch preparations made at the time of specimen removal can then be used.

2. Materials

2.1. Preparation of Cell Smears or Touch Preps

1. Gloves.
2. Clean glass slides or positively charged slides.
3. Beveled edge slide.
4. Small glass transfer pipette.
5. Sterile swabs.
6. 0.1% Poly-L-lysine solution (Sigma Chemical Co., St. Louis, MO).
7. Staining racks and dishes.
8. Stirring block with stir bars.
9. Cyto Prep spray fixer (Fisher Scientific, Pittsburgh, PA).
10. Methanol.

11. 10% neutral buffered formalin (NBF).
12. Gauze.
13. Coplin jar.
14. Forceps.

2.2. Preparation of Cytospin Slides

1. Cytocentrifuge.
2. Slide holder apparatus for cytocentrifuge.
3. Sample chambers for cytocentrifuge.
4. Filter cards for use with cytocentrifuge.
5. Fixative solution of 95% ethanol, 5% glacial acetic acid which should be prepared in advance and kept in the cold (4°C).

2.3. Immunostaining of Cytological Specimens

1. Phosphate buffered saline (PBS): 0.01 M sodium phosphate, 0.89% sodium chloride, pH 7.40 ± 0.05.
2. 0.25% Triton X-100, and 5% dimethylsulfoxide (DMSO) in PBS.
3. Endogenous enzyme blocking solution: 1.5% Hydrogen peroxide (H_2O_2) in PBS prepared from a dilution of 30% H_2O_2.
4. Serum blocking solution, 10% animal serum in PBS (the species of serum should match the detecting system antibody, *see* Note 1).
5. Acetone, refrigerated.

3. Methods

3.1. Preparation of Coated Slides (Unless Charged)

1. Position clean glass slides in a staining rack (*see* Note 2).
2. Immerse the slides for 30 min in a large staining dish containing a 1:10 dilution of 0.1% poly-L-lysine solution in deionized water.
3. Remove the slides and oven dry for 1 h at 60°C.

3.2. Preparation of Cytology Smears

3.2.1. Cell Film Preparation

1. Add a drop of cell material (blood, cell suspension, etc.) to the end of a coated glass slide (*see* Note 3).
2. Hold the beveled edge slide at a 45° angle to the plane of the coated slide, gently touch the surface of the slide, and back the edge over the drop of cells so that they spread within the 45° angle, the width of the slide (Fig. 1).
3. Slide the beveled edge slide toward the other end of the preparation slide (in the direction of the 135° angle) with a rapid uniform motion (*see* Note 4).

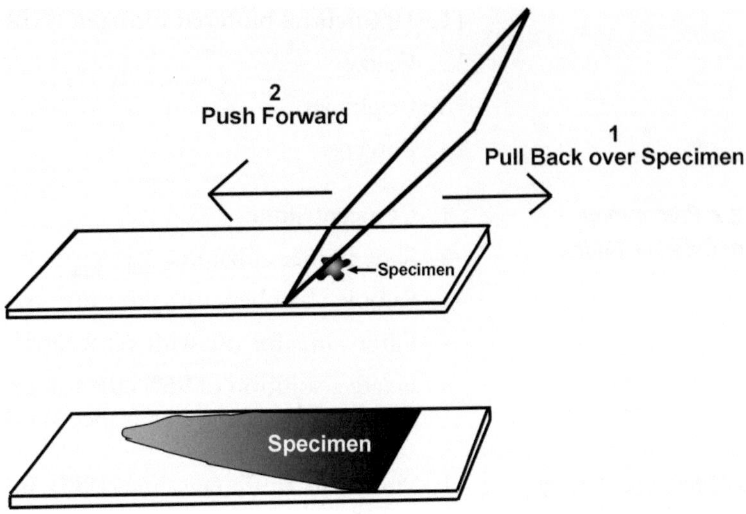

Fig. 1. Preparing a smear.

4. Allow to air dry for 30 min.
5. Immerse in methanol for 30 s to fix the cells.
6. Rinse slides three times with deionized water.
7. Incubate the slides in the solution of 0.25% Triton X-100, 5% DMSO in PBS for 10 min to make the membranes permeable (*see* Note 5).
8. Rinse three times in deionized water for 5 min each to remove detergents.
9. Block endogenous peroxidase and peroxidase-like activity by incubation in 3% H_2O_2 in methanol solution for 45 min with constant stirring (*see* Note 6).
10. Rinse three times with deionized water for 5 min each to remove hydrogen peroxide and methanol.
11. Block charged sites in the cell preparation with an incubation in the 10% animal serum in PBS overnight at 4°C (*see* Note 1).

3.2.2. Swabbed Slide Preparation

1. Obtain sample on sterile swab.
2. Smear the sample onto the glass slide using the majority of the surface area to distribute the specimen (*see* Note 3).
3. Spray fix the material with Cyto Prep.
4. Allow to air dry.
5. Postfix the slides in 10% neutral buffered formalin for 30 s.
6. Rinse three times with deionized water for 5 min each to remove the fixative.

7. Incubate the slides in the solution of 0.25% Triton X-100, 5% DMSO in PBS for 10 min to make the membranes permeable (*see* Note 5).
8. Rinse three times in deionized water for 5 min each to remove the detergents.
9. Incubate in 3% H_2O_2 in methanol for 45 min with constant stirring (*see* Note 6).
10. Rinse three times with deionized water for 5 min each to remove hydrogen peroxide and methanol.
11. Incubate in 10% normal serum of secondary species overnight at 4°C (*see* Note 1).

3.3. Preparation of Cytospin Specimens

1. Position slides in slide holders with filter cards and sample chambers and attach to cytocentrifuge rotor.
2. Prepare cell suspension of 500 cells/mm^3 (μL) with PBS (*see* Note 7).
3. Add 0.1 mL cell suspension to the chamber and centrifuge at 82 *g* for 5 min (*see* Note 8).
4. Remove the slide and immediately dip in 95% ethanol, 5% glacial acetic acid fixative for 2 min (*see* Notes 9 and 10).
5. Rinse three times with deionized water for 5 min each to remove the fixative.
6. Incubate the slides in a solution of 0.25% Triton X-100, 5% DMSO in PBS for 10 min to make the membranes permeable (*see* Note 5).
7. Rinse three times in deionized water for 5 min each to remove detergents.
8. Incubate in 1.5–3% H_2O_2 in methanol for 30 min (*see* Note 6).
9. Rinse three times with deionized water for 5 min each to remove hydrogen peroxide and methanol.
10. Incubate in 10% normal serum of secondary species overnight at 4°C (*see* Note 1).

3.4. Preparation of Touch Prep Specimens

1. Take the refrigerated acetone and add to a coplin jar.
2. Holding the tissue with forceps, position the excised tissue directly above the slide with the best side facing the slide (*see* Note 10).
3. Align the slide horizontally on a flat surface (*see* Note 11).
4. Gently touch the selected exposed tissue surface down onto the slide (*see* Note 12).
5. Apply slight pressure and then remove the tissue after a few seconds (*see* Note 12).

6. Immerse slide in the cold acetone solution with minimum disturbance (*see* Note 9).
7. Remove slide after 10 min and air dry.
8. Rehydrate the imprints with three changes of deionized water, for 5 min each.
9. Incubate the slides in a solution of 0.25% Triton X-100, 5% DMSO in PBS for 10 min to make the membranes permeable (*see* Note 5).
10. Rinse three times in deionized water for 5 min each to remove detergents.
11. Block endogenous peroxidase and peroxidase-like activity by incubation in 1.5–3% H_2O_2/PBS solution for 15 min with constant stirring (*see* Note 6).
12. Rinse in water with three changes for 5 min each to remove all the hydrogen peroxide.
13. Block charged sites on tissue surface with incubation in the 10% serum in PBS serum blocking solution overnight at 4°C (*see* Note 1).

4. Notes

1. The cells exist in a sometimes mucoid, often electrostatic, extracellular fluid. To prevent antibodies from binding due to excess surface charges or mucus, a proteinaceous solution is allowed to bind to these sites in advance of the antibody incubations. The charged protein molecules of the serum will bind to the charged sites or stick to the mucoid fluid preventing the antibody reagents from binding to these areas nonspecifically. A normal animal serum from the same species as that providing the secondary or detecting system antibody is used, 10% in PBS. Since these preparations are of individual cells and not tissues, the extent to which serum proteins are used to block nonspecific charged adherence of antibodies is variable. Sometimes no protein is needed at all, while at other times, the use of a 2% bovine serum albumin solution will be needed. As in the case of frozen sections (*see* Chapter 10) there is also a danger of exogenous antigen addition when dealing with whole cells on slides. How the preparation is made depends to a large extent on what antigen is being studied. This is especially true when assaying for a compound present in high concentrations in the serum. When applying serum to a section the desired antigen is also being applied and it may bind to areas which would be unavailable in a formalin-fixed, paraffin-embedded

section. If the antibody to be used has a broad spectrum of reactivity and can detect the antigen in various species, the antigen could be identified where it has bound inadvertently. If these are potential concerns, charged sites on individual cell preparations may be blocked with the use of 2% bovine serum albumin. An overnight incubation at 4°C is best for the complete removal of available charged sites for nonspecific binding, but a 2-h room temperature incubation will suffice.

2. Immunocytochemical procedures require the sections to be in buffers and solutions for hours or days and they can float off of the slides during that time if not affixed properly. Many manufacturers sell positively charged slides that are ideal for these applications. Sometimes, though, extra coating is desired and it is quite simple to create your own charged slides in the laboratory. Some charged slides and some slide coatings like poly-L-lysine can create background staining with certain techniques. Experimentation can determine the slide, or slide coating, which provides clean backgrounds with the technique of choice.
3. As always, when handling fresh blood or body fluids, it is imperative to wear gloves and protective clothing.
4. In the preparation of smears it is necessary to get a nice thin film to avoid cells bunching up in layers. Start with a smaller amount of sample if this is occurring. The cells will spread out over the surface of the slide and form a film with a feathered edge if done properly.
5. Swabs which are heavily mucoid such as gynecological specimens present a problem in physically locating the antibody near the antigen. These specimens need some additional treatments in the form of cell membrane disruption with DMSO or detergents to ensure that intracytologic components are available for testing (3). Also, the intact nature of cell touch preps may require detergent incubation. It is important to completely dissolve the Triton X-100 in the phosphate buffered saline before adding the DMSO. While each of the procedures outlined here calls for the pretreatment step with Triton X-100 and DMSO, it should be pointed out that this may not be necessary in all cases. The accessibility of any one antigen for any one antibody is due to many factors, including location, structure, and concentration of the antigen to be identified. The use of detergents and other solutions to gain access to an antigen are only necessary if the antigen is difficult to detect. Obviously, it is best to use the fewest steps possible to analyze the cells so as not to cause undue manipulation. These protocols are intended as a guideline, and as templates with which to examine individual systems, subject to experimentation.

6. If a peroxidase marker molecule is to be used for immunostaining, endogenous peroxidase or peroxidase-like activity should be blocked. Due to the large amount of red blood cells in blood preparations, some remaining endogenous enzyme and enzyme-like activity may occur, if using a peroxidase system. Even though the standard 3% solution is recommended, it may be necessary to increase the amount of hydrogen peroxide or increase the time of incubation. The amount of red blood cells present may cause a visible bubbling action on the surface of the slide. This is not detrimental but should be monitored in case the oxidation is violent enough to remove cells from the slide. In the case of cytospins, though, sometimes the cell suspension is free of endogenous enzyme or enzyme-like material and the amount of H_2O_2 needed can be reduced. Wear gloves and exercise caution when handling the 30% H_2O_2 as it is caustic and can cause burns. Touch preps often require slightly different handling. Because these preparations are more fragile than a fixed, embedded, sample, and do not share the support of a surrounding mucoid environment, endogenous enzyme is inactivated with a weaker blocking solution than would otherwise be used. The standard endogenous oxidation blocking solution when using peroxidase enzymes is a solution of 3% hydrogen peroxide in methanol. For these fresh cells though, PBS is substituted for the same reason for which formalin is avoided. The compound of interest should not be subjected to any more denaturing agents than is necessary. Also the amount of H_2O_2 can be reduced; a 1.5% solution is usually sufficient.
7. Preparations which are too dilute for cytocentrifugation may be dropped with a pipette using the location of the filter card as a guide, and allowed to dry (4).
8. It is important to get just the right amount of speed for cytocentrifugation, as too much speed will flatten the cell, and too little will not allow the cells to adequately bind to the slide.
9. For touch preps, the slide should be immersed in acetone as soon as possible, but the cells need a moment to adhere to the plane of the glass. Slowly dip the slide into the acetone as a violent action at this point could wash off some of the cells. As is the case with frozen sections, fixation is a matter of choice. In this instance the use of acetone is preferred because the cells are still whole and the membranes require disruption in order for the contents to be accessible for later analysis. However, an ethanol/acid fixative (95% ethanol, 5% glacial acetic acid) is perfectly acceptable if desired. For the other cytology specimens, experimentation within individual systems is necessary. There is no right or wrong way to make these preparations. There is a fine balance struck between the

need for good morphology and the need for antigen preservation. Alcohol (ethanol or methanol) is a mild fixative that preserves protein epitopes for antibody recognition. Yet, with some whole cell preparations, a short postfixation (fixing a second time) in an aldehyde cross-linking fixative sometimes better stabilizes antigenic determinants. This method can only be used in cases where antigen is not destroyed by formaldehyde fixation (5). Other possible fixatives to try may include methanol or Bouin's fluid. Some have had success with methanol and acetone mixed in a 1:1 ratio (6). A large number of antibodies are being generated against acid precipitated proteins and the presence of acid denaturation in the tissue preparations is often required for antibody recognition. This is the reason for the ethanol/acetic acid fixation protocol being featured in this chapter. However, simple acetone fixation is best in order for cells to remain as close to an in vivo state as possible. Formalin fixation, if attempted, should be brief; 30 s to 1 min.

10. In preparing cells for cytospin slides there are times when immediate fixation is necessary. For these instances the cells can be fixed before centrifugation. Starting at step **2** for the cytocentrifuged specimen (*see* Subheading 11.3.3), continue with the following steps:
    (a) Prepare cell suspension by diluting to 1,000 cells/mm^3 with PBS.
    (b) Add 0.25 mL of cell suspension to 0.25 mL of 95% ethanol, 5% glacial acetic acid and mix immediately.
    (c) Incubate for 2 min and add to sample chambers.
    (d) Centrifuge at 325 *g* for 5 min.
    (e) Continue with the above procedure (*see* Subheading 11.3.3) from step 4.

    Caution: If the cells are fixed before centrifugation they may aggregate and require more vigorous mixing prior to centrifugation.
11. The purpose for the preparation of these types of slides is to examine the cells of a tissue quickly with no need for tissue preparation and cutting. It is important to work quickly since the tissue will start to deteriorate the moment it is obtained. Therefore, it is important to have all the preparations ready for the rapid handling of the excised tissue. As soon as a surface of the tissue is decided upon, it should immediately be touched to a waiting slide, oriented properly and ready to be fixed.
12. Excess tissue fluid may be absorbed with a little gauze but touching any wet cells should be avoided. Also, gentle pressure is required but if too forceful, some cells may be destroyed.

The opinions or assertions contained herein are the private views of the author and are not to be construed as official or as reflecting the views of the Department of the Army or the Department of Defense.

References

1. Kobayashi T, Ueda M, Araki H, Toyoda K, Ohmori K, Sawaragi I (1987) Immunocytochemical demonstration of chlamydia infection in the urogenital tracts. Diagn Cytopathol 3:303–306
2. Masood S (1989) Use of monoclonal antibody for assessment of estrogen receptor content in fine-needle aspiration biopsy specimen from patients with breast cancer. Arch Pathol Lab Med 113:26–30
3. Li C, Lazcano-Villareal O, Pierre R, Yam L (1987) Immunocytochemical identification of cells in serous effusions. Am J Clin Pathol 88:696–706
4. Janssens P, Kornaat N, Tieleman R, Monnens L, Willems J (1992) Localizing the site of hematuria by immunocytochemical staining of erythrocytes in urine. Clin Chem 38: 216–222
5. Tse J, Goldfarb S (1988) Immunohistochemical demonstration of estrophilin in mouse tissues using a biotinylated monoclonal antibody. J Histochem Cytochem 36:1527–1531
6. Bein G, Bitsch A, Hoyer J, Kirchner H (1991) The detection of human cytomegalovirus immediate early antigen in peripheral blood leucocytes. J Immunol Methods 137:175–180

Chapter 12

Processing of Tissue Culture Cells

Gary L. Bratthauer

Abstract

Live cells are often studied, in vitro, bathed in nutrient growth media. It is sometimes necessary to study individual compounds produced by these cells and antibodies work well for this purpose. These cells must first be concentrated and fixed before testing. There are a couple of ways to study cells in culture using antibodies. One is to fix the cells in place as they adhere to a solid surface and then test them as though they were cells on a slide. Another is to retrieve them and pellet the cells, fixing them in a test tube and then embedding and sectioning them as though they were a solid tissue. Fixatives can be mild to moderate depending on the antigens to be studied. Sectioned cells can be tested following mild pretreatment steps. Cells fixed in the culture dish can be tested following mild pretreatment steps in buffers containing 0.25% Triton X-100 and 5% dimethylsulfoxide (DMSO) to allow for easier antibody penetration. The endogenous peroxidase enzyme or oxidative compounds can be quenched in a mild hydrogen peroxide solution. The sections are then ready to test with antibody after an incubation in a normal serum solution blocks any available charged sites.

Key words: Cell culture, Fixation, DMSO, Antibody penetration, Cell pellets

The opinions or assertions herein represent the personal views of the author and are not to be construed as official or as representing the views of the Department of the Army or the Department of Defense.

1. Introduction

In research, a technique which has evolved in importance is the analysis of the living cell as seen in cell culture. It is within the special boundaries of cell culture that conditions can be manipulated in order to examine living cells and to better understand their behavior (1). The fact that transformed or malignant cells grow very nicely in rather simple conditions of chemical formulation make these cells ideal laboratories to study cellular processes. Immunocytochemistry as applied to cell culture has allowed

C. Oliver and M.C. Jamur (eds.), *Immunocytochemical Methods and Protocols*, Methods in Molecular Biology, Vol. 588,
DOI 10.1007/978-1-59745-324-0_12, © Humana Press, a part of Springer Science+Business Media, LLC 1995, 1999, 2010

experiments on living cells to be examined through the detection of products produced as a result of those experiments *[2]*. Also, the immunocytochemical analysis of cell cultures can be used to examine viral infections before obvious cytopathic effect *[3]*. It becomes important, therefore, to prepare these cells adequately in order to fully understand the implications of the various experiments or inoculations. There are many ways of doing so, with and without cell removal, from the culture flask. Once the cells are ready to be evaluated by immunocytochemical means, there are several preparative procedures available, each effective for a slightly different set of conditions. Cells are grown in culture to confluence (or in suspension in the case of non-adherent cells). The techniques for growing cells are beyond the scope of this text; most cell culture protocols are readily available in the literature. When the cells have grown confluent to the point of study, they can be removed from culture by digestion and centrifugation or allowed to remain adherent and assayed directly. They may be obtained in solution and treated in the same manner as cells from aspirates or they can be concentrated and prepared in a cell block as described for whole tissue in Chapter 13.

2. Materials

2.1. Culture Slide or Block Preparation

1. Gloves.
2. Lab-Tek™ slides (Nunc Inc., Naperville, IL).
3. Cell scraper.
4. 15-mL Polystyrene conical centrifuge tube.
5. 50-mL Polypropylene centrifuge tubes.
6. Vortex.
7. Centrifuge (3,000 *g*).
8. 3-mL Syringe with 22 gauge needle.
9. Forceps.
10. Trypsin, 0.1% in culture medium.

2.2. Immunostaining of Specimens

1. Fixative solution: 95% ethanol, 5% glacial acetic acid.
2. Phosphate buffered saline (PBS): 0.01 M sodium phosphate, 0.89% sodium chloride, pH 7.40 ± 0.05.
3. 0.25% Triton X-100 and 5% dimethylsulfoxide (DMSO).
4. Endogenous enzyme-blocking solution, 1.5% hydrogen peroxide (H_2O_2) in PBS prepared from a dilution of 30% H_2O_2.

5. Serum-blocking solution, 10% animal serum in PBS (the species of serum should match the detecting system antibody, *see* Note 8).
6. 10% Neutral buffered formalin (NBF).

3. Methods

3.1. Preparation of Cell Culture Slides (Method 1)

This method is only appropriate for cells that adhere to the flask.

1. Transfer 200 μL of cell culture to the wells of a Lab-Tek™ slide chosen to facilitate the experiment (*see* Notes 1 and 2).
2. Allow cells to grow to confluence with the addition of fresh media.
3. Wash the cells thoroughly with five changes of PBS for 2 min each (*see* Notes 3 and 4).
4. Drain the PBS and add fixative directly to the cells. Fix cells for 3 min (*see* Note 5).
5. Wash away excess fixative with five changes of water for 2 min each.
6. Incubate the slides in the solution of 0.25% Triton X-100, 5% DMSO in PBS for 10 min to make the membranes permeable (*see* Note 6).
7. Rinse three times in deionized water for 5 min each to remove detergents.
8. Block the endogenous enzyme or enzyme-like activity, if necessary, by incubation in 1.5% H_2O_2 in PBS solution for 15 min (*see* Note 7).
9. Rinse three times with deionized water for 5 min each to remove hydrogen peroxide.
10. Incubate in the 10% animal serum in PBS overnight at 4°C. The charged protein molecules of the serum will bind to available sites preventing the antibody reagents from binding to these areas non-specifically (*see* Note 8).

3.2. Preparation of Cell Culture Cell Blocks (Method 2)

If the desire to examine cells in culture is to relate the findings to solid tissues, then the investigator may opt to test the cultured cells as though they were a solid tissue by embedding and sectioning them.

1. Grow cells in flask to confluence, or to a heavy suspension if non-adherent (*see* Note 1).
2. Remove confluent cells by the addition of 0.1% trypsin in media solution for 2 min, followed by extensive media washing and decanting to a 50-mL centrifuge tube. Cells grown

in suspension are merely decanted to a 50-mL centrifuge tube (*see* Note 9).

3. Centrifuge at 800 × *g* for 5 min to remove cells from the media (*see* Note 10).
4. Gently decant the media from the cells and add 20 mL of PBS, vortexing slowly.
5. Centrifuge at 800 × *g* for 5 min to remove cells from the PBS.
6. Gently decant the media from the cells and add 20 mL of PBS, vortexing slowly.
7. Centrifuge at 800 × *g* for 5 min to remove cells from the PBS.
8. Gently decant the PBS from the cells and add 10 mL of PBS to the tube and vortex.
9. After the suspension is thoroughly mixed, decant to a 15-mL polystyrene centrifuge tube.
10. Centrifuge at 1,500 × *g* for 10 min to pellet the cells.
11. Decant the PBS and carefully add 4 mL of 10% neutral buffered formalin down the side of the tube, overlaying the pellet without causing turbulence (*see* Note 11).
12. Incubate overnight at 4°C.
13. Decant the formalin, and GENTLY overlay pellet with 5 mL water.
14. Using the syringe and needle, gently enter the water down the side of the tube and draw 2 mL into the syringe.
15. Carefully undermine the pellet with the needle along the wall of the tube and face the bevel toward the plastic face on the inside of the tube.
16. Rapidly express the syringe and the cells will dislodge as a solid pellet. The undermining action may have to be repeated several times to dislodge the pellet depending on the type of cells and the force of centrifugation. Also, even if some of the pellet breaks off and is lost, this should not affect the bulk of the cells which should still be in the form of the pellet (*see* Note 12).
17. Add 5 mL of water slowly and swirl the pellet in the liquid being careful not to disrupt the cells.
18. As the pellet is in motion within the tube, quickly pour water and pellet into a wide mouth glass container easily accessible with forceps.
19. When pellet has settled, decant the water and add enough 70% ethanol to cover the pellet.

20. The pellet is now ready for processing in an automated tissue processor. If a processor is not available, the pellet can be embedded in paraffin by hand, gradually replacing the ethanol with xylene and then gradually replacing the xylene with paraffin.
21. Once the pellet is embedded in paraffin, it can be treated as any tissue specimen would be treated.

4. Notes

1. Care must be taken while handling live cells in culture because potential biohazards exist. Personal precautions should be followed to include the wearing of gloves and protective clothing.
2. Choice of slide design is often dictated by the experiment. Some slides have four wells, some have eight, some are glass, and some are plastic. Glass is recommended simply because the slide becomes more versatile, acetone can be used as a fixative, and finished slides can be dehydrated in ethanol and cleared in xylene. Slides with individual culture wells make the examination of more than one cell area possible on the same slide and are good for the study of different conditions. If these slides are not available a cell culture flask can be used by cutting out the bottom and assaying as if it were a slide. Different conditions can be tested by using a cutout template of thickened cardboard and confining solutions to prescribed areas on the flask bottom.
3. When assaying individual wells differently, it is necessary to keep the plastic well cover in place. However, when the specific individual treatments are finished, all of the wells can be assayed together as an entire slide. In order to do this, the rubber gasket separating the chambers should be removed using forceps. This may be difficult depending on fixation used and step in the protocol. Usually the use of alcohol softens the rubber sufficiently to allow for easy removal. This must be done prior to coverslipping. Simply pull on one end of the gasket and tear the whole piece off. If the gaskets are left in place, there will be a bit of background associated with the edge where the gasket was positioned. Since these culture slides must be sterile, and are sold in sealed packages, the cells are not fixed to the surface with any special compound. This makes these preparations a bit more fragile and generally prohibits the use of enzymatic digestion protocols.
4. One problem unique to these slides is the closed system in place in the cell culture well. As these cells grow their metabolites

are shed into the surrounding medium. If a particular analyte is in high enough concentration to be contained in the spent medium it could also be left behind attached to some cells because of inadequate washing. It is very important to wash the spent medium away with many buffer washes before fixation. This way, no extracellular constituent will cause aberrant reactions due to its remaining on the cell inappropriately.

5. The assay of cells grown on slides becomes very much like the assay of cells described in Chapters 10 and 11. The style and use of fixative is up to the investigator. The limitations when using plastic surfaces involve the use of acetone or xylene in the preparations. Acetone would have deleterious effects, so 95% ethanol, 5% glacial acetic acid can be used as a mild yet competent fixative. When using a multiwell type of slide, different conditions of fixation can easily be tested confined to separate wells on the slide. Generally though, with the advantage of freshly fixed cells to work with, the mildest fixative that preserves adequately will be best for an immunocytochemical study.
6. Depending on the desired antigen to be identified and its location within the cell, the cells could be subjected to a detergent incubation (4). A pretreatment of DMSO, Triton X-100 in PBS can be employed for better immunoglobulin penetration. It is important to completely dissolve the Triton X-100 in the phosphate buffered saline before adding the DMSO.
7. Depending on the cells being analyzed, the removal of endogenous enzyme prior to immunostaining may not be necessary. With some cell lines there are no endogenous enzyme or enzyme-like substances present and this step would be unnecessary. If that is the case, it is best to avoid the additional treatment. Cells grown and tested like this provide a system which is close to what might be seen in vivo. Therefore, the fewest manipulations necessary to allow the detection of the desired analyte is preferred in order to enhance the accuracy of that detection. If a peroxidase marker molecule is to be used and the cells have either the enzyme or a high level of oxidative function, the endogenous peroxidase or peroxidase-like activity should be blocked with 1.5% hydrogen peroxide in PBS. The enzyme or the chromogen detection system determines whether any endogenous material must first be destroyed. Depending on the type of cells assayed, the concentration and duration of the hydrogen peroxide step may be altered. If necessary, only the concentration and incubation time needed to effectively quench endogenous enzyme is advised. Since these preparations are

more fragile than a fixed embedded sample, endogenous enzyme is inactivated with a weaker blocking solution than would otherwise be used. The standard endogenous oxidation blocking solution, when using peroxidase enzymes, is a solution of 3% hydrogen peroxide in methanol. For cell culture slides, though, PBS is substituted for the same reason formalin is avoided. The compound of interest should not be subjected to any more denaturing agents than is necessary *[5]*. Also the amount of H_2O_2 may be reduced; a 1.5% solution is usually sufficient. Sometimes even 1.5% H_2O_2 will cause visible bubbles of gas to develop, and if too intense, may succeed in lifting cells off of the slide. Careful monitoring and gentle tapping of the container will help to prevent this from happening. Wear gloves and exercise caution when handling the 30% H_2O_2, as it is caustic and can cause burns.

8. The cells exist in a formulated medium containing serum. If washing is incomplete or if the medium is a little viscus, non-specific antibody binding may occur. To prevent antibodies from binding non-specifically, a proteinaceous solution is used to bind to these sites in advance of the antibody incubations. A 10% normal animal serum in PBS is used from the same species as that providing the secondary or detecting system antibody. The use of other species' serum may cause the antibodies to adhere non-specifically or cross-react. A problem which sometimes occurs when dealing with fresh material is that the cells, being less denatured, are often more prone to protein binding to functionally preserved receptors *[6]*. In this case the use of serum may cause a problem by functionally reacting with the cells and creating "exogenous antigen." This is especially true when assaying for a substance present in high concentrations in the serum. When applying serum to the cells, the antigen of interest is also being applied, and may bind to areas which would be unavailable in a paraffin-embedded section. If the antiserum has a broad spectrum of reactivity, and can detect the antigen in various species, the antigen could be identified where it has bound inadvertently. If this is a potential concern, charged sites on cell culture cells may be blocked with the use of 5% bovine serum albumin in PBS. An overnight incubation at 4°C is best for the complete removal of available sites for non-specific binding, but a 2-h room temperature incubation will suffice.

9. Avoid over-trypsinizing, as too much will not only destroy some cells but may alter the antigen in those remaining. If trypsin presents a problem, the cells could be scraped off with a cell scraper.

10. Proper centrifugation speed is necessary to avoid crushing the cells together.

11. The fixative used is again a matter of preference. However, the main reason for preparing this type of specimen is usually to compare fresh cells to the cells found in tissue specimens. Therefore, it is recommended that formalin fixation is used since this is the fixative of choice for most tissue protocols and the crosslinking that develops helps to hold the cells together as a pellet. Specimens can be fixed in 95% ethanol/5% glacial acetic acid but will be more fragile in pellet form.
12. Technique is the major factor in successfully extricating a pellet from the tube. Sometimes it is necessary to practice with a few samples. The nice part about cell culture is that there are numerous cells available to study. It is wise to set up several tubes to obtain a decent pellet to embed. Sometimes the cells are in short supply or conditions indicate more fortification is needed for the pellet to stick together. In these instances, after step 10, Subheading 12.3.2, an equal volume of 2% gelatin (warmed to liquid) is added to the pellet and the pellet is re-suspended. The sample is placed at –70°C to speed up gelatin solidification. The sample is then fixed as in step 11. This provides a matrix in which the cells will adhere. It can be easier to dislodge a more intact pellet this way.

References

1. Carone F, Nakamura S, Schumacher B, Punyarit P, Bauer K (1989) Cyst-derived cells do not exhibit accelerated growth or features of transformed cells *in vitro*. Kidney Int 35: 1351–1357
2. Silverman T, Rein A, Orrison B, Langloss J, Bratthauer G, Miyazaki J, Ozato K (1988) Establishment of cell lines from somite stage mouse embryos and expression of major histocompatibility class I genes in these cells. J Immunol 140:4378–4387
3. Weber B, Harms F, Selb B, Doerr H (1992) Improvement of rotavirus isolation in the cell culture by immune peroxidase staining. J Virol Methods 38:187–194
4. Li C, Lazcano-Villareal O, Pierre R, Yam L (1987) Immunocytochemical identification of cells in serous effusions. Am J Clin Pathol 88:696–706
5. Van Bogar L (1985) Present status of estrogen-receptor immunohistochemistry. Acta Histochem 76:29–35
6. Ditzel H, Erb K, Nielsen B, Borup-Christensen P, Jensenius J (1990) A method for blocking antigen-independent binding of human IgM to frozen tissue sections when screening human hybridoma antibodies. J Immunol Methods 133:245–251

Chapter 13

Processing of Tissue Specimens

Gary L. Bratthauer

Abstract

In order to test tissue specimens with antibody, they first have to be preserved in fixative, embedded in paraffin, and sectioned very thinly onto glass microscope slides. Any piece of tissue, immediately after excision, must be placed into an adequate volume of fixative. Fixatives vary, but the standard one is 10% buffered formalin. After an optimum fixation time (for formalin, about 16 h), the sample must be embedded in paraffin and sectioned on a microtome. Paraffin-embedded sections placed on positively charged slides (either coated or commercially prepared) are then ready for various pretreatment steps. First, the paraffin must be replaced with water through a series of rehydration steps. Then, depending on the antigen to be tested, the section can be proteolytically digested with enzymes or heat-treated in low or high pH solutions. Following that, the endogenous peroxidase enzyme or oxidative compounds can be quenched in a hydrogen peroxide solution. The sections are then ready to be tested with antibody after an incubation in a normal serum solution blocks any available charged sites.

Key words: Tissue, Fixative, Paraffin-embedded, Antigen retrieval, Pressure cooker, Microwave, Enzymatic proteolytic digestion, Charged slides

The opinions or assertions herein represent the personal views of the author and are not to be construed as official or as representing the views of the Department of the Army or the Department of Defense.

1. Introduction

One of the areas in which the use of immunocytochemistry has had the greatest impact is in the examination of tissue in the medical pathology laboratory. Immunocytochemistry, or actually, immunohistochemistry, in the pathology laboratory, enhances the study of diseased tissue. It is important, when studying disease, to obtain and process the tissue as quickly as possible. The reason for this is so that the cellular constituents can be preserved as completely as possible. As is the case with any solid piece of

C. Oliver and M.C. Jamur (eds.), *Immunocytochemical Methods and Protocols*, Methods in Molecular Biology, vol. 588
DOI 10.1007/978-1-59745-324-0_13, © Humana Press, a part of Springer Science+Business Media, LLC 1995, 1999, 2010

tissue, the smaller the piece, the easier it is to preserve the cellular constituents. The varied types of tissue also determine, to an extent, preparation protocols because some types require a more specialized form of preservation than others do. Some specimens such as bone require many days for proper fixation, while other looser connective tissues are preserved in a matter of hours by simple immersion fixation. It should be mentioned, though, that depositing large organs such as whole brains in buckets of fixative may provide fine cellular detail but will probably result in the loss of some labile brain proteins desired for study (1). The individual who actually obtains the specimen is an important aspect of tissue processing. This individual needs to quickly remove the sample and immediately place the correctly sized (small) sample into the desired fixative before much autolysis occurs. It is then incumbent upon the laboratory to process this specimen into paraffin as soon as possible after the requisite fixation time has passed. Aberrant immunoreactivity often is the result of improper fixation time (2). This chapter deals with the intricacies involved in preparing a tissue sample for analysis with antibodies.

2. Materials

2.1. Production of Tissue Slides

1. Gloves.
2. Small wide mouth vials.
3. Process/embedding cassettes.
4. Tissue processor.
5. Paraffin.
6. Clean positively charged glass slides.
7. Microtome.
8. Flotation water bath.
9. Dissecting needle and brush.
10. Staining racks and dishes.
11. 60°C oven.
12. Stirring block with stir bars.
13. Microwave oven.
14. Electric pressure cooker.

2.2. Processing of Tissue

1. Neutral buffered formalin: add 100 mL 37–40% formalin to 900 mL deionized water, then add 4 g monobasic sodium phosphate and 6.5 g dibasic sodium phosphate.
2. Bouin's fluid: Combine 1,500 mL picric acid (saturated in deionized water at 21 g/L), 500 ml formalin, and 100 mL glacial acetic acid.

3. Ethanol/acid fixative: Add 50 mL glacial acetic acid to 950 mL ethanol.
4. B5 fixative: Add 12 g mercuric chloride to 200 mL of deionized water; add 2.5 g sodium acetate; add 20 mL formalin.
5. Phosphate buffered saline (PBS): 0.01 M sodium phosphate, 0.89% sodium chloride, pH 7.40 ± 0.05, or Tris-buffered saline (TBS) (TBS plus, Biocare Medical Corporation, Concord, CA).
6. Xylene.
7. Ethanol.
8. Digestion solution: 0.05% protease VIII (*see* Note **1**) in 0.1 M sodium phosphate buffer, pH 7.8, kept at 37°C.
9. Endogenous enzyme blocking solution: 3–6% hydrogen peroxide (H_2O_2) in methanol (10–20% solution of 30% hydrogen peroxide).
10. Nonspecific binding blocking solution: 10% normal serum of the secondary antibody generating species in PBS or TBS.
11. Sodium phosphate buffer: 0.1 M sodium phosphate, pH 7.80 ± 0.05.
12. Methanol.
13. 30% hydrogen peroxide.
14. Antigen recovery solution – 0.01 M citric acid in dH_2O, pH 6.0.
15. Commercially available combination rehydration/recovery solutions.

3. Methods

3.1. Common Fixation

1. Add approximately 5–10 times the volume of the appropriate fixative (*see* Chapter 8) to the sample in a small wide mouth vial and incubate for 4–24 h depending on the optimum time for the fixative selected (i.e., formalin, 6–12 h; Bouin's, 4 h; ethanol/acid, 24 h) (*see* Note 2).
2. Rinse in three changes of 70% ethanol and place in embedding cassettes in 70% ethanol.

3.2. Preparation of Tissue Blocks

1. Place the processing cassette with the tissue in 70% ethanol into the tissue processor for dehydration and infiltration with paraffin (*see* Note 3).
2. Orient the specimen in the embedding cassette, embed it in paraffin, and cool it to a solid block.

3.3. Preparation of Slides

1. Fasten the tissue block in the block holder of the microtome and adjust the knife.
2. Slice 6-μm sections repeatedly so that a ribbon forms and gently transfer the paraffin ribbon to the surface of a flotation water bath containing only water.
3. With a dissecting needle and brush, tease the ribbon apart into separate floating sections.
4. Holding a charged or coated slide by the label end, enter the water bath under the desired section. Maneuver the slide under the section and lift it up, retrieving the section on the slide surface (*see* Note 4).
5. Keep the slides flat and allow them to dry overnight at room temperature.

3.4. Preparation of Sections for Immunostaining

1. Place the slides into a slide rack and heat in the oven for 1 h at 60°C.
2. Remove and air dry for 30 s only.
3. Place the slide rack into xylene and incubate for 2 min to remove the paraffin. Repeat through four changes of fresh xylene. Alternatively, and to save time, one may use a rehydration/recovery reagent (*see* Note 5).
4. After the final xylene incubation, place the slides in ethanol for 2 min. Repeat through four changes of fresh ethanol.
5. Move slides into deionized water and wash for 2 min. Repeat through three changes of deionized water.
6. Place the slides receiving proteolytic digestion in digestion solution at 37°C for 3 min. Slides not being digested may remain in deionized water (*see* Note 6).
7. Place the slides receiving microwave irradiation in plastic slide holders in the citric acid solution. These solutions are also commercially available (Dako Inc., Carpinteria, CA; Biogenex Corporation, San Ramon, CA; or Biocare Medical, Concord, CA) (*see* Note 5).
8. Microwave for 20 min at near boiling temperatures. When using a pressure cooker for this purpose, 3–10 min will provide optimal results (*see* Note 6).
9. Remove from oven and allow to cool in the citric acid buffer for 45 min (*see* Note 6).
10. Following enzyme digestion, microwave irradiation, or pressure cooker heating, rinse the slides in deionized water for 2 min. Repeat through three changes of water.
11. Combine with slides not being digested and place in ethanol for 2 min. Repeat through three ethanol changes.

12. Place the slides in endogenous enzyme blocking solution and incubate with stirring for 30 min (*see* Note 7).
13. Remove the slides and wash in deionized water for 2 min.
14. Repeat through three changes of water.
15. Place the slides in nonspecific binding blocking solution and incubate at 4°C overnight (*see* Note 8).

4. Notes

1. Since these sections are cut, the intracellular constituents are generally available for detection without the need for special pretreatments. However, some antigens are masked by the use of certain fixatives and cannot be recognized by the antibody (3). Unique to fixed paraffin embedded samples is the flexibility to treat the tissue a bit more aggressively in trying to enhance immunoreactivity (*see* Chapter 14). This is usually accomplished either with some proteolytic enzyme digestion which perturbs the tissue enough to unmask these antigens or with heat enhanced retrieval methods. These heated methods are effective, and with certain antigen/antibody combinations necessary, however, there are still antigen/antibody combinations, which react optimally following enzyme digestion. Obviously, any of these treatments should be done cautiously so as not to destroy the section. Protease type VIII has been used for this purpose and is a quick acting enzyme. Careful control of concentration, temperature, and time will provide good reproducible results. A standard treatment is possible although each tissue and each antigen–antibody combination will have an optimal digestion protocol that can be experimentally determined. Samples fixed in milder fixatives such as ethanol may not need to be digested with proteolytic enzymes. Also, depending on the antigen and antibody used, some specimens fixed in formalin need not be digested either, although some form of digestion, whether it be with enzymes, or with heat, is required more often than not.
2. As always, when handling fresh tissue, it is imperative to wear gloves and protective clothing. Proper fixation is the most important aspect for obtaining successful results. Strive for small samples properly fixed for the optimum time. A small sample allows for quick and thorough penetration and using, at a minimum, 5 volumes of fixative should help to ensure proper fixation. Penetration and time are the biggest variables in fixing samples. It is important to optimize the time for best results. Process the tissue as soon as possible after adequate fixation.

The type of fixative used does not matter as much as the quality of the fixation, but different antigens may be fixative dependent (4) (*see* Chapter 8). In working with fixatives, one should be reminded of the hazardous nature of the materials and protective clothing such as gloves should be worn. The neutral buffered formalin fixative is preferred for pathology specimens due to the superior morphologic preservation, although the others are also effective. These can be treated the same as formalin, but the immunostaining results may differ depending on the fixative used. For instance, samples fixed in the mercurial fixatives often show mercurial pigments under the microscope. These pigments are often confusing and distracting and can be removed by using a solution of alcoholic iodine or Lugol's iodine (5):

(a) Prepare solution of 1% iodine in 80% ethanol or Lugol's iodine of 1% iodine, 2% potassium iodide in distilled water.

(b) Incubate slides for 10–15 min.

(c) Wash with water and incubate a few minutes in 5% sodium thiosulfate in distilled water before a final water wash.

This treatment may result in less reactivity due to the chaotropic nature of the solution.

3. There are numerous instruments that automatically process specimens for embedding in paraffin. The processor dehydrates to 100% ethanol and then infiltrates the tissue with xylene. Xylene saturated tissue is then infiltrated with melted paraffin at 60–70°C. The tissue processor accomplishes this quickly with heat and pressure. The processor should not be heated above 65°C to avoid destroying heat-labile antigens. Once the block is formed, it must be sectioned with a good sharp knife properly oriented in the microtome. Good histologic slide preparation will provide a good immunohistochemical test sample.

4. The sections should be cut as thin as possible on glass slides that are coated with a substance promoting adherence to prevent the tissue from coming off later in the process. Immunohistochemical procedures require the sections to be in buffers and solutions for hours or days, and if not affixed properly they mightfloat off of the slides during that time. Also, slides need to be coated for these samples owing to the enzyme digestion or microwave treatment that is normally required. The commercially available charged slides provide adequate section adherence with limited background in immunohistochemical analyses. Some positively charged slides may inhibit antibody binding to all areas of the section, however. If necessary, slides may be coated with poly-L-lysine, a simple means of binding a section to the surface of a slide, but it can cause nonspecific staining with some chromogens:

(a) It is very important that the slides be precleaned. Clean glass slides should be placed in a staining rack.

(b) Immerse the slides for 30 min in a 1:10 dilution of 0.1% poly-L-lysine solution in distilled water in a large staining dish.

(c) Remove the slides and oven dry for 1 h.

When using poly-L-lysine or silane-coated slides in enzyme digestion protocols, the method of their preparation determines the success of section adherence. The slides must be clean, and specimens must be heated prior to deparaffinization. Experimentation can determine the slide coating that provides clean backgrounds with the technique of choice.

When drying these sections, it is necessary to allow them to dry at room temperature. The use of a warming plate or oven while the sections are still wet can result in the loss of some antigens proportional to the drying temperature. Once the slides are dry, though, they must be heated in an oven prior to the immunoassay. There is no adverse effect associated with heating dried sections.

Elmer's Glue-All is an older and less expensive method of section adherence that does not cause nonspecific binding when used properly. However, Elmer's Glue-All used in high concentrations can cause artifacts when viewed under the microscope in the form of a refractile, cracked appearance. It is necessary to use no more than 15% v/v of the glue. It is usually recommended that the section be allowed to dry as the glue dries (attach a wet section to a wet glued slide). Predried glued slides can be used with success; however, occasionally, sections drying on predried slides may wash off in subsequent steps.

There are instances when glue coatings are not acceptable. Certain automated instruments for immunostaining require capillary action in the process. These instruments are dependent on slides with painted surfaces which are assayed in tandem creating a gap of determined width for reagents to traverse. In order for the flow of reagents to be uniform and consistent, the slides must have a smooth surface which withstands antigen recovery techniques as can best be provided by commercially available charged slides, poly-L-lysine, or silane. In preparing slides for automation, it is mandatory that the slide surface not be touched, since skin oils inhibit capillary action, and that the section be located near the bottom of the slide. This is to enable the reagents, by capillary action, to cover the entire section.

5. Deparaffinization is a very important part of the procedure as well. The slides must be deparaffinized in xylene after they are oven heated. The heat helps to anneal the section a bit before it is subjected to the rigors of the procedure, but also dissolves the paraffin slightly, making it easier for it to go into solution in the xylene. When the slides are removed from the oven, the paraffin will be clear and wet. As soon as the paraffin starts to solidify, the slides should be placed in the xylene.

   Alternatively, rehydration and antigen recovery may be accomplished in a single step. There are commercially available solutions now that can serve this purpose. Declere or Trilogy from Cell Marque Corporation (Hot Springs, AR) and Reveal from Biocare Medical (Concord, CA) are acceptable reagents to name just a few. From the oven, the slides are put into 1× solutions of these reagents and heated in a pressure cooker for 3–10 min. This accomplishes both rehydration and heated antigen recovery. After pressure cooker heating, the sections are allowed to continue heating in a fresh solution of 1× reagent for 30 min (warm pressure cooker setting) and then endogenous peroxidase-like reactivities are quenched (step 12) (6).

6. The use of Protease VIII is not exclusive. Trypsin may also be used as it is milder and will take longer to show the same effect (30 min to 3 h). This can be beneficial when dealing with antigens that are less stable. Other enhancing enzymes include other protease types such as proteinase K, pronase (a very rigorous enzyme), and ficin (7). Saponin, Triton X-100, and Tween 20 are detergents that can have as much effect as some of the enzymes in enhancing antibody–antigen interactions (8). Also, some have used acids such as formic acid to denature the antigens and make them more accessible to antibody (9). All of the pretreatments are designed to either perturb the section surface enough to allow recognition of antigen or to make the section more permeable to immunoglobulin by reducing surface charges. If an assay is not working properly with a given enzyme or detergent, another pretreatment regimen may yield better results. Also, the time of digestion may be varied to enhance the effect.

   Another pretreatment that is being more widely used with formalin fixed samples is heat induced antigen recovery (10). This technique makes use of high heat coupled with a slightly acidic solution to denature available proteins and enhance antigen detectability. A microwave can be used for this purpose. It can be calibrated by consistently using the same containers, filled in the same manner, with a constant number of slides for every use (11). If not enough sections are to be processed, blank slides should be used instead. The oven is heated on high power with the containers in place, covers slightly askew to permit steam escape (microwaves with turntables work the best, however, if one is not available, the exact same location of the container within the oven should be used every time). The time to full boiling is noted and subtracted from 20 min. For the remaining time, the microwave is operated at a lesser power setting. For most applications, 30% power for the remaining time is adequate. The desired effect is for the solution to begin boiling for a few seconds after the microwaving starts. When only the fan is running, the solution should stop boiling. In this way, the solution is kept at a near boiling temperature, and there is no loss due to evaporation. After 20 min, the sections are removed from the oven, the lids of the containers are replaced, and the slides are allowed to cool in the buffer for at least 45 min. This cooling period appears to be important in the detection of the desired antigen. Alternatively, this process can be performed at high power for 5 min, three times, each time adding back some buffer lost through evaporation. This process, though, often yields inconsistent results. An electric pressure cooker can also be used for 3 min to add pressure to the heat, or for a milder treatment, steam can be used.

Some newer monoclonals detect antigens only after heating, while others are greatly enhanced after using this method. Among them are tests for the estrogen, progesterone, and androgen receptors in the nucleus, some cycling proteins such as PCNA, MIB I, or the cyclins, and some cytoplasmic or surface proteins as well, such as inhibin or CD15. There are also antigens which are less likely to be detected when using the heat induced methods. Also, artifacts and unwanted cross-reactivity can be induced using these more sensitive techniques.

It is difficult to use proteolytic enzyme digestion with this treatment, but if needed, the sections should be digested following the microwave heating because boiling enzymatically digested tissue results in tissue loss. A milder form of this method is to boil the citric acid buffer only and incubate the sections in the preheated solution or steam for 15 min. Alternatively, sections can be heated to 80°C in this buffer and kept overnight with similar results (12). Finally, in addition to citric acid (pH 6) solutions, there are commercially available recovery solutions at pH 10 or containing EDTA that can be employed. Certain antigen–antibody combinations may be enhanced by the use of one of these solutions.

7. The enzyme or the chromogen detection system determines whether any endogenous material must first be destroyed. Wear gloves and exercise caution when handling the 30% H_2O_2, since it is caustic and can cause burns.
8. Cells exist in an electrically charged environment. To prevent antibodies from binding due to excess charges on the tissue

surface, a proteinaceous solution is used to bind to these sites in advance of the antibody incubations. A 10% normal animal serum from the same species that provides the secondary or detecting system antibody in PBS or TBS is used. The use of other species' serum may cause the antibodies to adhere nonspecifically or cross-react. The charged protein molecules of the serum will bind to the charged areas on the section, preventing the antibody reagents from binding to these areas nonspecifically. An overnight incubation at 4°C is best for the complete removal of available charged sites for nonspecific binding, but a 2-h room temperature incubation could nearly suffice if desired. When using the newer rehydration/ recovery solutions (*see* Note 5) along with TBS plus buffer, this step may not be needed. Sections can remain in the TBS plus until antibody application.

References

1. Guntern R, Vallet P, Bouras C, Constantinidis J (1989) An improved immunohistostaining procedure for peptides in human brain. Experientia 45:159–161
2. Battifora H (1991) Assessment of antigen damage in immunohistochemistry. Am J Clin Pathol 96:669–671
3. Login G, Schnitt S, Dvorak A (1987) Rapid microwave fixation of human tissues for light microscopic immunoperoxidase identification of diagnostically useful antigens. Lab Invest 57:585–591
4. Baumgartner W, Dettinger H, Schmeer N, Hoffmeister E (1988) Evaluation of different fixatives and treatments for immunohistochemical demonstration of *Coxiella burnetii* in paraffin-embedded tissues. J Clin Microbiol 26:2044–2047
5. Ambrogi LP (ed) (1957) Manual of histologic and special staining techniques. Armed Forces Institute of Pathology, Washington, DC
6. Bratthauer GL, Moinfar F, Stamatakos MD, Mezzetti TP, Shekitka KM, Man YG, Tavassoli FA (2002) Combined E-cadherin and high molecular weight cytokeratin immunoprofile differentiates lobular, ductal, and hybrid mammary intraepithelial neoplasias. Hum Pathol 33:620–627
7. Taschini P, MacDonald D (1987) Protease digestion step in immunohistochemical procedures: ficin as a substitute for trypsin. Lab Med 18:532–536
8. Stirling J (1990) Immuno- and affinity probes for electron microscopy: a review of labeling and preparation techniques. J Histochem Cytochem 38:145–157
9. Kitamoto T, Ogomori K, Tateishi J, Prusiner S (1987) Formic acid pretreatment enhances immunostaining of cerebral and systemic amyloids. Lab Invest 57:230–236
10. Shi S, Key M, Kalra K (1991) Antigen retrieval in formalin-fixed, paraffin-embedded tissues: an enhancement method for immunohistochemical staining based on microwave oven heating of tissue sections. J Histochem Cytochem 39:741–748
11. Tacha DE, Chen T (1994) Modified antigen retrieval procedure: calibration technique for microwave ovens. J Histotechnol 17:365
12. Man Y-g, Tavassoli FA (1996) A simple epitope retrieval method without the use of microwave oven or enzyme digestion. Appl Immunohistochem 4:139–141

Chapter 14

Heat-Induced Antigen Retrieval for Immunohistochemical Reactions in Routinely Processed Paraffin Sections

Laszlo Krenacs, Tibor Krenacs, Eva Stelkovics, and Mark Raffeld

Abstract

The development of heat-induced antigen (epitope) retrieval (HIER) technologies has led to dramatic improvements in our ability to detect antigens in formalin fixed, archival tissues. Paradoxically, wet heat treatment at temperatures greater than 95°C in appropriate buffer solutions can reconstitute the antigenicity of many proteins that have been rendered nonreactive during the fixation and paraffin embedding process, which heretofore could only be identified in fresh or frozen tissues. The reason for this effect is unclear, but it has been suggested that the vigorous heat treatment partially reverses or disrupts the aldehyde cross-links occurring in proteins during formalin fixation and restores the original conformation of antigenic epitopes. The great success of antigen/epitope retrieval technologies further emphasizes the importance of preanalytical steps in immunohistochemistry. Over the past several years, since this technology was first reported, there have been numerous modifications to the original formulation. It is the purpose of this chapter to discuss the critical issues required for optimal HIER and to provide guidelines for the use of popular HIER buffers and heating devices used for routine immunohistochemical detection.

Key words: Heat-induced epitope retrieval, Archived tissues, Restoring epitope conformation, Paraffin sections, Time and temperature control, Microwave, Pressure cooker, Citrate buffer pH 6.0, Tris buffer pH 8.0, Tris–EDTA buffer pH 9.0

1. Introduction

Immunohistochemistry has become an essential adjunct of modern diagnostic pathology. However, successful staining is highly dependent on the preparation of the tissues prior to immunohistochemical staining. Traditionally, most pathological tissue samples are fixed in formaldehyde and embedded in paraffin wax in preparation for examination of microscopic morphology. Unfortunately, many potentially interesting antigens become altered during tissue fixation and processing, interfering with their immunohistochemical detection.

C. Oliver and M.C. Jamur (eds.), *Immunocytochemical Methods and Protocols*, Methods in Molecular Biology, Vol. 588, DOI 10.1007/978-1-59745-324-0_14,

To overcome this obstacle, snap-frozen tissue sections had been a preferred alternative to formalin-fixed paraffin-embedded tissue sections. However, the morphology of frozen section immunohistochemistry is relatively poor, the use of frozen tissue necessitates additional equipment for freezing and storing frozen tissues, and the pathologist must decide in advance which tissues to freeze for immunohistochemical studies. By contrast, paraffin sections offer well-preserved tissue architecture and cytomorphology, are routinely prepared and readily available in every pathology department, and require no special handling or additional equipment. Furthermore, formalin-fixed paraffin-embedded tissues represent an invaluable source of human tissues for retrospective immunohistochemical studies (1). As a result of these considerations, pathologists and other investigators have continually sought methods for recovering the antigenicity of fixed tissues.

Alterations of antigens in paraffin-embedded tissues are related to a variety of changes in the three-dimensional structure (conformation) of proteins due to cross-linking by formaldehyde and to a lesser extent to heating and dehydration during paraffin embedding (2). As a consequence, the antigenic determinants (epitopes) are destroyed, denatured, or masked, which may diminish or abrogate their detection. The earliest attempts to retrieve antigenicity utilized proteolytic enzymes (3, 4), which presumably act by breaking formaldehyde-induced methylene cross-links in the antigenic molecules. Although proteolytic methods have been especially useful for retrieval of cytokeratins, they are difficult to control, and careful attention is needed to optimize their retrieval effect and avoid tissue destruction. Other approaches using coagulative agents such as heavy metals, alcohols or acid solutions with or without formaldehyde for tissue fixation, and pretreatments with cold 20% sucrose-saline or with sodium methoxide solutions have also been tested to improve immunostaining of specific antigens (5, 6).

1.1. Wet Heat-Induced Epitope Retrieval

Despite some successes with the above pretreatments, the development of *wet heat-induced epitope retrieval (HIER)* procedures, which involves heating the fixed tissue sections in dilute metal–salt or buffer solutions at or above 100°C, for several minutes to 1/2 h, was the critical breakthrough in paraffin section immunohistochemistry (2, 7–9). Today, there are many variations of the original HIER technique. These differ primarily in the recommended buffer solutions and/or the source or mode of heating, but the basic formula of wet heat treatment over a fixed time period is similar. The most popular HIER technologies use microwave ovens, stainless steel or plastic pressure cookers, autoclaves, vegetable steamers or water-baths as the heat sources and low molarity buffers with acidic or alkaline pH (8, 9, 11–14).

HIER methods have dramatically expanded the universe of antibodies that react in formalin-fixed paraffin-embedded tissues. Antibodies that never before reacted in paraffin section show specific staining following HIER pretreatment. Moreover, HIER substantially increases the sensitivity of reactions of the majority of antibodies directed to formaldehyde-resistant antigens as well. Additionally, appropriate HIER minimizes the problem of overfixation, reducing the immunostaining differences found between the 24-h fixed material and tissues that have been kept in formalin for days or even weeks (*see* Note 1). HIER technology has also enabled immunohistochemists to routinely stain a wide spectrum of antigens in etched, epoxy resin-embedded sections for bone marrow diagnosis (10).

The exact mechanism by which HIER works is unknown. Hydrolytic cleavage of formaldehyde-related chemical groups and cross-links, unfolding of inner epitopes, and the extraction of calcium ions from coordination complexes with proteins are among the hypothesized mechanisms (15–17). Antigens that are hidden in 4% formaldehyde-fixed tissues may become available without HIER, if a coagulative agent such us acetic acid or mercuric chloride is added to the formaldehyde or coagulative agents are used for fixation without formaldehyde (*see* Fig.1). Coagulative agents reduce the cross-linking potential of formaldehyde, suggesting the possible involvement of formaldehyde cross-links in the antigen masking effect (2). The involvement of formaldehyde cross-links in antigen masking is also supported by the observation that tissues fixed in coagulative or mixed (formaldehyde and coagulant) fixatives need substantially shorter HIER times for antigen recovery than for tissues fixed in 4% formaldehyde alone. On the other hand, as a result of its cross-linking ability, formaldehyde fixation alone provides better antigen definition and morphological preservation after HIER than does mixed or neat coagulative fixatives (*see* Fig.1).

In addition to ongoing efforts to refine pathologic diagnoses, the rapid development of molecularly targeted therapies and the need to identify these targets or their surrogate markers in pathologic tissues have continued to drive the demand for improvements in antigen identification and the development of new antibodies. New generations of highly specific antibodies directed against peptide sequences of lymphocyte subset antigens (e.g. CD4, CD10, CD79a), oncoproteins (i.e. bcl-2, cyclin D1, p53), or molecules of prognostic and/or predictive relevance in cancer (i.e. CD117, Her2/c-erbB2, Her1/EGFR, estrogen and progesterone receptors) that require or benefit from HIER have been introduced, and their number is expanding rapidly. As a consequence, immunophenotyping of paraffin-embedded tissues, coupled with an appropriate HIER technique, has attained a central role in the modern immunohistochemistry laboratory.

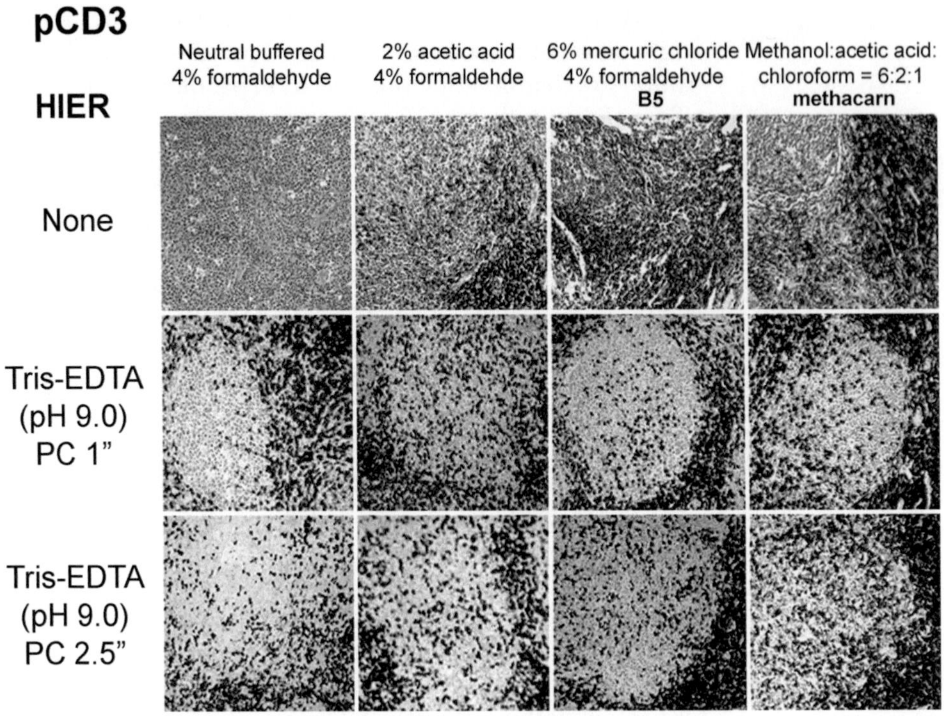

Fig.1 Detection of CD3 T-lymphocyte antigen in 16-h formalin-fixed, paraffin-embedded reactive human tonsil sections. In the absence of HIER the antigen is not detectable in the tissue fixed in neat formaldehyde, but it is stained in tissues fixed either in mixed (formaldehyde and coagulant) or in coagulative fixatives. Increasing the HIER treatment time (PC 2.5′) does not substantially improve immunostaining, but adversely affects tissue morphology.

In this chapter, we briefly summarize the current principles of HIER and offer protocols for its reliable use in paraffin-embedded tissues. The broad methodological repertoire now available provides great latitude for laboratories using HIER, but also underscores the need for standardization to achieve better intra and interlaboratory reproducibility. There are several quality assurance organizations that offer proficiency testing programs and provide valuable technical information on their websites designed to promote standardization (*see* Note 2).

1.2. Factors that Influence HIER

1.2.1. Composition of Retrieval Buffer

Experimental data suggest that the amount of heat and the duration of heating followed by the pH and chemical composition of the retrieval buffers are the most important factors for efficacy of HIER (7, 8, 15–18). Citrate buffer (sodium citrate–citric acid) at pH 6.0 is a very popular retrieval medium and has been used at molarities between 0.01 and 0.1 M (7, 8). Detergents (e.g., 0.1% Tween 20) added to the standard citrate buffer may improve the performance (14), but more prominent tissue deterioration and foaming may also be experienced. Other widely used antigen retrieval buffers are Tris–HCl at various concentrations (0.1–0.5 M) at alkaline pH (8.0–10.0) (7, 11, 14, 17, 19), EDTA–NaOH (0.1 M) at pH 8.0, and the mixture of 0.1 M Tris and 0.01 M EDTA at pH 9.0 (15, 16, 19). The EDTA-containing solutions provide excellent antigen recovery, but treated tissues may show enhanced tissue damage as compared to citrate-based retrieval buffers. Other HIER solutions have also been tested, but are not as widely used as those described above (7, 8).

There are a number of companies that offer prepared "proprietary" antigen retrieval buffers. Of the commercially available citrate-based antigen retrieval buffers, we have used the pH 6.0 Target Retrieval Solution (TRS) from Dako (Carpinteria, CA) with excellent results (20, 21). TRS can be used to retrieve epitopes that are not otherwise detectable in formalin-fixed, paraffin-wax sections (i.e., CD5/Leu1; CD35/To5), and it can substitute for enzymatic digestion in the detection of other antigens, e.g. CD21/1F8; CD35/Ber-MAC-DRC and BerEP4 (20, 22) (*see* Fig.2).

1.2.2. Heating Devices

A wide variety of heating devices have been adapted for use in HIER, including microwave ovens (MWO), pressure cookers, vegetable steamers, autoclaves, and water-baths. The most reproducible results may be achieved with MWOs that incorporate time and temperature control even above the atmospheric boiling point (combined with a plastic pressure cooker). The archetypes are the professional laboratory microwave instruments, which

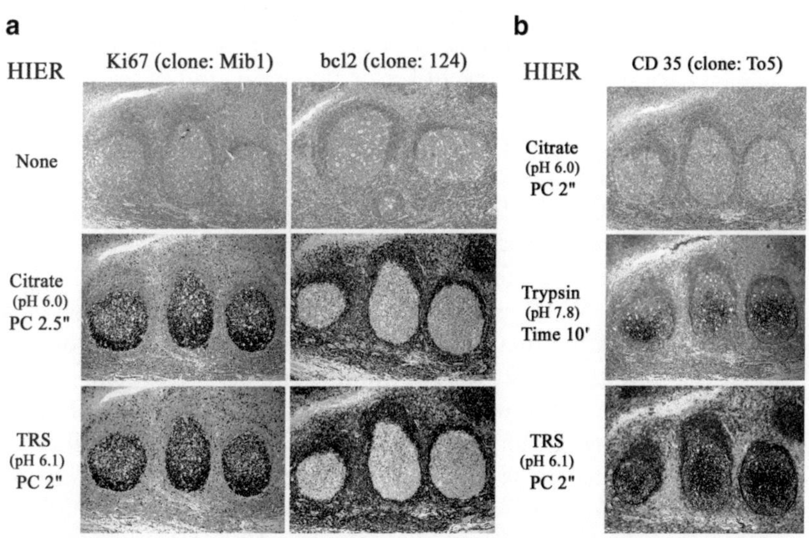

Fig.2 Detection of antigens in 16-h formalin-fixed, paraffin-embedded reactive human tonsil. (**a**) Demonstrates retrieval of Ki67 and bcl2 antigenicity following HIER treatment using standard citrate buffer and a commercial citrate-based buffer (TRS; DakoCytomation). The TRS buffer shows slightly better retrieval. (**b**) Poor retrieval for CD35 using standard citrate buffer and excellent retrieval using the TRS buffer. Trypsin (0.1%) shows intermediate level of antigen retrieval. Use of "higher efficiency" buffers Tris pH 8.0 and Tris–EDTA pH 9.0 did not provide significant retrieval (not shown).

allow the full control of time/temperature/power and vacuum (*see* Note 3). Owing to of the high cost of these instruments, most immunohistochemistry laboratories utilize simpler consumer type microwave ovens. The most important factors to be considered in choosing a commercial MWO are the presence of (1) a *digital* timer for precise time adjustment and (2) a *turntable* for uniform heating of the retrieval solution. MWOs can either be used at their maximum power of 700–1,200 W, or at a reduced power of 250–300 W. The advantage of using reduced power is that heavy boiling and evaporation can be avoided, while maintaining the buffer temperature near 100°C. However, the duration of treatment should be extended by ~40% of the corresponding treatment time at maximum power. MWO-mediated HIER can also be performed in plastic pressure cookers designed for household kitchen applications (*see* Subheading 3.2), which appear to eliminate some of the drawbacks (e.g., heavy boiling and evaporation) of the standard MWO protocols. Metallic tools should never be used in the MWO, therefore, heat-resistant plastic Coplin jars or containers and heat-resistant plastic slide holders with a capacity of 15 sections and above are required for this application.

The use of stainless steel kitchen pressure cookers (PC) is another simple instrument for achieving reproducible HIER (*see* Subheading 3.4) (*see* Note 4). The heating device is usually an inexpensive commercial electric hotplate with at least 1 kW of power. Careful use of a PC provides uniform heating without heavy boiling and allows one to treat large batches of slides (9, 13, 19). The PC method eliminates the need for careful monitoring during the retrieval that is necessary in full-power MWO method to prevent accidental drying out of the sections as a result of evaporation. Recently, time and temperature controlled electric heating devices have been commercialized to achieve more standard results, which work either at atmospheric pressure such as the PT (LabVision, Fremont, CA) or under supra-atmospheric pressure such as the Pascal (Dako) and the Decloaking chamber (Biocare Medical, Concord, CA).

Wet (hydrated) autoclave treatment represents a uniform heating method and is preferred over MWO irradiation by some authors (12, 17) (*see* Subheading 3.5). The main disadvantages of the autoclave method are availability and prolonged procedure time. In an effort to standardize heating conditions of HIER, water-baths have recently been recommended (*see* Subheading 3.6), e.g. for the FDA-approved Herceptest. However, water-baths are necessarily limited to 100°C. Vegetable steamers (e.g., Model HS900; Black and Decker, Towsen, MD) have also been employed successfully for HIER and represent yet another inexpensive heat source. Like water-baths, their maximum temperature is limited to 100°C.

1.2.3. Temperature and Duration of Treatment

The power of the heating device, the composition, pH, the volume of buffer, and the degree of tissue fixation are the major factors that determine the duration of a particular HIER protocol. The efficacy of antigen retrieval is also influenced by the duration and conditions of cooling following heat treatment (*see* Subheadings 3.1–3.6) (*see* Note 5). The recent technique using heated buffer solutions (without organic solvent) for dewaxing and rehydration of sections (e.g. Trilogy; Cell Marque, Hot Springs, AR) will also contribute to the retrieval effect and should be considered when HIER is designed. Automated immunostainers combining dewaxing with additional HIER pretreatment followed by the full immunostaining sequence (e.g., BenchMark; Ventana Medical Systems, Tucson, AZ) provide highly reproducible and standard results.

Most methods employ temperatures near or above 100°C. Heating above the atmospheric boiling temperature is possible in traditional or in microwavable pressure cookers as well as in autoclaves (*see* Subheading 1.2.2). The best commercial PCs can reach an operating pressure of about 103 kPa/15 psi, resulting in ~120°C temperature (19, 21). It is important to emphasize that the maximal temperature achievable in pressure cookers depends upon the particular model used (*see* Note 4). When utilizing autoclaves as the heat source, 120°C is easily achievable and is the recommended standard (12, 17, 21).

Under identical heating conditions, i.e. temperature and duration, buffers of alkaline pH (pH 8–10) such as the common Tris or EDTA-containing HIER buffers generally result in more efficient antigen retrieval than the conventional citrate buffer at pH 6.0. The performance of both buffer types can be improved using higher temperatures or extending the time of treatment. However, there is a point at which no significant additional benefit can be achieved and at which continued treatment will begin to result in tissue deterioration. Generally, maximal antigen recovery is reached well before significant tissue damage occurs, but this time point can be influenced by the degree of tissue fixation. As a general rule, the high pH and EDTA-containing buffers reach their optimal treatment time much faster than do the lower pH citrate-containing buffers. It is important to be aware that prolonged treatment with EDTA-containing buffers may attack soda-lime glass below the adhesive layer, facilitating tissue detachment. Table 1 lists some of the popular HIER buffers according to their efficiency/aggressiveness under the same heating conditions. Guidelines on the use of some of these popular HIER buffers and heating devices are summarized in Table 2.

Firm attachment between the tissue and the glass slide is crucial to prevent detachment of the section during HIER. Mounting the sections on 3-amino-propyltriethoxysilane (APES)-coated glass slides creates suitable adhesion to withstand the HIER procedure.

Table 14.1
Common antigen retrieval buffers grouped according to their HIER efficiency and aggressiveness on tissue morphology

Group 1 Higher efficiency buffers Shorter incubation times Most tissue destructive	– EDTA, pH 8.0 (1–100 mM) – TRS high, pH 9.9 (DakoCytomation) – Tris–EDTA, pH 9.0 (10 mM/1 mM) – TRIS, pH 10.0 (10–200 mM)
Group 2 Lower efficiency buffers Longer incubation times Less tissue destructive	– TRS, pH 6.1 (DakoCytomation) – Boric acid, pH 7.0 (20 mM) – Citrate, pH 6.0 (10 mM)

Alternatively, charged glass slides, such as *SuperFrost (Ultra) Plus* (e.g. Fisher Scientific), provide highly standard adhesion even under extreme HIER conditions. Heat activation of the binding between the adhesive layer and the tissue section by melting the wax, for at least 30 min, is crucial before dewaxing.

If unacceptable tissue deterioration occurs, reducing the duration of heating and/or the subsequent cooling period or decreasing the ionic strength of the retrieval buffer may improve the cytomorphological preservation. In some cases, inferior nuclear morphology, due to partial loss of histone proteins, can be compensated with extended counterstaining. Some antigens may be destroyed or washed out by the higher temperature, i.e. extracellular antigens, glycophorin C, and surface immunoglobulin light chains. Therefore, careful titration of HIER is needed when a new antibody is tested in these applications.

The most rapid HIER procedures utilize the standard MWO or the household pressure cooker, whereas the more time-consuming procedures use the MWO/pressure cooker combination, the autoclave, vegetable steamer, and the water-bath. In the full-power MWO procedures, treatment is performed in 2–4 heating cycles of 5 min each. Each cycle is interrupted to replenish evaporated buffer in the Coplin jars containing the slides. MWO can also be used without disruption either with larger buffer volumes of 600–800 mL at full power or with a Coplin jar volume of buffer but at limited power (~300 W). The duration of treatment should be extended in the latter case. The household pressure cooker procedure may take up to 40 min, while the combined use of MWO and pressure cooker can exceed 60 min (*see* Subheadings 3.1 and 3.2). "Hot start" modifications of the latter method, in which buffer is preheated before placement of the slides within the pressure cooker (*see* Subheading 3.3), can shorten the treatment time considerably. Wet autoclave HIER is probably the most time-consuming method, since the total time required from start-up to cool-down of the autoclave might be up to 2 h

Table 2 Guidelines for the use of HIER buffers and heading devices

Heat source	Buffer type	Buffer volume	Temperature	Time of exposure[a,b]	Comments
Professional-type MWO with temp. control	Group 1Group 2	1,000 mL	98°C (set)	15–20 min 20–25 min	Total heating time (from room temp.)
Professional-type MWO with temp. control	Group 1Group 2	1,000 mL	120°C (set)	1.5–2 min 2–4 min	Time at working temperature
Consumer-type MWO at full power	Group 1Group 2	90–150 mL	100°C (boiling)	2–3 × 5 min 3–4 × 5 min	Total heating time (from room temp.)
Consumer-type MWO at full power 700–1,200 W	Group 1Group 2	600–800 mL	100°C	18–20 min 24–30 min	Total heating time (from room temp.)
Consumer-type MWO at low power 300 W	Group 1Group 2	100–150 mL	100°C	28–30 min 30–35 min	Total heating time (from room temp.)
Traditional PC (5 L)	Group 1Group 2	3,000 or 150 mL in plastic slide container	~120°C	1.5–2 min 2–4 min	Time at full pressure
Microwave PC (NordicWare)	Group 1Group 2	1,500 or 150 mL in plastic slide container	~110°C	25–30 min 30–40 min	Total heating time (from room temp.)
Autoclave	Group 1Group 2	Autoclavable container with buffer	120°C (set)	12–15 min 15–20 min	Total heating time (from room temp.)
Water-bath	Group 1Group 2	Coplin jars with preheated buffer	95–99°C	25–30 min 40–45 min	Time at working temperature

[a]The duration of HIER within the indicated range depends on the duration of formaldehyde fixation
[b]Extending HIER beyond the indicated duration, particularly with *Group 1* buffers, may be tissue destructive

(*see* Subheading 3.5) (17). The water-bath method operating just below 100°C may also take 40 min or more (*see* Subheading 3.6).

2. Materials

1. Tissue sections mounted on adhesive glass slides, e.g. *SuperFrost (Ultra) Plus* (Fisher Scientific) and heat activated at 60°C (3–5-μm thick paraffin sections) or at 85°C (1–2-μm thick epoxy resin sections) for at least 30 min.
2. Standard domestic microwave oven at 700–1,200 W, with a turntable for constant temperature and an electronic timer control.
3. Plastic Coplin jars or other microwaveable slide containers and suitable slide racks.
4. Microwaveable pressure cooker of 3-L volume (MWPC) (Nordic Ware, Minneapolis, MN).
5. Stainless steel commercial pressure cooker of 5.5-L volume (e.g., Prestige Model 6193, Prestige Group UK Plc., Lancashire, UK).
6. Electric hot plate rated at 1,000 W.
7. Laboratory autoclave, e.g. Sanyo MAC 235 EX (Sanyo, Osaka, Japan).
8. Standard laboratory water-bath rated at 100°C.
9. Antigen retrieval buffer solutions (*see* Table 1).
10. Post-HIER blocking buffer: 0.05 M Tris-buffered saline (TBS pH 7.6) containing 2% low-fat milk powder.
11. Immunostaining buffer: TBS containing 1% BSA or normal goat serum.
12. Test antibodies: mouse monoclonal anti-Ki67/Mib1 (1:150), anti-bcl2/124 (1:100), anti-CD35/To5 (1:100), and rabbit polyclonal anti-CD3 (all from Dako). Incubation: 60 min at room temperature. (For immunostaining protocols, *see* Chapters 25, 26, 28, and 29)).
13. Antimouse Ig-s polymer-conjugate, EnVision+™ detection system (Dako; K4001). Incubation: 30 min at room temperature.
14. DAB+/H_2O_2 chromogen-substrate kit (Dako; K3468). Incubation: 10 min at room temperature.

3. Methods (*See* Note 6)

3.1. Standard MWO Antigen Retrieval: Basic Method (7, 8, 17, 19, 21)

1. Transfer the dewaxed or deplasticized (*see* Note 7) rehydrated and methanolic peroxide blocked slides into plastic Coplin jars or containers filled with a HIER buffer (*see* Table 1 and Note 8).
2. Fill remaining positions in the Coplin jars or plastic slide racks with blank slides (*see* Note 9).
3. Place the Coplin jars or plastic containers in the center of the microwave's turntable, cover containers with loose-fitting lids or screw caps, and heat at maximum power (700–1,200 W). The time of irradiation depends upon the power setting of the microwave, the type of container used, and the volume of buffer (*see* Table 2). The solution should boil for 3–5 min. A large capacity microwaveable plastic container filled with 600–800 mL of HIER buffer may require a ~30–45 min continuous heating cycle (13).
4. After the heat cycle, add distilled water into the container to replenish any evaporated buffer (*see* Note 10). Repeat the heat cycle up to three times. Alternatively, uninterrupted heating at low power (250–300 W) for ~30 min may be performed without the risk of unwanted drying out of sections due to vigorous boiling and evaporation.
5. Following the necessary number of heating cycles, allow the slides to cool for approx. 20 min (*see* Notes 5, 11, and 12).
6. Proceed immediately with the immunostaining protocol (*see* Notes 13–17 and Chapters 25, 26, 28, and 29).

3.2. Microwave Pressure Cooker Method (14)

1. Place the dewaxed/deplasticized and rehydrated sections (*see* Notes 7 and 8) in an MWPC filled with 1,500 mL HIER buffer (*see* Tables 1 and 2 and Note 18).
2. Place the MWPC inside the MWO. Heat at maximum power (700–1,200 W) for 30–40 min with a standard buffer volume and slide number (*see* Notes 9 and 19). Under these conditions, it will take about 15–20 min to reach maximum temperature. The slides should then remain at maximum temperature for less than 20 min (*see* Notes 20 and 21).
3. Release the pressure carefully and cool the sections immediately in post-HIER blocking buffer (*see* Subheading 2, step 10) for 15–20 min before immunostaining (*see* Note 10). Alternatively, the slides can be allowed to cool down in the open pressure cooker (approx. 20–30 min) and then transferred into the post-HIER buffer (*see* Notes 5, 11, and 12).
4. Proceed immediately with the immunostaining protocol (*see* Notes 13–17 and Chapters 25, 26, 28, and 29).

3.3. "Hot Start" Variation for Microwave Pressure Cooker (14)

This variation is performed as described above in Subheading 14.3.2., except that the sections are placed into buffer preheated to about 95°C, and irradiation is performed for only 8–15 min in the closed MWPC. Under these conditions, maximum heat is attained in 3–5 min.

3.4. Standard Pressure Cooker Method (9, 13)

1. Preheat 3 L of HIER buffer (*see* Tables 1 and 2) to a boiling point in a stainless steel 5.5 L capacity pressure cooker (Prestige) without sealing the lid, using an electric hot plate as a heat source. Alternatively, to conserve buffer, the pressure cooker may be filled with distilled water, and a small loosely covered container filled with the selected buffer may be placed into the pressure cooker to hold the slides (*see* Note 18).
2. Place the dewaxed/deplasticized and rehydrated slides in metal slide racks and immerse in the hot buffer (*see* Notes 7 and 8). Seal the PC and bring to full pressure, which is attained when both the "rise-n-time" indicator and the safety plug are in the upright position. Treat the sections at full pressure for 2–3 min (*see* Note 4).
3. Release the pressure and cool the PC under running tap water for approx. 10 min (*see* Note 5).
4. Transfer slides into post-HIER blocking buffer for 15–20 min (*see* Notes 10–12) and continue with the immunohistochemical staining procedure (*see* Notes 13–17 and Chapters 25, 26, 28, and 29).

3.5. Autoclaving (12, 21)

1. Place the dewaxed/deplasticised and rehydrated slides into metal or heat-resistant plastic slide racks (*see* Notes 7 and 8) and immerse in an autoclavable incubation container filled with 250 mL HIER buffer (*see* Tables 1 and 2). Cover the container with a loose-fitting lid to avoid evaporation.
2. Autoclave at 120°C (2 atm) for a maximum time of 20 min.
3. As soon as the autoclave can be opened, the slides should be washed in the post-HIER blocking buffer (*see* Notes 10–12) for 15–20 min, then proceed with the immunostaining (*see* Notes 13–17 and Chapters 25, 26, 28, and 29).

3.6. Water-Bath Heating (21)

1. Immerse the Coplin jar(s) into the water-bath and preheat HIER buffer (*see* Table 1) to the required temperature (95–99°C).
2. Immerse the dewaxed/deplasticised and rehydrated slides into the preheated HIER buffer and cover the Coplin jar with a loose-fitting lid to avoid evaporation (*see* Notes 7 and 8).
3. Continue with HIER for the required time, which is usually 40 min (*see* Table 2).

4. Incubate the slides in the post-HIER blocking buffer for 15–20 min (*see* Notes 10–12) then proceed with the immunostaining (*see* Notes 13–17).

4. Notes

1. One may compensate for over-fixation of tissues by increasing either the duration of HIER by 20–30% of the standard protocol or by increasing the temperature at which epitope retrieval is performed.
2. Information from international external quality assurance organizations and databases is freely available through the Internet. Highly recommended sources are UK NEQAS for Immunocytochemistry: http://www.uknequasicc.ucl.ac.uk and NORDIQC: http://www.nordiqc.org.
3. In most professional microwave ovens, power is regulated according to the set temperature, which is measured inside the HIER buffer. Some of these are complete histological microwave workstations and incorporate both large scale, rapid tissue processing under vacuum as well as HIER applications. Such instruments include, e.g. the Hostos Pro from Milestone Srl. (Sorisole, Italy) and the Meditest 800-3 series from Meditest Kft. (Budapest, Hungary).
4. Since the achievable pressure and temperature in commercial pressure cookers vary among different models, the optimum duration of HIER must be determined for each instrument. Stainless steel pressure cookers usually allow heating up to 120°C and are more durable than those made of aluminum alloys which can be damaged by acidic or alkaline buffer solutions. Timer-controlled electric pressure cookers made of stainless steel are available at low price, e.g. Farberware Programmable Pressure Cooker, 4.5 L, and allow for easy standardization of HIER duration.
5. The cool-down time following the actual high temperature HIER treatment contributes to the overall antigen retrieval effect and should be considered and standardized when testing new antibodies.
6. The procedures described represent guidelines; optimal methods should be determined in individual laboratories. This is due to the variability of tissue fixation and processing and the variety and stability of antigen targets.
7. Deplasticize epoxy resin sections by immersing them in sodium eth(meth)oxide (alcohol saturated with NaOH pellets), for 15 min (10). Wash the sections twice with equal

parts of methanol (or IMS) and xylene, then twice with methanol for 3 min each and rehydrate. Afterwards the same HIER and immunostaining can be employed as for paraffin sections.

8. Optional endogenous peroxidase blocking with methanolic hydrogen peroxide can be performed either before or after HIER.
9. For reproducibility, the slide number and buffer volume should be standardized.
10. Sections should *never* be allowed to dry during or after the HIER procedure because it will result in artifactual staining or loss of staining. A rim of unstained area around the periphery of sections usually indicates drying artifact, which may occur when sections are transferred from the boiling HIER buffer into the room temperature post-HIER blocking buffer. This can be avoided by allowing sections to cool down before transferring them to the post-HIER buffer.
11. APES has some protein binding capacity and may rarely bind the immunoglobulin reagents utilized for IHC. This may result in nonspecific background staining and a reduced signal to noise ratio. Such nonspecific background staining can be avoided by allowing the slides to cool down in protein blocking buffer (e.g. TBS containing 2% low-fat milk or 1% bovine serum albumin) immediately following the HIER procedure for 15–20 min.
12. APES may interfere with silver salt solutions used in the intensification step of immunogold–silver staining techniques. Protein blocking before applying the silver salts or the use of poly-L-lysine or gelatin coated slides for these applications can be beneficial.
13. Some damage to tissue sections is inevitable with HIER, which may influence the morphological assessment. This is most prominent in tissues rich in connective tissues, e.g., skin and breast. More extensive damage is expected at higher temperatures achieved using the pressure cooker or autoclave methods, with longer retrieval times, and when detergents are added to the retrieval buffer.
14. HIER treatment efficiently exposes endogenous biotin. This effect can lead to high background staining in tissues rich in mitochondria (e.g. the epithelia of kidney, liver, and gastrointestinal tissues). For this reason, we recommend the use of one of the newer nonbiotin-based polymer conjugate detection systems such as EnVision+™ (Dako).
15. Diffuse, false positive cytoplasmic staining after HIER, due to endogenous biotin, may be eliminated with commercial

blocking reagents (e.g. Biotin Blocking System, X0590; Dako) or by using a nonbiotin polymer conjugate system, e.g. EnVision+ (Dako). False positive staining may also originate from over-treatment by HIER and is usually accompanied by tissue damage. Reducing the time of antigen retrieval or the temperature and/or increasing the dilution of the primary antibody may be helpful.

16. Weak, false positive nuclear staining may occur with some monoclonal or polyclonal antibodies. Careful assessment of the reaction pattern, correlated with the biology and the expected distribution pattern of the target molecule in normal cells, is always recommended. Nonspecific nuclear staining may be accentuated if slides are allowed to dry during the staining procedure.

17. The combination of HIER and proteolytic enzyme digestion has also been reported; however, this increases the risk of tissue disintegration and nonspecific background staining (23). Significant shortening of the digestion time and/or reduction of the enzyme concentration should be considered when testing such protocols. Furthermore, reproducible proteolytic enzyme treatments require optimal conditions for individual tissues, which make these protocols difficult to standardize.

18. To reduce the use of costly commercial retrieval buffers (e.g. TRS) a small plastic container filled with the appropriate HIER buffer may be immersed within distilled water filling the MWPC chamber.

19. Standardization of the conditions of HIER procedures is prudent. The power setting of the MWO, the number of the slides, the composition and volume of the retrieval medium, and the duration of the treatment are all interrelated. Always use standard power settings, either at a maximum or at limited power and titrate the procedure by adjusting the duration of retrieval or the buffer conditions. We would recommend using one or, at most, two HIER buffers for general applications and other buffer(s) only when absolutely necessary.

20. Tissue deterioration will occur with prolonged exposure to high heat. This effect is particularly pronounced in the group of high pH buffers (*Group 1* in Table 1). Reducing heating time and/or employing the "hot start method" (*see* Subheading 3.3) or using the lower pH citrate containing buffers may help avoid this risk.

21. Commercial MWPO do not reach the operating pressures and temperatures attained by traditional pressure cookers.

References

1. Mason DY, Gatter KC (1987) The role of immunocytochemistry in diagnostic pathology. J Clin Pathol 40:1042–1054
2. Shi S-R, Gu J, Turrens JF, Cote RJ, Taylor CR (2000) Development of the antigen retrieval technique: philosophical and theoretical bases. In: Shi S-R, Gu J, Taylor CR (eds) Antigen retrieval techniques. Eaton Publishing, Natick, MA, pp 17–39
3. Huang SN, Minassian H, Moore JD (1976) Application of immunofluorescent staining on paraffin sections improved by trypsin digestion. Lab Invest 35:383–390
4. Battifora H, Kopinski M (1986) The influence of protease digestion and duration of fixation on the immunostaining of keratins. A comparison of formalin and ethanol fixation. J Histochem Cytochem 34:1095–1100
5. Krenacs T, Stiller D, Krenacs L, Bahn H, Molnár E, Dux L (1990) Sarcoplasmic reticulum (SR) Ca^{2+}-ATPase as a marker of muscle-cell differentiation: immunohistochemical investigations of rhabdomyosarcomas and enhancement of immunostaining after sodium methoxide treatment. Acta Histochem 88:159–166
6. Krenacs L, Tiszlavicz L, Krenacs T, Boumsell L (1993) Immunohistochemical detection of CD1a antigen in formalin-fixed and paraffin-embedded tissue sections with monoclonal antibody O10. J Pathol 171:99–104
7. Shi S-R, Key ME, Kalra KL (1991) Antigen retrieval in formalin-fixed, paraffin embedded tissues: an enhancement method for immunohistochemical staining based on microwave oven heating of tissue sections. J Histochem Cytochem 39:741–748
8. Cattoretti G, Pileri S, Parravicini C, Becker MHG, Poggi S, Bifulco C, Key G, D'Amato L, Sabattini E, Feudale E, Reynolds F, Gerdes J, Rilke F (1993) Antigen unmasking on formalin-fixed, paraffin-embedded tissue sections. J Pathol 171:83–98
9. Norton AJ, Jordan S, Yeomans P (1994) Brief, high-temperature heat denaturation (pressure cooking): a simple and effective method of antigen retrieval. J Pathol 173:371–379
10. Krenacs T, Bagdi E, Stelkovics E, Bereczky L, Krenacs L (2005) How we process trephine biopsy specimens-epoxy resin-embedded bone marrow biopsies. J Clin Pathol 58:897–903
11. Beckstead JH (1994) Improved antigen retrieval in formalin-fixed, paraffin-embedded tissues. Appl Immunohistochem 2:274–281
12. Bankfalvi A, Navabi H, Bier B, Bocker W, Jasani B, Schmid KW (1994) Wet autoclave pre-treatment for antigen retrieval in diagnostic immunohistochemistry. J Pathol 174:223–228
13. Miller K, Auld J, Jessup E, Rhodes A, Ashton-Key M (1995) Antigen unmasking in formalin-fixed routinely processed paraffin wax-embedded sections by pressure-cooking: a comparison with microwave oven heating and traditional methods. Adv Anat Pathol 2:60–64
14. Krenacs L, Harris CA, Raffeld M, Jaffe ES (1996) Immunohistochemical diagnosis of T-cell lymphomas in paraffin sections. J Cell Pathol 1:125–136
15. Morgan JM, Navabi H, Schmid KW, Jasani B (1994) Possible role of tissue-bound calcium ions in citrate-mediated high-temperature antigen retrieval. J Pathol 174:301–307
16. Morgan JM, Jasani B, Navabi H (1997) A mechanism for high temperature antigen retrieval involving calcium complexes produced by formalin fixation. J Cell Pathol 2:89–92
17. Taylor CR, Shi S-R, Cote RJ (1996) Antigen retrieval for immunohistochemistry: status and need for greater standardization. Appl Immunohistochem 4:144–166
18. Shi S-R, Imam SA, Young L, Cote RJ, Taylor CR, Key ME, Kalra KL (1995) Antigen retrieval immunohistochemistry under the influence of pH using monoclonal antibodies. J Histochem Cytochem 43:193–201
19. Pileri SA, Roncador G, Ceccarelli C, Piccioli M, Briskomatis A, Sabattini E, Ascani S, Santini D, Piccaluga PP, Leone O, Damiani S, Ercolessi C, Sandri F, Pieri F, Leoncini L, Falini B (1997) Antigen retrieval techniques in immunohistochemistry: comparison of different methods. J Pathol 183:116–123
20. Leong AS-Y, Milios J, Leong FJ (1996) Epitope retrieval with microwaves. A comparison of citrate buffer and EDTA with three commercial retrieval solutions. Appl Immunohistochem 4:201–207
21. Key M, Boenisch T (2006) Antigen retrieval. In: Key M (ed) Immunohistochemical staining methods. DAKO, Carpinteria, CA, pp 41–46
22. Bagdi E, Krenacs L, Krenacs T, Miller K, Isaacson PG (2001) Follicular dendritic cells

in reactive and neoplastic lymphoid tissues: a re-evaluation of staining patterns of CD21, CD23 and CD35 antibodies in paraffin sections after wet-heat induced epitope retrieval. Appl Immunol Mol Morphol 9:117–124

23. Krenacs T, Rosendaal M (1995) Immuno histological detection of gap junctions in human lymphoid tissue: Connexin43 in follicular dendritic and lymphoendothelial cells. J Histochem Cytochem 43:1125–2237

Part III

Light Microscopic Detection Systems

Chapter 15

Fluorochromes: Properties and Characteristics

J. Michael Mullins

Abstract

Immunofluorescence microscopy provides a sensitive means by which antigens can be localized within tissues or individual cells. For the most effective use of this technique the researcher can draw upon basic information on factors that affect the brightness of the fluorescence image, and how well that image can be distinguished from background fluorescence or interfering fluorescence signals. A wide variety of fluorochromes are available, with emitting wavelengths that range from the blue-violet end of the visible spectrum to the infrared. Individual fluorochromes are characterized by their extinction coefficients, quantum yields, susceptibility to photobleaching, the wavelengths at which they maximally absorb excitatory and emit fluorescent light, and how far apart those wavelength maxima are separated. Additional choices for fluorescent labeling of antibodies are provided by the availability of fluorescent quantum dots®. Informed choices of fluorochromes can obviate many problems, particularly with regard to situations in which two or more antigens are to be localized simultaneously within a specimen.

Key words: Fluorescence, Immuofluorescence, Fluorochrome, Photobleaching, Multiple labeling

1. Introduction

Since its inception in the 1940s, the technique of immunofluorescence microscopy has provided a sensitive, high-resolution method for determining the presence and distribution of an antigen within a specimen. Fluorescent molecules, termed fluorochromes, can be conjugated directly to antibodies by covalent linkage, or coupled indirectly to antibodies via conjugation to proteins A and G, or through an avidin–biotin bridge (*see* Chapters 6 and 7). A fluorochrome that is coupled to an antibody or other probe is often termed a fluorophore; here, the term fluorochrome is used to refer to both the free and conjugated forms of these molecules. The basic features of immunofluorescence are straightforward, but a working knowledge of the commonly used fluorochromes is of value for obtaining maximum performance from

C. Oliver and M.C. Jamur (eds.), *Immunocytochemical Methods and Protocols*, Methods in Molecular Biology, Vol. 588, DOI 10.1007/978-1-59745-324-0_15,

immunofluorescence microscopy and flow cytometry. The discussion below focuses on the fluorochromes commonly used for immunolabeling, and does not encompass fluorochromes that provide direct, molecule- or organelle-specific labeling without the use of antibodies.

2. Fluorescence

Fluorescence, a form of photoluminescence, occurs in response to absorption of light by a fluorochrome, producing an excited state in which an electron from the highest occupied orbital is elevated to a higher energy state in an unoccupied orbital. Some of the absorbed energy is dissipated through rotational or vibrational changes, and so does not contribute to photon emission. Return of the electron to its ground state, however, results in emission of a photon whose wavelength is determined by the wavelength of the absorbed photon. Since some of the energy absorbed by the fluorochrome is dissipated in nonfluorescent ways, the emitted photon will be of longer wavelength and lower energy than the one that was absorbed. Fluorescence is distinguished by the immediate dissipation of the absorbed energy, as opposed to phosphorescence, in which the excited state persists for some interval before photon emission.

Representative absorption (excitation) and emission spectra of a fluorochrome are provided in Fig. 1. Some degree of overlap

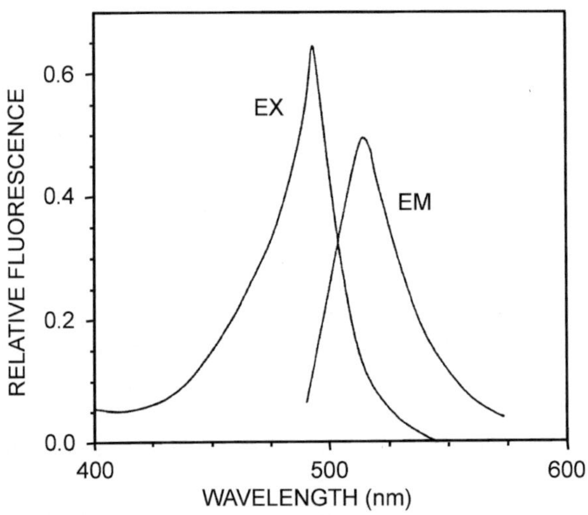

Fig.1 Excitation and emission spectra of the fluorescein derivative DTAF. Modified from ref. 1. *EX* excitation spectrum; *EM* emission spectrum.

between the two spectra is typical, and often the excitation and emission spectra are mirror images of each other.

3. Brightness and Detection of the Fluorescence Signal

Specific detection of a fluorochrome depends primarily on the brightness, or intensity, of its fluorescence, and on the ability of the detection system to distinguish the emitted wavelengths from background. Mathematically, fluorescence intensity is proportional to the product of the extinction coefficient (ε units: $M^{-1}\,cm^{-1}$), a measure of the capture of excitation light by the fluorochrome, and the quantum yield (*A*; maximum value of 1.0), a ratio of photons fluoresced to photons absorbed (2). In actual practice, however, a number of factors may diminish the fluorescence intensity of a fluorochrome or limit its detection. Quantum yield, for instance, decreases noticeably for many fluorochromes on conjugation to an antibody, producing a concomitant decrease in brightness.

The Stokes shift, or separation between the wavelengths corresponding to the excitation and emission maxima, is an important factor that influences both brightness and detection of a fluorochrome. Scattering of the intense, excitation light, which can interfere with the dim fluorescence image, is minimized with a longer Stokes shift. Additionally, the decreased overlap of excitation and emission spectra that attends a longer Stokes shift allows wider band pass optical filters to be employed in the microscope. The use of wider segments of the excitation and emission spectra provides greater light intensity and, therefore, a brighter image. By contrast, for a fluorochrome with a short Stokes shift and considerable overlap of the excitation and emission spectra, clean detection of the weak fluorescence signal requires the use of narrow band pass optical filters to limit excitation and emission wavelengths to nonoverlapping portions of the spectra. Use of such narrow segments of the two spectra diminishes the brightness of the fluorescence signal.

Brightness can be augmented by increasing the numbers of fluorochromes conjugated to each antibody, but there are modest limits to such increases. Interactions between closely positioned fluorochromes on an antibody may reduce fluorescence intensity through selfquenching. In the case of fluorescein, for example, maximum brightness is attained with 2–4 fluorochromes per antibody (2). An additional consequence of an increased fluorochrome-to-antibody ratio is a greater nonspecific binding of the antibody, leading to background fluorescence that degrades the contrast of the fluorescence image.

Naturally occurring fluorescent compounds in cells and tissues provide another source of background fluorescence. Such autofluorescence in mammalian cells arises principally from the excitation of the flavin compounds FAD and FMN (excitation at 450 nm, emission at 515 nm) and NADH (excitation at 340 nm, emission at 460 nm) (3, 4). Porphyrin compounds, including hemoglobin and chlorophyll, also fluoresce, absorbing in the UV-to-blue range and emitting in the orange-to-red range. Additional tissue fluorescence may arise from interactions of additive fixatives, such as glutaraldehyde, with cell constituents to produce fluorescent compounds. Interference from autofluorescence background can be minimized by an appropriate selection of fluorochromes and optical filters to avoid overlap with the spectra of autofluorescing compounds (e.g., ref. 5). Fluorescence arising from glutaraldehyde fixation can be minimized by treating fixed cells with the reducing agent sodium borohydride (6).

In practical application, the intensity of the fluorescence image depends also on the configuration of the fluorescence microscope or other detection system. The light source, the selection of filters to limit excitation and emission wavelengths, and the choice of objectives have major influences on the brightness of the microscope image (7). Similarly, for confocal microscopy or flow cytometry, excitation light is restricted to the wavelengths produced by a given laser. In such cases fluorescence intensity will often be limited to that which can be obtained by exciting fluorochromes at wavelengths other than their excitation maxima (8, 9).

Photobleaching of fluorochromes on exposure to high-intensity excitation light progressively reduces image brightness. This situation presumably arises from the fact that a fluorochrome in an excited state tends to be more chemically reactive, and so may be altered by oxidative or other processes. Susceptibility to photobleaching varies among fluorochromes, and so may be a factor in the choice of a fluorochrome for a given application. Reagents that retard photobleaching are discussed in Chapter 20.

4. Characteristics of Commonly Employed Fluorochromes

Of the many known fluorochromes a relative few are routinely employed for immunofluorescence. Spectral maxima for several fluorochromes are provided in Table 1. Conjugation of fluorochromes to antibodies is typically achieved through isothiocyanate, sulfonyl chloride, succinimidyl ester, or other reactive groups

Table 1
Spectral properties of some representative fluorochromes (arranged by ascending order of emission wavelengths)

Fluorochrome	Excitation max (nm)	Emission max (nm)
Cascade Blue	396	410
SITS	335	438
DAMC	354	441
Alexa Fluor 350	346	442
AMCA	355	450
Cy2	489	506
BODIPY FL	505	513
Oregon Green 488	490	514
FITC	494	519
Alexa Fluor 488	495	519
Fluor X	494	520
Alexa Fluor 430	433	539
Alexa Fluor 532	532	554
Cy3	550	570
TRITC	547	572
Alexa Fluor 546	556	573
BODIPY TMR	542	574
B-PE	545	575
R-PE	565	578
Cy3.5	581	596
XRITC	582	601
Alexa Fluor 568	578	603
Texas Red	589	615
BODIPY TR	589	617
Alexa Fluor 594	590	617
Alexa Fluor 633	632	647
Cy5	649	670
Alexa Fluor 660	663	690
Cy5.5	675	694

AMCA 7-amino-4-methylcoumarin; *B-PE* B phycoerythrin; *Cy* cyanine; *DAMC* diethylaminocoumarin; *FITC* fluorescein isothiocyanate; *R-PE* R phycoerythrin; *SITS* 4-acetamido-4′-isothiocyanato-stilbene-2,2′-disulfonic acid; *TRITC* tetramethyl rhodamine isothiocyanate; *XRITC* rhodamine X isothiocyanate

Information obtained from refs. 2, 9, 10

that provide bonding to protein amines. Fluorescein isothiocyanate, for example, is coupled to antibodies by its reactive isothiocyanate group. Since most investigators purchase fluorochromes already conjugated to antibodies, the chemistry of these and other reactive groups will not be further addressed here (*see* Chapter 6, for details).

The following sections describe some of the fluorochromes that are commonly used for immunofluorescence labeling. Categorization of the fluorochromes is done by the approximate color of their emitted light. Since color varies continuously across the visible spectrum it is obviously somewhat arbitrary to assign a given wavelength to one color range or another (i.e., orange vs. red). Nonetheless, arranging the fluorochromes by the approximate color of their emitted light provides a reasonable means to organize discussion.

Some manufacturers offer families of fluorochromes with emission wavelengths that span most of the visible spectrum and into the near infrared, providing an ample selection of fluorochromes for situations in which multiple labeling is to be done, or under conditions in which background autofluorescence in a specimen needs to be minimized. Notable fluorochrome families include the BODIPY and Alexa Fluor series, and the cyanine (Cy) fluors. Some of these fluorochromes are listed in Table 1. Quantum dots®, discussed in Subheading 4.5, also offer a broad range of emission wavelengths, in addition to several other interesting properties.

4.1. Violet- to Blue-Emitting Fluorochromes

Violet- to blue-emitting fluorochromes absorb in the ultraviolet range, providing good separation from the absorbance and emission spectra typical of the green- and orange/red-emitting fluorochromes routinely used for immunofluorescence. They are, thus, useful for multiple labeling procedures, and their application for that purpose is discussed in Subheading 5.

4.2. Green- to Yellow-Emitting Fluorochromes

The pioneering immunofluorescence studies of Albert Coons and colleagues in the 1940s and 1950s (reviewed in ref. 11) established the effectiveness of fluorescein for immunofluorescence microscopy. The green emission of fluorescein isothiocyanate (FITC) was shown to provide a strong signal, well separated from blue cellular autofluorescence. Continued wide use of fluorescein attests to its utility. Conjugation of fluorescein to an antibody reduces its quantum yield by half (from 0.85 to 0.5–0.3) (2). Nonetheless, conjugated fluorescein provides good fluorescence intensity, and fluorescein's small size and hydrophilic nature are advantageous. Drawbacks include a short Stokes shift and a susceptibility to photobleaching (8). Fluorescein is also pH-sensitive, fluorescing maximally in the range of pH 8.0–9.0. This is not a problem for immunofluorescence of fixed cells, since buffers of optimal pH can be used, but does limit fluorescence intensity in procedures by which fluorescein-labeled molecules are introduced onto or into living cells.

Fluorochromes have been introduced that offer excitation and emission spectra similar to those of fluorescein, but that overcome some of fluorescein's limitations. These include the cyanine fluors Cy2 and FluorX, that are said to offer greater brightness and photostability than fluorescein. BODIPY FL has a short Stokes shift, but offers higher fluorescence intensity, and is claimed to be more photostabile and less pH-sensitive than is fluorescein. Oregon Green 488, a fluorescein derivative, and Alexa Fluor 488 have nearly identical spectra to fluorescein, but are more photostabile and produce less quenching of fluorescence with higher numbers of fluorochromes per antibody. Additionally, other fluorochromes are now available that give a greater breadth of green-emitting choices as well as emission into the yellow region. These range from shorter wavelength maxima (e.g. Cy2 at 506 nm) to the yellow-green 539 nm emission of Alexa Fluor 430, and the yellow-emitter Alexa Fluor 532.

4.3. Orange- to Red-Emitting Fluorochromes

The orange- to red-emitting rhodamine derivatives, especially tetramethylrhodamine isothiocyanate (TRITC), have been widely employed for immunofluorescence. Rhodamine is constructed around the same basic xanthene framework as is fluorescein (2). Additional derivatives of rhodamine available for conjugation to antibodies include lissamine rhodamine sulfonyl chloride (RB-200-SC), rhodamine B isothiocyanate (RBITC), rhodamine X isothiocyanate (XRITC), and Texas Red. The spectra of XRITC and Texas Red are shifted to longer wavelengths compared to those of other rhodamines, making them particularly useful for dual labeling procedures in combination with fluorescein or other green emitters (*see* Subheading 5). Of the two, Texas Red, which is more hydrophilic and so less likely to precipitate proteins upon conjugation (12), is more commonly employed.

Rhodamine conjugates are less sensitive to pH and are less prone to photobleaching than are those of fluorescein. Their fluorescence intensity is generally lower than that of fluorescein conjugates under comparable conditions of excitation, but the intense 546 nm excitatory light provided by the mercury arc lamp of a fluorescence microscope may make rhodamine appear brighter (7).

The family of cyanine (Cy) fluorochromes includes orange- and red-emitters (13, 14). The red-emitting cyanine 3.18, for example, which was shown to give a significantly brighter image than TRITC, lissamine rhodamine, Texas Red, or fluorescein under specific conditions of microscopy (7), provides a useful alternative to the rhodamines. Other useful substitutes for rhodamines include the Cy3 and 3.5, BODIPY TMR and TR, and

Alexa Fluor 546, 568, and 594 fluorochromes. Both the cyanine and Alexa Fluor series are offered as fluorochromes with enhanced photostability, decreased pH sensitivity, and good brightness. Both series include far red emitters as well as those that emit fluorescence wavelengths in the near infrared range above 700 nm. Some of these fluorochromes are listed in Table 1. The rapidly declining sensitivity of the eye to the middle-to-far red wavelengths makes detection by electronic sensors necessary, as does the use of fluorochromes emitting in the near infrared region.

4.4. Phycobilliproteins

Phycobilliproteins, components of algal photosynthetic systems, are naturally occurring, fluorescent molecules (15, 16). Each phycobilliprotein has several (as many as 30) tetrapyrrole groups covalently bonded to it. In living algae the tetrapyrrole groups contribute to photosynthesis by absorbing light, and then transferring the absorbed energy to chlorophyll through fluorescence. The presence of several tetrapyrrole groups per protein, coupled with high extinction coefficients and quantum yields, gives the phycobilliproteins high fluorescence intensities. Fluorescence of some phycobilliproteins is said to equal that resulting from comparable excitation of 30 fluorescein or 100 rhodamine molecules (2).

Three major groups of phycobilliproteins, termed phycoerythrins, phycocyanins, and allophycocyanins, are available for conjugation to antibodies. Their fluorescence is insensitive to pH, and is characterized by emission maxima at relatively long wavelengths and by short Stokes shifts (Table 1). Excitation spectra of the phycobilliproteins span a broad range of wavelengths. This feature, coupled with their high fluorescence intensity, has proven useful for flow cytometry and confocal microscopy, techniques in which excitation wavelengths are limited to those of the laser light source and so may be far from the maximum for a given fluorochrome.

Most use of phycobilliproteins has involved B and R phycoerythrins, which yield the highest fluorescence intensities. They are also the largest phycobilliproteins, with respective molecular weights of 1,960 and 2,410 kDa (2). Such large size poses problems of stearic interference with binding of antibody to antigen, and the possibility of background fluorescence due to inadequate washing of large, unbound antibody conjugates from fixed cells and tissues. Nonetheless, phycoerythrins have been successfully used for immunofluorescence microscopy. Phycoerythrin-conjugated antibodies have been used, for example, to identify T-cell subsets in lymph nodes (17). Corsetti et al. (5) used R phycoerythrin to localize apolipoprotein B in cultured rat hepatocytes. Phycoerythrin was chosen for this work since, unlike fluorescein, its spectral properties allowed minimal interference from the strong, green autofluorescence of hepatocytes.

4.5. Quantum Dots®

The fluorochromes discussed so far have been either small organic molecules or proteins with fluorescence properties. Recently, a new type of fluorescence system that is a very different sort of molecular beast has been adapted for biological use. In this system the fluorescent entity consists of nanocrystals, or quantum dots, that are formed from semiconductor materials such as CdSe, CdS, and CdTe (reviewed in ref. 18). As indicated by the nanocrystal designation, quantum dots range in size from about 2 to 10 nm, placing them in the size range between green fluorescent protein and phycobilliproteins. The basic structure consists of a semiconductor crystal core, typically spherical or rod-like, that is continuous with a protective shell of another material, often ZnS. Quantum dots, thus formed, have some appealing fluorescence properties (19). (1) For quantum dots of the same composition and shape, the emission wavelengths are determined by the size of the dot. Thus, the emission spectrum can be tuned from blue to red by rigorously controlling dot size. (2) Unlike conventional fluorochromes, fluorescence does not depend upon the specific absorption of a relatively small band of excitatory wavelengths. Instead, excitation can be achieved with any wavelengths shorter than that of the emitted light. (3) Quantum dot fluorescence is characterized by high extinction coefficients and brightness. (4) Unlike typical fluorochromes, quantum dots appear to be virtually impervious to photobleaching.

Properties (1) and (2), combined with the fact that quantum dot emission spectra are characteristically narrow and symmetrical compared to those of conventional fluorochromes, offer considerable potential for clean, multiple fluorescence labeling of specimens. With appropriate emission filters in place, the same excitation wavelengths can be used to produce fluorescence from carefully selected quantum dots of different sizes, resulting in the emission of closely spaced, but nonoverlapping colors.

The major obstacle to the employment of quantum dots for biological detection stemmed from the fact that the dots are hydrophobic, and so tend to cluster nonspecifically in aqueous conditions. This problem was overcome by adding an outer silica layer that provides hydrophilic properties and provides reactive groups that allow the quantum dots to be conjugated to antibodies, avidin, biotin, etc. (20). Such modification allowed successful employment of biotin-conjugated quantum dots to label actin filaments, via streptavidin, to phalloidin–biotin, in 3T3 fibroblasts (19), and quantum dots coupled to transferrin to track receptor-mediated endocytosis in HeLa cells (21). Since such initial demonstrations of the utility of quantum dots conjugated to biological probes a number of investigators have employed quantum dots for fluorescence labeling. For example, the breast cancer marker Her2, and actin filaments, microtubules, and nuclear antigens were all labeled via quantum dots that were conjugated to antibodies or to streptavidin (22). A variety of quantum dot conjugates are now available commercially. Given the fact that quantum dots are relatively large compared to organic fluorochromes, there may be some situations for which they will be unsuited. Otherwise, their use for immunofluorescence labeling is likely to expand considerably.

5. Multiple Fluorescent Labeling of Antigens

The sensitivity and high resolution of immunofluorescence microscopy can be exploited to advantage through techniques that allow more than one antigen to be localized simultaneously in the same cell or tissue section. This is possible when two or more primary antibodies differ in some basic characteristic, such as species of origin or isotype, allowing secondary antibodies of corresponding specificities to deliver different fluorochromes to each primary antibody. The distribution of each antigen is thus revealed by a different color of fluorescence. Alternatively, the primary antibodies can be conjugated directly to the fluorochromes of choice, but that approach typically delivers lower fluorescence intensity and involves the possibility of unwanted alterations to the specificity of the primary antibody. Recently, discrimination between two primary antibodies raised in the same species (e.g. rabbit polyclonal sera) was achieved by coupling the high dilution of one of the antibodies in conjunction with its detection via a fluorescence catalyzed reporter deposition (CARD) method (23).

Effective multiple labeling requires that the excitation and emission spectra of each fluorochrome have minimal overlap with those of the other fluorochromes. If this is not so, then discrimination of the distribution of one fluorochrome from that of another may be impossible. Double labeling using a fluorochrome combination of fluorescein and rhodamine, or other green and orange-red emitters, is a common multiple-labeling technique. Although the excitation and emission spectra of fluorescein and rhodamines overlap to some extent, proper selection of optical filters to limit bandwidth provides readily distinguishable red and green signals. Texas Red has the advantage of less spectral overlap with fluorescein (12). As seen in Table 1, a variety of fluorochromes with emission maxima spanning the visible spectrum are now available for use in multiple labeling.

Localization of more than two antigens in the same cell is possible if a set of fluorochromes with minimal spectral overlap can be assembled. Successful triple labeling has been achieved by the addition of violet- or blue-emitting fluorochromes to the green-orange/red combination typically used for double labeling. Initially, SITS was employed as this fluorochrome (24). Subsequently, improved results were obtained by replacing SITS with the coumarin derivatives diethylaminocoumarin, DAMC (25–27), or 7-amino-4-methylcoumarin-3-acetic acid, AMCA (28). Cascade Blue (29), which has less spectral overlap with fluorescein than the coumarins, and the more recently introduced Alexa Fluor 350 provide additional possibilities for triple labeling combinations.

Typically, the distribution of each fluorochrome is viewed and photographed separately by selection of the appropriate filter set. The production of images displaying multiple emission patterns simultaneously is now commonly done by taking digital color or monochrome photographs for each separate fluorochrome, and then combining the separate images, with color reintroduced as necessary, using a graphics program. Alternatively, filter sets are available that allow simultaneous excitation and observation of two to four different fluorochromes. With such filters the brightness of the fluorescence for a given fluorochrome is less than that obtained with filters optimally matched to its spectra only. In combination with color photography, however, the simultaneous localization of two or more fluorescence signals can provide striking and informative photographs provided care is taken to balance the intensities of the different fluorescence signals. Additionally, simultaneous detection obviates any problems that might arise from small changes in the alignment of different filter cubes and the attendant shifts in the position of the fluorescence images.

The extent to which multiple fluorescence signals can be distinguished in a single specimen was demonstrated by resolution of five separate fluorochromes within individual, living 3T3 cells (30), and by the simultaneous detection of nine separate fluorochromes in immuno-phenotyping of murine B cells by flow cytometry (31).

References

1. Blakslee D, Baines MG (1976) Immunofluorescence using dichloro-triazinylaminofluorescein (DTAF). I. Preparation and fractionation of labelled IgG. J Immunol Methods 13: 305–320
2. Hemmila IA (1991) Applications of fluorescence in immunoassays. Wiley, New York, NY
3. Aubin JE (1979) Autofluorescence of viable cultured mammalian cells. J Histochem Cytochem 27:36–43
4. Benson RC, Meyer RA, Zaruba ME, McKhann GM (1979) Cellular autofluorescence: is it due to flavins? J Histochem Cytochem 27:44–48
5. Corsetti JP, Way BA, Sparks CE, Sparks JD (1992) Immunolocalization, quantitation and cellular heterogeneity of apolipoprotein B in rat hepatocytes. Hepatology 15:1117–1124
6. Bacallao R, Morgane B, Stelzer EHK, DeMey J (1989) Guiding principles of specimen preservation for confocal fluorescence microscopy. In: Pawley JB (ed) Handbook of biological confocal microscopy. Plenum, New York, NY, pp 197–205
7. Wessendorf MW, Brelje TC (1992) Which fluorophore is brightest? A comparison of the staining obtained using fluorescein, tetramethylrhodamine,

lissamine rhodamine, Texas red, and cyanine 3.18. Histochemistry 98:81–85

8. Haugland RP (1990) Fluorescein substitutes for microscopy and imaging. In: Herman B, Jacobson K (eds) Optical microscopy for biology. Wiley-Liss, New York, NY, pp 143–157
9. Tsien RY, Waggoner A (1989) Fluorophores for confocal microscopy: photophysics and photochemistry. In: Pawley JB (ed) Handbook of biological confocal microscopy. Plenum, New York, NY, pp 169–178
10. The handbook – a guide to fluorescent probes and labeling technologies (2008) Invitrogen, Molecular Probes, http://probes.invitrogen.com/handbook/
11. Kasten FH (1989) The origins of modern fluorescence microscopy and fluorescent probes. In: Kohen E, Hirschberg JG (eds) Cell structure and function by microspectrofluorometry. Academic, San Diego, CA, pp 3–50
12. Titus JA, Haugland R, Sharrow SO, Segal DM (1982) Texas Red, a hydrophilic, red-emitting fluorophore for use with fluorescein in dual parameter flow microfluorometric and fluorescence microscopic studies. J Immunol Methods 50:193–204
13. Mujumdar RB, Ernst LA, Mujumdar SR, Waggoner AS (1989) Cyanine dye labeling reagents containing isothiocyanate groups. Cytometry 10:11–19
14. Southwick PL, Ernst LA, Tauriello EW, Parker SR, Mujumdar RB, Mujumdar SR, Clever HA, Waggoner AS (1990) Cyanine dye labeling reagents: carboxymethylindocyanine succinimidyl esters. Cytometry 11:418–430
15. Kornick MN (1986) The use of phycobilliproteins as fluorescent labels in immunoassay. J Immunol Methods 92:1–13
16. Oi VT, Glazer AN, Stryer L (1982) Fluorescent phycobiliprotein conjugates for analyses of cells and molecules. J Cell Biol 93:981–986
17. Pizzolo G, Chilosi M (1984) Double immunostaining of lymph node sections by monoclonal antibodies using phycoerythrin labeling and haptenated reagents. Am J Clin Pathol 82:44–47
18. Chan WC, Maxwell DJ, Gao X, Bailey RE, Han M, Nie S (2002) Luminescent quantum dots for multiplexed biological detection and imaging. Curr Opin Biotechnol 13:40–46
19. Bruchez MJ, Moronne M, Gin P, Weiss S, Alivisatos AP (1998) Semiconductor nanocrystals as fluorescent biological labels. Science 281:2013–2016
20. Liz-Marzan LM, Giersig M, Mulvaney P (1996) Synthesis of nanosized gold-silica core-shell particles. Langmuir 12:4329–4335
21. Chan WC, Nie S (1998) Quantum dot bioconjugates for ultrasensitive nonisotopic detection. Science 281:2016–2018
22. Wu X, Liu H, Liu J, Haley KN, Treadway JA, Larson JP, Ge N, Peale F, Bruchez MP (2003) Immunofluorescent labeling of cancer marker Her2 and other cellular targets with semiconductor quantum dots. Nat Biotechnol 21:41–46
23. Uchihara T, Nakamura A, Nakayama H, Arima K, Ishizuka N, Mori H, Mizushima S (2003) Triple immunofluorolabeling with two rabbit polyclonal antibodies and a mouse monoclonal antibody allowing three-dimensional analysis of cotton wool plaques in Alzheimer disease. J Histochem Cytochem 51: 1201–1206
24. Rothbarth PH, Tanke HJ, Mul NA, Ploem JS, Vliegenthart JF, Ballieux RE (1978) Immunofluorescence studies with 4-acetamido-4′-isothiocyanatostilbene2-2′-disulphonic acid (SITS). J Immunol Methods 19:101–109
25. Meister B, Hokfelt T (1988) Peptide- and transmitter-containing neurons in the mediobasal hypothalamus and their relation to GABAergic systems: possible roles in control of prolactin and growth hormone secretion. Synapse 2:585–605
26. Small JV, Zobeley S, Rinnerthaler G, Faulstich H (1988) Coumarin–phalloidin: a new actin probe permitting triple immunofluorescence microscopy of the cytoskeleton. J Cell Sci 89:21–24
27. Staines WA, Meister B, Melander T, Nagy JI, Hokfelt T (1988) Three-color immunofluorescence histochemistry allowing triple labeling within a single section. J Histochem Cytochem 36:145–151
28. Wessendorf MW, Appel NM, Molitor TW, Elde RP (1990) A method for immunofluorescent demonstration of three coexisting neurotransmitters in rat brain and spinal cord, using the fluorophores fluorescein, lissamine rhodamine, and 7-amino-4-methylcoumarin-3-acetic acid. J Histochem Cytochem 38: 1859–1877
29. Whitaker JE, Haugland RP, Moore PL, Hewitt PC, Reese M (1991) Cascade blue derivatives: water soluble, reactive, blue emission dyes evaluated as fluorescent labels and tracers. Anal Biochem 198:119–130
30. DeBiasio R, Bright GR, Ernst LA, Waggoner AS, Taylor DL (1987) Five-parameter fluorescence imaging: wound healing of living Swiss 3T3 cells. J Cell Biol 105:1613–1622
31. Bigos M, Baumgarth N, Jager GC, Herman OC, Nozaki T, Stovel RT, Parks DR, Herzenberg LA (1999) Nine color eleven parameter immunophenotyping using three laser flow cytometry. Cytometry 36:36–45

Chapter 16

Direct Immunofluorescent Labeling of Cells

Maria Veronica Dávila Pástor

Abstract

In the direct immunofluorescent labeling technique, fluorochrome-labeled antibodies are used as probes for particular antigens or biomolecules. Cells, usually after appropriate fixation, are incubated with the antibodies to which fluorochromes have been directly conjugated. Following incubation, excess antibody is washed off with PBS and the cells are mounted on coverslips with antifade mounting medium. Immunofluorescent labeled cells are analyzed using a conventional fluorescence microscope or by confocal microscopy. Direct labeling has two major advantages: it requires only a single incubation with the labeled reagent, decreasing the number of steps in the staining procedure; and more importantly, provides minimal nonspecific staining and less background. Additionally, the direct labeling technique allows the use of two or more primary antibodies of the same species or isotype, avoiding the problems with secondary antibody staining. This method has multiple applications: to label simultaneously two or more antigens within the same cell or tissue sections; to characterize the subcellular distribution of biomolecules of interest, by concurrently labeling with antibodies to both the antigen of interest and to a known organelle; to investigate whether several antigens of interest are colocalized; and to phenotype cells, for which no specific markers are available, using an appropriate panel of antibodies.

Key words: Immunoassays, Fluorochromes, Fluorescent antibody, Direct immunolabeling, Labeled antibodies, Immunofluorescent labeling, Primary antibodies, Immunofluorescence, Antibodies, Fluorescence

1. Introduction

Fluorochromes absorb energy when exposed to incident light of a particular wavelength, causing excitation of electrons to higher energy levels. As the energized or excited electron returns to its original ground state, fluorescent light is emitted at a wavelength longer than that of the original excitation light (1, 2). This principle has applications in the measurement of analytes in immunoassays. Antibodies labeled with fluorochromes can be employed both in direct and indirect detection methods and have applications in flow cytometry and immunomicroscopy. In the direct

C. Oliver and M.C. Jamur (eds.), *Immunocytochemical Methods and Protocols*, Methods in Molecular Biology, Vol. 588,
DOI 10.1007/978-1-59745-324-0_16, © Humana Press, a part of Springer Science+Business Media, LLC 1995, 1999, 2010

immunofluorescence labeling technique, described originally by Coon and collaborators (3, 4), labeled primary antibodies were used to demonstrate the distribution of an antigen throughout a tissue and within isolated cells. Direct immunolabeling has the advantage of requiring only a single incubation with the labeled reagent and provides minimal nonspecific staining and less fluorescent background. The direct labeling technique can be employed to identify two different antigens in the same preparation simultaneously, using antisera conjugated to dyes which emit fluorescence at different wavelengths. Therefore, this method can be used to prevent the crossreaction of two indirect immunolabeling sequences, which is common in double-labeling experiments. Alternatively, in double-labeling experiments cross-reaction of secondary antibodies can be avoided by using a direct labeling step to apply the second fluorochrome. In addition, multiple primary antibodies of the same isotype or derived from the same species can easily be used in the same experiment when they are directly labeled. Despite these factors, the direct labeling technique has some disadvantages: each primary antibody must be fluorescently labeled and, since only one labeled primary antibody binds to each antigen, the resulting fluorescence may be weaker than with an indirect method. In the indirect labeling technique, an unlabeled antibody is applied directly to the tissue and can be visualized by treatment with a fluorochrome-conjugated antiimmunoglobulin. Labeled secondary antibodies for various species of immunoglobulin classes are available commercially and are relatively inexpensive. Indirect immunolabeling also has the advantage of amplifying the fluorescent signal. Since several fluorescent immunoglobulins bind to each of the primary antibody molecules, the fluorescence is higher than with the direct method. However, the technique of coupling biotin to the primary antibody and finally staining with fluorescent streptavidin can be employed in order to increase signal strength (Fig. 1),

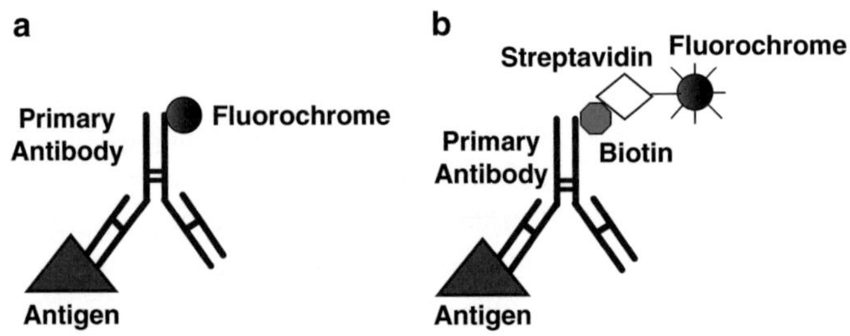

Fig. 1 Diagram illustrating the molecular interactions of direct immunofluorescent labeling method. The fluorochrome-labeled antibody reacts with the cell or tissue antigen in a one-step staining procedure (**a**). Alternatively, the primary antibody, labeled with biotin, can be used with a secondary fluorochrome–streptavidin reagent to increase signal strength (**b**).

when the direct labeling method is required by the experimental circumstances described above.

The selection of specific fluorochromes depends on: the availability of light sources, filter sets, and detection systems; the sensitivity required; and the degree of color separation desired for multiple labeling. For example, Fluorescein isothiocyanate (FITC) and Texas Red® (Fig. 2) are commonly used in wide-ranging applications including microscopy and flow cytometry. Cy3 and Cy5 and Alexa fluors are brighter than other fluorophores and therefore may be selected for increased labeling intensity. Examples of fluorochromes used as labels for immunoassays and their properties are shown in Table 1. Finally, primary antibodies can be coupled with fluorescent nanocrystals (quantum dots or Q Dots®), or with fluorescent microspheres. This method has been applied for the immunofluorescent labeling of cell surface or intracellular antigens (5–7).

The efficiency of any fluorescent antibody conjugate in immunoassays is largely dependent upon the specificity and the concentration of the antibody involved. Monoclonal primary antibodies exhibit better performance in an assay or for detecting antigens in cells or tissue, because of their specificity and will often give significantly less background staining than polyclonal antibodies. Otherwise, suboptimal concentrations of the antibody can lead to poor fluorescence intensity, whereas excessive conjugation can lead to either higher nonspecific binding or selfquenching.

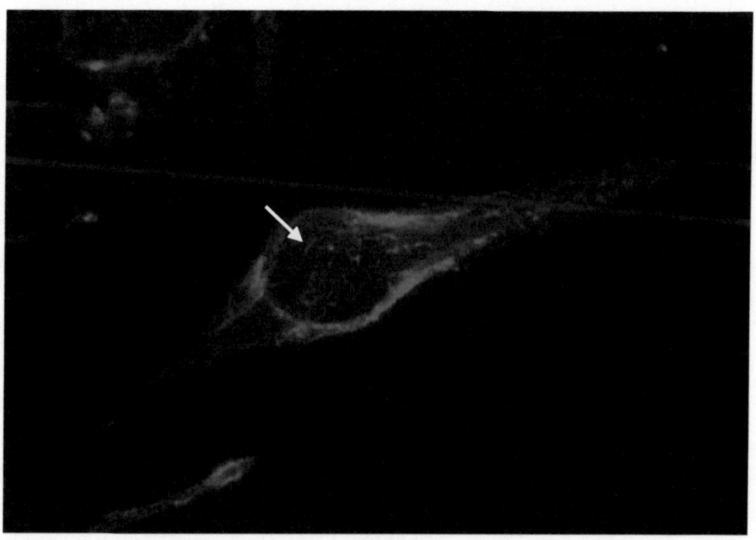

Fig. 2 RBL-2H3 cell labeled in vitro with mAb AA4 directly conjugated to Texas Red® after fixation. The plasma membrane is labeled by the antibody. Microvilli (*arrow*) can be seen on the cell surface.

Table 1
Approximate peak wavelengths of excitation and emission, and appearance of commonly used fluorochromes

Fluorochrome	Excitation peak (nm)	Emission peak (nm)	Appearance
Aminomethylcoumarin (AMCA)	350	450	Blue
Cyanine (Cy2)	492	510	Green
Fluorescein isothiocyanate (FITC)	492	520	Green
Alexa Fluor 488™	495	519	Green
Rhodamine	525	555	Red
Indocarbocyanine (Cy3)	550	570	Orange, red
Tetranethyl rhodamine (TRITC)	550	570	Red
Alexa Fluor 594™	590	617	Red
Texas Red™ (TR)	596	620	Red
Indocarbocyanine (Cy5)	650	670	Red

Two different protocols for the direct labeling of a cell surface antigen are described next: one for unfixed cells in suspension and another for fixed cells adhered to coverslips (Fig. 2). A permeabilization step (*see* Chapter 9) must be added for staining intracellular antigens with fluorescent antibodies or their fragments.

2. Materials

1. Cells in the appropriate medium: for this example isolated peritoneal lavage mast cells resuspended in PBS at approximately 1×10^6 cells/mL.
2. Phosphate buffered saline (PBS) 1×. For 1 L, 10× stock solution: dissolve 2 g KH_2PO_4, 21.6 g Na_2HPO_4, 80 g NaCl and 2 g KCl in 500 mL distilled H_2O by stirring. Adjust the pH to 7.4 and bring to a final volume of 1 L. Store the stock solution at 4°C. Dilute tenfold with distilled water for use. Warm the stock solution to dissolve salt crystals before dilution, if necessary.
3. 0.1 M glycine in PBS.

4. Bovine Serum Albumen (BSA).
5. Fluorophore-conjugated primary antibody diluted 1:20–1:100 in PBS containing 1% BSA (*see* Notes 1–3).
6. Pipetors: 10–1,000 μL with tips.
7. 12-mm round coverslips.
8. Microscope slides.
9. 15-mL Conical centrifuge tubes.
10. Antifade mounting medium such as Fluoromount G (Electron Microscopy Sciences, Hatfield, PA).
11. Ice bath.
12. Additional material for fixed mounted cells: 2% paraformaldeyde in PBS, 24-well culture microplates or Petri dish, 12-mm round coverslips coated with an adhesive agent (*see* Note 4).

3. Methods

3.1. Unfixed Cells in Suspension

1. Add 1 mL of the cell suspension to a 15-mL conical centrifuge tube and pellet the cells by centrifugation for 5 min at 200 × *g*.
2. Decant the supernatant and resuspend the cells with 100 μL of the blocking buffer (1% BSA in PBS), for 15 min at room temperature (RT).
3. Pellet the cells by centrifugation for 5 min at 200 × *g*.
4. Incubate the cells with 150–200 μL of the fluorophore-conjugated primary antibody solution, for one h in the dark at RT (*see* Note 5).
5. Rinse the cells three times in 5 mL of PBS, centrifuging for 5 min at 200 × *g* and decanting the supernatant. After the last centrifugation, resuspend the cells in 90 μL of PBS.
6. Mount approximately 30 μL of the cell suspension on an adhesive coated coverslip (*see* Note 4) and mount on slide with antifade mounting medium. Examine with a fluorescent microscope equipped with the appropriate filters (*see* Notes 6–9).

3.2. Fixed Cells Adhered on Coverslips

1. Place the coated coverslip, coated side up, in 24-well culture microplates (*see* Note 10).
2. Cover the dried, coated coverslips with the cell suspension (30 μL/coverslip) and incubate for 15–30 min at RT (*see* Note 11).

3. Rinse the cells attached to coverslips twice with PBS, removing liquid by gentle aspiration in this and all the subsequent steps, being careful not to let the cells dry.
4. Fix the cells with 2% paraformaldehyde in PBS (200 µL/coverslip), for 10 min at RT (*see* Notes 12–14).
5. Rinse the cells twice with PBS and once in PBS containing 0.1 M glycine (*see* Note 14).
6. Incubate the cells with 200 µL of the blocking buffer, for 30 min at RT.
7. Remove the blocking buffer. Do not rinse.
8. Distribute 150–200 µL of the fluorophore-conjugated primary antibody on each coverslip and incubate for one h in the dark at RT.
9. Rinse the cells five times with PBS.
10. Gently rinse the coverslips with dH_2O from a wash bottle.
11. Invert each coverslip onto a slide containing 10 µL of mounting media.
12. Remove the excess mounting media with fiber-free paper, without disturbing the coverslip. Seal the edges of each coverslip with formaldehyde-free transparent nail polish (*see* Note 15) and allow to dry for 3 min. This will provide semi-permanent preparations. The cells are now ready for microscopic viewing.

4. Notes

1. When using an antibody for the first time, it is advisable to try a dilution series (i.e., 1:50, 1:100, 1:500, 1:1,000) to determine the optimal antibody dilution for the system in which it is being employed. Datasheet protocols may be used as a guide for dilution series starting points.
2. The antibody may not bind well to the antigen if the diluent's pH is incorrect. Generally TBS or PBS, pH 7.0–8.2 is recommended.
3. Antibodies must not be stored for extended periods at their working dilutions, unless a stabilizing protein such as BSA has been added. Storing undiluted antibody in aliquots eliminate the need for repeated freeze/thaw, which may cause antibody aggregation or denaturation.
4. Coverslips may be coated with an adhesive such as Cell-Tak™ (Becton Dickinson, Franklin Lakes, NJ), Biobond (Electron

Microscopy Sciences, Hatfield, PA), or poly-L-lysine (Sigma-Aldrich, St. Louis, MO). Cells are resuspended in PBS or other buffer free of protein and fixatives, ~30 μL drops of the cell suspension are placed on the coated coverslip, and the cells allowed to adhere to the coverslip for 10–30 min. The coverslips are then rinsed in PBS, rapidly in distilled water and mounted on slides.

5. Incubation times may range from 30 to 90 min on ice, overnight at 4°C, or from one to six h at RT. If antibody binding will activate the cells or induce endocytosis of the antibody–antigen complex, all steps should be done at 4°C.
6. Cells must be maintained cold to prevent redistribution of antigens–antibody complexes.
7. Photobleaching (fading) may be reduced with mounting media containing antifading reagents such as N-propyl gallate.
8. Several approaches can be considered in case of low signal: use a different fixative; permeabilize cells; extend the incubation time of the antibody to overnight at 4°C; or test different antibody concentrations.
9. If background staining occurs, use the following controls: use an alternative blocking agent; reduce the primary antibody concentration; be sure tissue sections are kept moist during all steps in the procedure. A commercially available blocking reagent such as Molecular Probes' (Invitrogen, Carlsbad, CA) Image-iT FX™ signal enhancer is particularly useful with tissue sections that have a high background.
10. Alternatively a Petri dish may be used. Place the coverslips cells-side-up in a moist environment to prevent drying.
11. Adherent cells may be grown directly on coverslips or in chamber slides; suspension cells may be adhered to coverslips coated with an adhesive agent.
12. Paraformaldehyde should be prepared fresh. It is toxic and should be handled appropriately in a fume hood.
13. After fixation the procedure can be interrupted. Depending on the antigen, formaldehyde-fixed coverslips can be stored in PBS at 4°C for several weeks.
14. Glycine, ammonium chloride or sodium borohydride may be used after fixation with formaldehyde to block free aldehyde groups.
15. Nail polishes containing formaldehyde are autofluorescent and will emit a strong fluorescence. Formaldehyde-free nail polishes are frequently sold as antiallergic nail polish.

References

1. Tiffany TO (2001) Light emission and scattering techniques. In: Burtis CA, Ashwood ER (eds) Tietz fundamentals of clinical chemistry. W. B. Saunders Company, Philadelphia, PA, pp 74–90
2. Carpenter AB (2002) Antibody-based methods. In: Rose NR, Hamilton RG, Detrick B (eds) Manual of clinical laboratory immunology. ASM Press, Washington, DC, pp 6–25
3. Coons AH, Creech HJ, Jones RN (1941) Immunological properties of an antibody containing fluorescent group. Proc Soc Exp Biol Med 47:200–202
4. Coons AH, Kaplan MH (1950) Localization of antigen in tissue cells. J Exp Med 91:1–13
5. Colton HM, Falls JG, Ni H, Kwanyuen P, Creech D, McNeil E, Casey WM, Hamilton G, Cariello NF (2004) Visualization and quantification of peroxisomes using fluorescent nanocrystals: treatment of rats and monkeys with fibrates and detection in the liver. Toxicol Sci 80:183–192
6. Sukhanova A, Devy J, Venteo L, Kaplan H, Artemyev M, Oleinikov V, Klinov D, Pluot M, Cohen JH, Nabiev I (2004) Biocompatible fluorescent nanocrystals for immunolabeling of membrane proteins and cells. Anal Biochem 324:60–67
7. Wu X, Liu H, Haley KN, Treadway JA, Larson JP, Ge N, Peale F, Bruchez MP (2003) Immunofluorescent labeling of cancer marker Her2 and other cellular targets with semiconductor quantum dots. Nat Biotechnol 21:41–46

Chapter 17

Fluorescence Labeling of Surface Antigens of Attached or Suspended Tissue-Culture Cells

Mark C. Willingham

Abstract

This chapter deals with the detection of antigens that are accessible on the surface of isolated living cells using fluorochrome labels. By incubating live cells at 4°C, to prevent endocytosis of bound molecules, the attached antibody can remain on the cell surface, and either be observed in the live state or subsequently fixed. This method yields the greatest sensitivity and best morphologic preservation for detection of surface molecules using antibodies for microscopy.

Key words: Fluorescence, Cell surface antigens, Living cells, Immunocytochemistry, Epitope

1. Introduction

The surfaces of living cells contain a wide variety of molecular species that are characteristic of the type and physiological role of the cell. These surface molecules mediate cell-recognition events, receptor–ligand interactions and hormonal signaling events, surface homeostasis and transport regulation, attachment to surrounding structures, and a host of other physiologically vital functions. The types of surface molecules present include integral, as well as peripheral elements, and include proteins, carbohydrate moieties, and lipids. The number of each molecular species that serves a physiological function can vary from only a few hundred molecules per cell on the surface to many millions of molecules per cell. The unique nature of many of these molecules was recognized early in the development of immunologic techniques for cell identification, and this serves as the basis for many highly useful diagnostic tools in clinical medicine. The identification of surface antigenic molecules

C. Oliver and M.C. Jamur (eds.), *Immunocytochemical Methods and Protocols*, Methods in Molecular Biology, Vol. 588,
DOI 10.1007/978-1-59745-324-0_17, © Humana Press, a part of Springer Science+Business Media, LLC 1995, 1999, 2010

using antibodies can be performed by several methods, including immunofluorescence microscopy, enzyme and discrete marker microscopy, enzyme and radioactive labeling of mass cultures, and flow cytometry using fluorescence dyes. In this chapter, methods will be described that concentrate on the immunofluorescence microscopy approach to surface antigen identification in cultured cells (1, 2).

The method described here assumes certain things about the nature of the antigen and the antibody reagents to be used. First, the epitope reactive with the antibody must be accessible on the exterior of the cell. Some transmembrane molecules have multiple epitopes that are present on the intracellular domains of the molecule, and these would not be applicable using the method described. Second, the antibody must react with this epitope when the molecule is in its native state, that is, when it is either alive or fixed in a way that preserves a native conformation. Some antibodies to surface antigens react only when the molecule is denatured or unfolded, such as the conditions of proteins after SDS gel electrophoresis and Western blotting. This type of epitope may not be detected by the protocol presented here, since the molecule will not be unfolded in this way by these methods. In addition, the epitope should not be rendered inaccessible by posttranslational modifications, such as addition of carbohydrate moities. Third, the number of molecules present on the cell surface must be high enough to be detected using microscopy. This generally means that the molecules must be present at over 1,000 sites/cell surface, at least in some cells in the culture, since below this level, fluorescence microscopy is not sensitive enough to allow detection of the surface reaction. Such low-level epitopes can be more easily detected using mass detection techniques, in which large numbers of cells are combined into a single detectable signal, or by flow cytometry (*see* Chapters 31–36), which can detect very low levels of surface reactivity.

Even though these points define the limitations of this method, it should be pointed out that direct visualization using immunofluorescence can detect surface antigens present in single cells that represent a minor population in a heterogeneous culture, and that the distribution of that antigen on that surface can be interpreted in the context of cell shape and surface morphologic domains, such as attachment points to substratum or surface patching and capping. Fluorescence detection, because of its point-light-source nature, also allows the visualization of very small objects, such as individual viral particles, that are below the resolution of light microscopy refractile methods. For these and other reasons, immunofluorescence microscopic detection of surface antigens is a powerful and frequently useful tool.

2. Materials

1. Use 35-mm plastic tissue-culture dishes such as Falcon (BD Biosciences, Bedford, MA) Corning-Costar (Corning, NY), Nunc (Nalge Nunc International, Rochester, NY), etc. Subculture cells onto these dishes at least 24 h before. For suspension cells, attach cells to plastic dishes using Cell-Tak™ (BD Biosciences, http://www.bd.com), or 1 mg/mL poly-L-lysine precoating and serum-free medium; cells can be forced against the plastic surface using a swinging bucket centrifuge at 800 × *g* for 5 min (*see* Note 6).
2. Dulbecco's phosphate-buffered saline (PBS) (with calcium and magnesium) (Invitrogen, GIBCO, Carlsbad, CA).
3. Crystalline bovine serum album (BSA) (Pentex, Miles Labs., Kankakee, IL; Sigma-Aldrich, St. Louis, MO). Prepare solution of BSA at 2 mg/mL in PBS (BSA–PBS) (*see* Notes 1 and 2).
4. Primary antibody: polyclonal or monoclonal of a specific species, e.g., mouse, diluted to 10 μg/mL in BSA–PBS (can be stored at –70°C for extended periods).
5. Secondary antibody: affinity-purified fluorescent antiglobulin conjugate reactive with the species globulin of the first step, e.g., affinity-purified rhodamine-conjugated goat antimouse IgG (H + L chains) (Jackson ImmunoResearch, West Grove, PA), diluted to 25 μg/mL in BSA–PBS can be stored at –70°C and reused (*see* Notes 3 and 4).
6. 3.7% Formaldehyde freshly diluted into PBS: 1:10 stock solution (37%) "Formalin" (Fischer Scientific, Pittsburgh, PA) into PBS.
7. Glycerol mounting medium (Difco) or 90% glycerol, 10% PBS.
8. Epifluorescence microscope equipped with appropriate filters (e.g., Zeiss Axioplan epifluorescence microscope with rhodamine filters).

3. Methods

1. Wash cultured cells attached to 35-mm plastic tissue-culture dishes in Dulbecco's PBS, then incubate in a blocking buffer consisting of BSA–PBS for 5 min, and cool to 4°C (see protocol flow chart in Fig. 1). Cooling prevents subsequent endocytosis of any added antibody reagents, as well as minimizing lateral mobility of bound antibody in the plane of the plasma membrane (*see* Notes 5 and 6).

Cells attached to 35 mm dish

↓

Wash away culture medium with PBS

↓

Incubate in BSA-PBS blocking solution

↓

Wash in PBS

↓

Incubate in primary antibody

↓

Wash

↓

Incubate in secondary fluorescent conjugated antiglobulin

↓

Wash

↓

Fix in formaldehyde

↓

Mount under coverslip in glycerol

Fig. 1. Flow

2. Add the primary antibody to the living cells at 4°C in BSA–PBS, and incubate for 30 min (1-mL vol. for a 35-mm dish). Do not pipet directly onto the cells, but add antibody solutions at the edge of the dish, and add wash solutions from a wide-mouth bottle or beaker to minimize the potential of removing cells by too vigorous fluid stream. Do not allow the cells to dry at any step. Rock the dish back and forth to maintain coverage over the cells if the antibody solution volume is too small (*see* Note 7).
3. Harvest the primary antibody solution from the dish using a Pasteur pipet and save. Wash the dish again in BSA–PBS at 4°C five times.
4. Add a secondary fluorescent conjugate antiglobulin in BSA–PBS at 4°C for 30 min.
5. Remove the indirect conjugate and save. Wash the dish with BSA–PBS at 4°C five times, followed by washing briefly in PBS alone at room temperature.
6. Fix the cells attached to the dish in 3.7% formaldehyde–PBS at room temperature for 15 min (*see* Note 8).

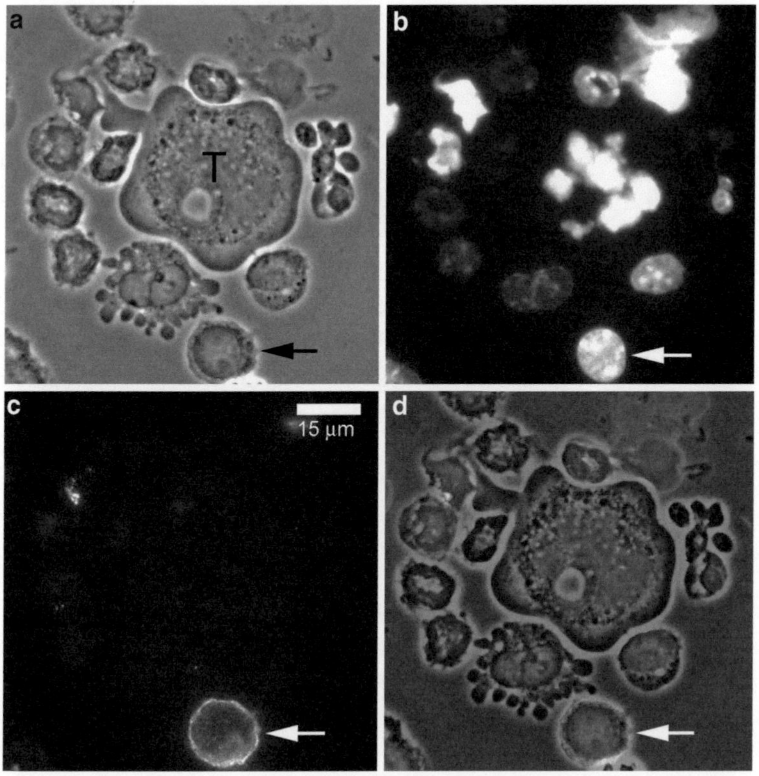

Fig. 2. Fluorescence detection of a CD45-positive mouse lymphocyte in a mixture of leukocytes from the peritoneal wash of an SR/CR mouse injected with S180 tumor cells (3). The cells were attached to a poly-L-lysine-coated surface using centrifugation. The *arrow points* to a single lymphocyte in this field which is shown by phase contrast in (**a**), using DAPI staining fluorescence to visualize nuclear DNA in (**b**), with fluorescence labeling of the surface with antiCD45 indirectly labeled with rhodamine (**c**), and in a color overlay of all three channels in (**d**). The large cell in the center is an S180 tumor cell undergoing necrosis in these cancer-resistant mice, which is in contact mainly with monocytes and neutrophils. The CD45-positive lymphocyte is not attached to the tumor cell, but is incidentally present in the field (bar = 15 μm).

7. Wash the dish in PBS at room temperature five times, cover the cells with mounting medium, and overlay with a no. 1 coverslip (*see* Fig. 2 in Chapter 18). Then view on an upright epifluorescence microscope (using rhodamine filters). Figure 2 demonstrates an example of the type of image seen for surface labeling of attached cells (*see* Notes 9–13).

4. Notes

1. The use of competitor proteins is important in these procedures to minimize nonspecific labeling owing to sticking of protein. Bovine serum albumin is a convenient, purified, inexpensive protein available for this purpose, but other proteins,

such as normal globulin of the same species as the second step, or normal calf serum or plasma, are also useful for this purpose.

2. The use of any detergent-like molecule is inappropriate for surface labeling, since it may remove portions of the surface membrane and dissolve the attachments for surface markers, as well as permeabilizing the cell to antibodies.
3. The use of an affinity-purified second-step reagent is important, since it dramatically reduces background. Although some other companies offer this reagent, Jackson ImmunoResearch, Inc. has a large series of speciality second-step reagents conjugated with several different labels that are all affinity-purified.
4. Rhodamine is a preferred fluorochrome over fluorescein because of its slower bleach rate and its emission in a spectrum that shows less cellular autofluorescence. Also, this spectrum produces less autofluorescence in plastic substrata (*see* Chapter 15). Rhodamine requires a mercury vapor light source, since other sources, such as xenon, do not have sufficient emission in the green spectrum.
5. Attached cultured cells are easiest to work with, since the wash steps can be performed directly on the dish without additional manipulation. For suspended cells, the cells can be incubated in suspension, and the wash steps performed using centrifugation in a microfuge (Eppendorf, Hamburg, Germany) to separate cells at each incubation and washing step. This is much more time-consuming and may lead to a significant loss of cell number during the procedure.
6. Another approach with suspended cells is to convert them into attached cells by either primarily culturing them on a highly adhesive surface, such as Cell-Tak™ (BD Biosciences, Bedford, MA, http://www.bd.com), when they are subcultured the day before, or to wash them free of protein-containing medium and attach them using poly-L-lysine to a dish surface. This is performed by incubating tissue-culture plastic dishes with 1 mg/mL poly-L-lysine (Sigma Aldrich, St. Louis, MO) of high molecular weight (>50,000) in PBS for 5 min at room temperature. The dish is then washed free of poly-L-lysine using PBS and left wet. The cell suspension in protein-free medium is then added, and the cells are either allowed to settle at 1 ×*g* or spun onto the coated surface in a large centrifuge on a swinging bucket adapted to hold dishes. This is analogous to the cytoprep approach (without drying) and works quite well. Unlike the routine "Cytoprep" (Cytospin Centrifuge, Thermo Electron Corporation, Waltham, MA) method, however, it is important to avoid drying of the cells

for good preservation of surface membrane integrity. The cells are then processed through the same protocol as if they were originally an attached cell type. Small amounts of surface labeling are sometimes more easily seen if the cells are rounded, in which the surface labeling appears as a "ring" around the cell periphery. For suspended cells, this labeling can be performed completely in suspension using a centrifuge to separate wash steps, or cells can be attached as above, but later disattached using mechanical means by vigorous pipeting. The observation is then performed while still in suspension in PBS under a coverslip. This method makes it more difficult to obtain photographs of the cells because of cell drift during exposure.

7. The most sensitive approach to surface antigen labeling is to incubate living cells at 4°C with antibodies. This prevents internal labeling background and also minimizes artifacts seen with some fixation. However, there are situations in which living cells are not available or the antigen of interest fails to react without some form of fixation. In these settings, formaldehyde fixation or other forms of fixation can be performed prior to incubation with antibodies. However, it should be noted that fixed cells are much more fragile and sticky compared to living cells, and some fixatives, such as ethanol or acetone, render the interior of the cell permeable, as well. This internal labeling results in background unrelated to the cell surface, as well as the chance of removing the elements of the cell membrane that stabilize the surface antigen of interest (*see* Chapter 8). As a result, prefixation of cells is best performed when cells are already attached to an immobile surface, such as in attached cultured cells or with suspended cells preattached to plastic or glass. Another point to note is that formaldehyde and glutaraldehyde fixation do not inherently permeabilize the plasma membrane, but they do induce a surface "blistering" artifact that produces random holes in the cell surface. Such artifactual holes can sequester antibody in a moth-eaten pattern that is nonspecific and not reflective of actual surface or intracellular distribution of the antigen.

8. The final formaldehyde fixation step links all of the antibody steps in place, preventing their dissociation. Immediate viewing of cells may not require this step, but after fixation, mounted cells can be kept at 4°C for several weeks with little loss of signal. Drying at any stage will severely affect the label, either causing it to be displaced or drastically altering morphology of the surface.

9. Weak fluorescence signals can be preserved for photography by using antioxidants in the mounting medium, such as *p*-phenylenediamine (4) or *N*-propyl gallate (5). This allows

long exposure times without loss of signal resulting from bleaching of the fluorochrome. Color film is not optimal for recording fluorescence images, since color film is usually less sensitive. Also, it shows an artifactual yellowing of localization in areas of higher intensity, which may be the result of background intensity and nonspecific signals. Further, color images are darker and harder to project for presentations and are much more expensive to process and print. The best films for recording fluorescence images are high-speed black and white films, such as Tri-X (Kodak) developed in Diafine (rated speed ASA 1600) (*see* Chapter 20). A more recent and better alternative is the use of direct digital image capture using a cooled CCD camera (e.g., SPOT camera, Diagnostic Instruments, Sterling Heights, MI; or Zeiss Axiocam).

10. The specificity of fluorescence localization is dependent on the specificity of the primary antibody, a property that must be tested and controlled by other methods, such as immunoprecipitation or immunoblotting. Controls for the labeling procedure described include deletion of the primary antibody step, which controls for the second-step reagent, or inclusion of a similar, but nonreactive antibody as a first step. In the case of the availability of purified primary antigen, competition controls can be used, but they only control for the reactivity of the antibody with one antigen, and do not rule out the possibility of a crossreactive, but unrelated antigen (*see* ref. 6).
11. In the case of cell-surface antigens, carbohydrate epitopes are very frequently present in large amounts that can produce highly reactive antibodies that will not necessarily appear on analysis for protein antigens. Thus, glycolipid and other carbohydrate antigens must be kept in mind in analysis of the specificity of a primary antibody. This is especially true of polyclonal or monoclonal antibodies raised to complex mixtures of antigens, such as whole cells. Also, in the case of polyclonal antibodies, affinity purification using purified antigen is a very useful step in preparing reagents for immunofluorescence, since it may eliminate many unwanted antibodies to highly immunogenic contaminants.
12. Several new fluorochromes are available in addition to the well-documented fluorescein or rhodamine labels and their derivatives. These include the highly useful Alexa dyes (7) (Invitrogen, Molecular Probes, Carlsbad, CA; http://www.probes.invitrogen.com). In addition, a new technology, quantum dots®, has become available for fluorescence labeling that promises some new advantages over conventional fluorochromes (8) and are available from Invitrogen (http://probes.invitrogen.com/products/qdot/) (these Q-dots® require special filter sets for optimal results).

13. Following the final fixation, one can also employ counterstain dyes to highlight specific organelles. An example of this is the use of DAPI (a UV-fluorescent dye that binds to DNA; Sigma) to label nuclei, as shown in Fig. 17.2. In this case the fixed cells are incubated for 1 min at room temperature in 0.01% DAPI dissolved in methanol, then washed with water prior to mounting under glycerol. DAPI fluorescence is visualized using UV excitation and visible light emission filters (also requires an objective lens that can transmit UV light for epi-illumination).

References

1. Willingham MC, Pastan I (1985) Immunofluorescence methods. In: An Atlas of immunofluorescence in cultured cells, Academic, Orlando, FL, pp 1–13
2. Willingham MC (1990) Immunocytochemical methods: useful and informative tools for screening hybridomas and evaluating antigen expression. FOCUS 12:62–67
3. Cui Z, Willingham MC, Hicks AM, Alexander-Miller MA, Howard TD, Hawkins GA, Miller MS, Weir HM, Du W, DeLong CJ (2003) Spontaneous regression of advanced cancer: identification of a unique genetically determined, age-dependent trait in mice. Proc Natl Acad Sci U S A 100:6682–6687
4. Platt JL, Michael AF (1983) Retardation of fading and enhancement of intensity of immunofluorescence by p-phenylenediamine. J Histochem Cytochem 31:840–842
5. Giloh H, Sedat M (1982) Fluorescence microscopy: reduced photobleaching of rhodamine and fluorescein protein conjugates by *N*-propyl gallate. Science 217:1252–1255
6. Willingham MC (1999) Conditional epitopes: is your antibody always specific? J Histochem Cytochem 47:1233–1235
7. Panchuk-Voloshina N, Haugland RP, Bishop-Stewart J, Bhalgat MK, Millard PJ, Mao F, Leung WY, Haugland RP (1999) Alexa dyes, a series of new fluorescent dyes that yield exceptionally bright, photostable conjugates. J Histochem Cytochem 47:1179–1188
8. Chan WC-W, Nie S (1998) Quantum dot bioconjugates for ultra-sensitive nonisotopic detection. Science 281:2016–2018

Chapter 18

Fluorescence Labeling of Intracellular Antigens of Attached or Suspended Tissue-Culture Cells

Mark C. Willingham

Abstract

This chapter deals with the detection of antigens located in the interior of isolated cells, in which antibodies can detect their antigens only after fixation and permeabilization of cell structure. Unlike surface antigens, cell structure must be preserved first with a fixative, and the lipid barrier of the plasma membrane must be permeabilized using solvents or detergents. Fluorescence detection enhances the sensitivity of detection of small objects in the cytoplasm of cells because the fluorochrome acts as a point source of light. Because many fixatives preserve the native conformation of fixed antigens, it is important to select antibody reagents that can react with undenatured antigen.

Key words: Membrane permeabilization, Fixation, Organelles, Lipid membranes, Immunocytochemistry

1. Introduction

Cells in culture offer a unique opportunity to visualize intracellular organelles. Because of the ability of some cultured cells to attach and spread on a substratum, the cell's cytoplasm can be spread over a large surface area, resulting in a thin, broad cytoplasmic layer. In this layer, optical methods can resolve details in much the same way as can be accomplished by sectioning of embedded cells, but without the need for embedding and sectioning, and yield detail similar to that available through the use of confocal fluorescence techniques. The patterns of different organelles are, in this setting, very easy to interpret using immunofluorescence, and the subcellular distribution of an antigen can frequently be more clearly and easily detected by this method than with any other. An important feature of this approach is the ease of performing the experiment, in that the organelle localization of an unknown antigen in a cultured cell can be revealed

C. Oliver and M.C. Jamur (eds.), *Immunocytochemical Methods and Protocols*, Methods in Molecular Biology, Vol. 588,
DOI 10.1007/978-1-59745-324-0_18, © Humana Press, a part of Springer Science+Business Media, LLC 1995, 1999, 2010

using a specific antibody in less than an hour by immunofluorescence, a result that might take weeks using cell fractionation methods (1, 2). On the other hand, there are several important methodological considerations that affect the accuracy and interpretability of the results.

One major problem area in immunofluorescence is the choice of the primary fixative. For intracellular antigens, unlike surface antigens, the access of a large protein, such as an antibody, requires permeabilizing the cell membrane, and the preservation of cell architecture and antigen distribution after membrane permeabilization requires precise structural preservation. This fixation step, usually a chemical treatment, will frequently determine the appearance and authenticity of organelle structure and antigen immobilization. Some fixatives, such as organic solvents, function by rendering molecules, such as proteins, insoluble. Others, such as aldehydes, result in specific crosslinking of some, but not all, molecular species in cytoplasmic, organelle, and nuclear matrices. The choice of fixative is often a compromise among structural preservation, accessibility of antibodies to antigen locations, and the preservation of antigen chemical structure in a form that can still react with antibody (*see* Chapter 8).

Antibodies recognize antigens, usually proteins or carbohydrates, generally in the state in which they were exposed to the immunized animal. Thus, proteins injected into an animal in their native conformation will produce antibodies that often react with this same native conformation. On the other hand, proteins that are originally denatured and unfolded, such as after SDS treatment, may result in antibodies that preferentially recognize these denatured forms. Frequently, commercially available antibodies react with proteins in one, but not both, of these situations. Antibodies produced to synthetic peptides will frequently recognize these small peptide region epitopes, often in unfolded proteins, but may fail to recognize them in the complex tertiary form of a native folded protein. This is usually indicated by reactivity of antibodies with antigen in Western immunoblots from denatured SDS gels, but not by immunoprecipitation of native protein from detergent cell extracts. In general, epitopes that are most readily utilized for immunofluorescence are those that represent the native, folded conformation of proteins, and not those that recognize only small peptide determinants in an unfolded, denatured preparation. There are, of course, exceptions to every rule, and some antibodies recognize epitopes in all situations. Suffice it to say that the type of epitope recognized and the quality of the antibody preparation are the single most important aspects of these procedures that determine the ability to interpret the distribution of an antigen in an intracellular site.

The patterns of antigen distribution in different organelles are quite characteristic in cultured cells, and examples of such patterns have been published in many journal articles and books (e.g., ref. (2)) From immunofluorescence images, antigens restricted to intracellular membranous organelles, cytoskeletal elements, cytosolic compartments, and nuclear components are readily identified. Such information is vital in the understanding of functional and biochemical potential roles of antigens. The procedure described here is an indirect immunofluorescence procedure that is both practical and simple, and results in the highest degree of structural preservation, especially for membranes, while still maintaining accessibility of antigens in most intracellular sites.

2. Materials

1. 35-mm plastic tissue-culture dishes such as Falcon (BD Biosciences, Bedford, MA) Corning-Costar (Corning, NY), Nunc (Nalge Nunc International, Rochester, NY), etc. Subculture cells into these dishes at least 24 h before use.
2. Dulbecco's phosphate-buffered saline (PBS) (without calcium and magnesium) (Invitrogen, GIBCO, Carlsbad, CA).
3. Fixative solution. (Formalin stock solution ["Formalin," Fischer, Pittsburgh, PA]) Freshly dilute formalin (37%) stock solution 1:10 in PBS (final concentration = 3.7% formaldehyde in PBS).
4. Prepare competitor protein buffer detergent solution: 4 mg/mL normal goat globulin or other competitor protein, (such as fetal calf serum, bovine serum albumin, bovine plasma, and so forth), and 0.1% saponin (Sigma-Aldrich, St. Louis, MO) in phosphate-buffered saline (NGG-sap-PBS).
5. Primary antibody (polyclonal or monoclonal of a specific species, e.g., mouse). Prepare solution (e.g., 10 μg/mL mouse monoclonal) in NGG-sap-PBS, minimum vol of 1 mL for each dish of cells to be examined. Diluted primary antibody in NGG-sap-PBS can be stored frozen, harvested back from the dish, and refrozen and reused several times.
6. Secondary antibody (affinity-purified fluorescent antiglobulin conjugate reactive with the species globulin of the first step, e.g., affinity-purified rhodamine-conjugated goat anti-mouse IgG (H + L chains) (Jackson ImmunoResearch, West Grove, PA) diluted in NGG-sap-PBS (25 μg/mL). This can be stored in this form, frozen, harvested back from the dish, and reused the same as the first antibody solution. Minimum volume = 1 mL for each dish to be incubated.
7. Glycerol mounting medium (90% glycerol, 10% PBS), or commercial glycerol mounting medium such as Fluoromount G (Electron Microscopy Sciences, Hatfield, PA).
8. Epifluorescence microscope equipped with appropriate filters (e.g., Zeiss Axioplan epifluorescence microscope with rhodamine filters).

3. Method

The sequence of steps is summarized in the flow chart in Fig. 1.

1. Cultured cells attached to 35-mm plastic tissue-culture dishes are washed in PBS, then fixed in 3.7% formaldehyde in PBS

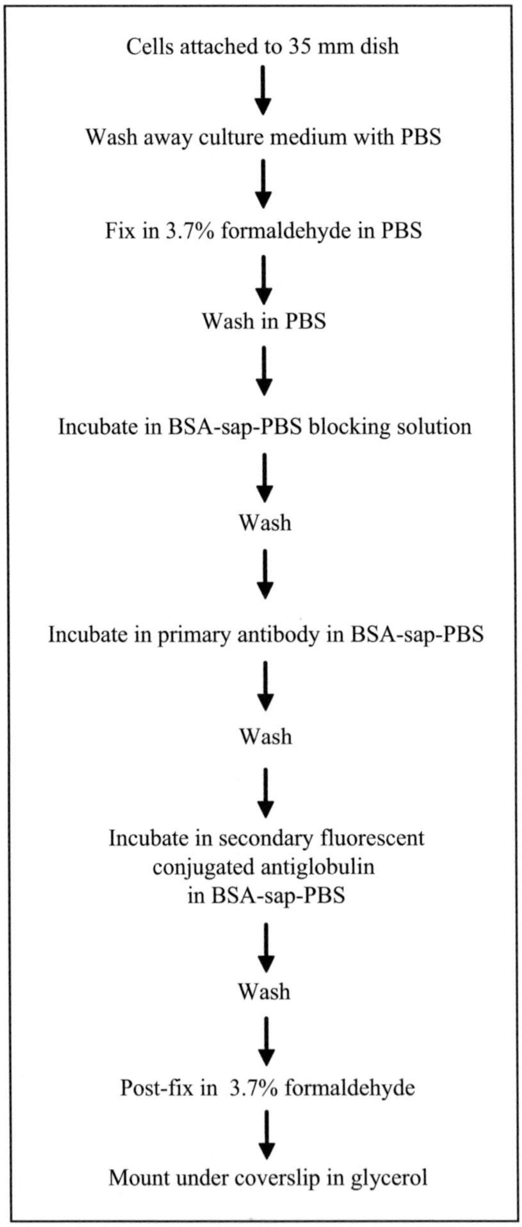

Fig. 1. Flowchart of an intracellular antigen labeling protocol. Abbreviations as in text.

for 10 min at room temperature. The dishes are then washed in PBS five times (*see* Notes 1–3).

2. Incubate dishes with NGG-sap-PBS solution for 10 min at room temperature. The normal goat globulin serves as a blocking protein to minimize nonspecific binding, and the 0.1% saponin renders the fixed cell membranes reversibly permeable to proteins (*see* Notes 4 and 5).
3. The primary antibody in NGG-sap-PBS (e.g., 10 μg/mL mouse monoclonal antibody) is then added to the fixed cells in NGG-sap-PBS and incubated for 30 min at room temperature. Do not pipet directly onto the cells, but add antibody solutions at the edge of the dish, and add wash solutions from a wide-mouth bottle or beaker to minimize cell disattachment. The minimum volume to cover a 35-mm dish surface completely is 1 mL.
4. Harvest and save the primary antibody solution, and immediately wash the dish with PBS five times. Do not let the cells dry at any step. Especially during washings, handle each dish individually, since leaving a washed dish without medium for even a few seconds can allow drying in the center of the dish.
5. Add NGG-sap-PBS competitor protein solution to the dish again briefly, and then pour off.
6. Add the secondary antibody conjugated to rhodamine in NGG-sap-PBS for 30 min at room temperature. Saponin does not render membranes irreversibly permeable, so it must be present in all antibody incubations.
7. Harvest the secondary antibody and save. Wash the cells in PBS five times.
8. Fix the cells again using 3.7% formaldehyde freshly made as performed in the initial fixation. The purpose of the second fixation is to crosslink the antibodies in place and prevent subsequent diffusion of label. If not postfixed in this way, the localization may not be stable for more than a few hours.
9. Wash the cells free of fixative using PBS.
10. Mount the cells under glycerol mounting medium under a no. 1 coverslip as shown in Fig. 2 (*see* Notes 6–9).

4. Notes

1. Physical methods of processing immunofluorescence samples other than plastic tissue-culture dishes are commonly used. The plastic tissue-culture dish is convenient in that cells can be easily grown and processed for immunofluorescence in the same container. Dishes have the slight disadvantage that they possess some autofluorescence, especially in the shorter wavelength

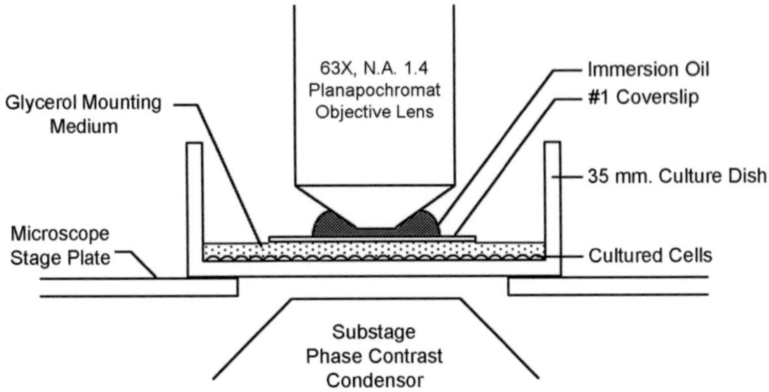

Fig. 2. Diagrammatic summary of the method of mounting and viewing cells in culture dishes on an upright microscope.

ranges, but this is rarely a real problem. Special chamber slides are available for creating separate wells on glass slides (Lab-Tek™ Chamber Slide™ System, Nalge Nunc International, Rochester, NY), and other devices for creating large number of small wells for use in immunofluorescence screening procedures have been devised (3). Coverslips or glass slides can also be placed in the bottom of individual tissue-culture dishes for cell growth when a slide format is desired. All of these approaches work well, but involve tradeoffs of convenience, size, or optical quality. For routine use, direct labeling in 35-mm plastic dishes seems to be the most practical approach. We utilize easily made aluminum plate dish holders that fit the slide clips of standard microscopes. Multiwell tissue-culture dishes often have dimensions that limit their ability to be used on a microscope, either because of too small an opening for large objectives or too large a base to fit easily on a microscope stage.

2. It is possible to label cells directly in suspension for intracellular antigens, but the detail of rounded cells for intracellular sites may be obscured by the cell shape, except for gross distributions, such as nuclear or cell-surface patterns. To discern the detail of intracellular distribution in suspended cells, it is best to attach them and, if possible, cause them to spread or flatten onto a substratum so that intracellular detail is visible. Otherwise, confocal microscopy is necessary. Such an approach is similar to that used for surface labeling, in which an adhesive substrate, such as poly-L-lysine (Sigma-Aldrich) or Cell-Tak™ (BD Biosciences), is fashioned to attach cells to the surface of a dish. The cells can then be handled the same as adherent cultured cells. For cells that do not spontaneously flatten, cytocentrifugation is useful, although the amount of intracellular detail is still somewhat limited. However, mitotic cells that are rounded in many cultured cell lines are an example of the pos-

sibility to visualize detailed intracellular structures even when cells are rounded. Tubulin localization in the mitotic spindle, for example, is very easy to visualize and has a characteristic appearance, even though the cell is completely round. Therefore, it is clear that the amount of detail obtainable in rounded cells will vary with the concentration and distribution of the antigen. The approaches to fixation and processing of such cells once attached to a substratum are essentially the same as for flattened cultured cells.

3. Formaldehyde works well as a primary fixative in this setting because it preserves cell morphology well and the time of exposure to the fixative is short. Formaldehyde fixation at room temperature is very effective, but at 4°C, it is a very poor fixative. Longer fixation times (30–60 min) may be helpful for some antigens that are difficult to preserve, but also may render some sites inaccessible.

   Fixation in glutaraldehyde produces better morphology, but induces a great deal of autofluorescence, and limits cytoplasmic and nuclear permeability. A protocol utilizing glutaraldehyde followed by borohydride treatment has been previously described that is applicable also for electron microscopy of cultured cells (4). Some areas of the cell are relatively impermeable with this approach, but this is an excellent choice of fixative protocol for microtubule morphology.

   Another fixative approach is the use of organic solvents, such as ethanol, methanol, and acetone. These precipitating fixatives also produce membrane permeability and generally yield a poorer quality of preservation, although with a high degree of permeability. Since pure acetone will dissolve styrene plastic dishes, this fixative is usable only with specially resistant plastic dishes (Permanox) or with glass substrates, such as glass coverslips. Acetone mixed with water (80% acetone, 20% water) will fix cells in styrene plastic dishes without dissolving the plastic. Methanol at –20°C is also a commonly used fixative for this purpose. Ethanol is generally a rather poor fixative for cultured cells.

   Other fixatives, such as water-soluble carbo-di-imides or di-imidates, have been used as fixatives, either alone or in combination with aldehydes, but except in special cases, they have no major advantage over aldehyde fixation (5) (*see* Chapter 8).

4. Since intracellular antigens are located inside the plasma membrane barrier, some treatment must be used in intact cells to permeabilize cell membranes. Organic solvent fixation produces permeability directly as a consequence of the fixation process. Formaldehyde and glutaraldehyde do not. Extended fixation in either of these aldehydes leads to fixation blister artifacts in the plasma membrane, which, if they pop, lead to artifactual holes in the cell surface and a moth-eaten appearance

in subsequent antibody labeling. A common approach to producing membrane permeability is the use of detergents after the primary fixative step. Triton X-100 (0.1%), NP40, or Tween-20 have been used to permeabilize fixed membranes. These detergents remove the cell's phospholipid barriers and usually render all membrane-limited compartments, including mitochondria and the nucleus, permeable. However, it is noteworthy that under some conditions, the inner nuclear envelope may require higher concentrations of detergent than the other membranes of the cell. Triton X-100 at 0.5% should permeabilize all mammalian cell membranes. Saponins are cholesterol-like sugar-containing detergents that intercalate into membranes that contain cholesterol. Such molecules surround antibody molecules and allow the transfer of antibody across fixed, cholesterol-containing membranes, as long as saponin is continuously present. Saponin-treated membranes are not permeable, however, to antibody molecules never exposed to saponin in solution. Therefore, for the protocol described above, saponin is present in all antibody incubation steps. The presence of saponin does not, however, render membranes permeable if they have no cholesterol. These include mitochondrial membranes and the inner nuclear envelope. Therefore, the protocol above is useful for cytoplasmic antigens in the cytosol or in membranous organelles that contain cholesterol, including lysosomes, the endoplasmic reticulum, and the Golgi, but will not be useful for antigens inside the nucleus or in mitochondria. For access to these sites, a treatment with a detergent, such as Triton X-100, is necessary. Saponin permeabilization, however, is the mildest form of membrane permeabilization and, as seen by electron microscopy, leaves an intact membrane structure at the cell surface into which many antigens are anchored. The effects of extraction of some membrane protein antigens by detergents other than saponin has been previously demonstrated (6).

5. The inclusion of normal goat globulin in this protocol is important in reducing nonspecific binding of globulins to fixed cell sites that are rendered sticky by chemical treatments. Thus, the high concentration of competitor protein that is not detected by the labeling method yields very low background levels in fixed cells. The globulin of the same species as the second step reagent would be the least likely protein to be detected by this antiglobulin reagent. Other proteins at high concentrations (1–10 mg/mL), such as bovine serum albumin, will also serve this purpose, and may be more available and cheaper. Care must be taken to minimize the content of proteases or other elements that might affect the preservation of the cell or the retention of the antigen of interest. A side

benefit of including high concentrations of carrier (competitor) protein is that the solutions may be harvested back from the dish and reused many times with little loss in specific antibody concentration. Also, the high concentrations of carrier protein allow freezing and thawing of these solutions without denaturation of the small amount of specific antibody present. Freezing is a much safer method of storage and does not require the presence of antibacterial agents to prevent overgrowth of organisms.

6. The pattern of organelles and their distribution in cultured cells of various types have been extensively studied, and books are available that demonstrate these patterns (e.g., ref. (1)). These patterns include membrane-associated antigens, organelle-selective antigens, cytoskeletal antigens, and diffusely distributed antigens. The information gained from these images can immediately categorize a particular antigen as being associated with a specific structure. These methods are also useful for detecting unique antigen expression in individual cells, such as those that express a transfected gene product, or that are generated during a pathologic event, such as apoptosis (*see* Fig. 3). By observing many cells at a time in a culture dish, one can also

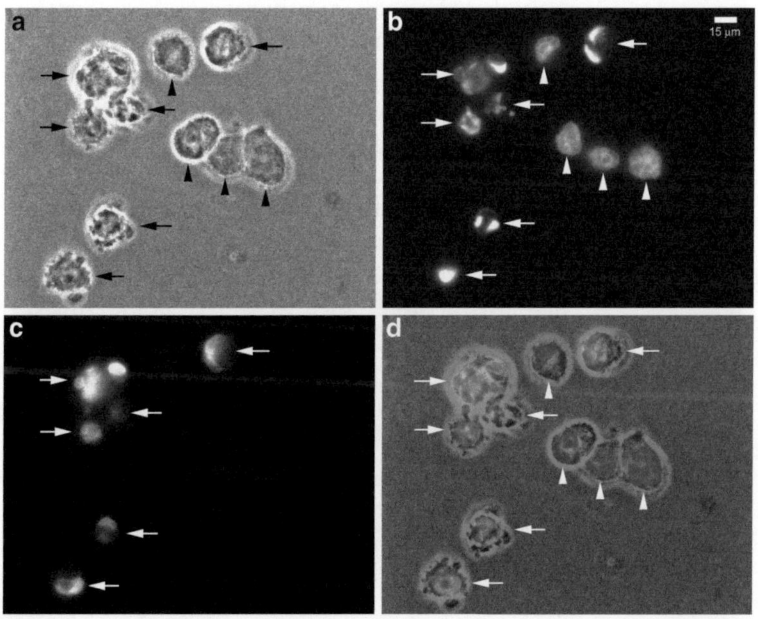

Fig. 3. Immunofluorescence localization of cleaved PARP in apoptotic cells. Cultured KB cells were incubated with ricin to induce apoptosis for 6 h, then fixed and permeabilized using Triton X-100 (0.2%) to permeabilize nuclear structures. An antibody to the neo-epitope generated by the caspase-mediated cleavage of PARP (a nuclear enzyme and caspase substrate) was detected using a specific antibody to cleaved PARP (Promega). Apoptotic cells are shown by the arrows by phase contrast (**a**), using DAPI staining for nuclear DNA in (**b**), and by anti-cleaved PARP indirectly labeled using rhodamine in (**c**). A color overlay of all of the channels is shown in (**d**). Note the normal nonapoptotic cells (*arrowheads*) that fail to show any cleaved PARP signal, whereas all of the apoptotic cells show a strong signal for cleaved PARP (Bar = 15 μm).

search for localization that indicates antigens expressed in only a small percentage of the cells in a culture or in different cellular conditions, such as during various stages of mitosis. It is this interpretive power that makes immunofluorescence such a useful tool. Because of its point-light-source nature, fluorescence can detect objects smaller than the limit of refractile resolution of light, such as individual viral particles. Difficulty in preservation of such objects and their infrequent location in a culture, for example, might make this detection impossible or impractical using electron microscopy.

7. The classical methods of demonstrating specificity of antibody reactions with antigens, such as immunodiffusion plates, are obsolete. Immunofluorescence is a very sensitive method that requires controls for specificity of equal sensitivity. The most important controls are not just those that demonstrate the presence of an antibody that reacts with the antigen of interest, but more importantly, the absence of antibodies that react with other things.

   Precise controls for the specificity of antibody reactions reside with other techniques, such as immunoprecipitation or immunoblotting. Controls for the labeling methodology include deletion of the first-step antibody (blank control), use of a nonreactive antibody in the first step (normal globulin control), or attempts to absorb the antibody if purified antigen is available (preabsorption control). Blank and normal globulin controls characterize the labeling system. Preabsorption controls can be problematic, require large amounts of purified antigen, and still depend on the purity of the antigen preparation. In the early days of these methods when affinity purification was not common and polyclonal sera were used, these preabsorption controls were the only specificity controls possible. With newer, more sensitive biochemical methods, such as Western blots, these preabsorption controls are sometimes not as useful. Controls in which a cell type completely lacks an antigen or in which the antigen's gene can be introduced into a negative cell type, serve as much better, although not perfect, demonstrations of specificity.

   Immunofluorescence frequently reveals crossreactions to other major molecular species that were not appreciated in biochemical isolation experiments because of lack of solubility, extractability, or stability of these crossreacting antigens. This is especially true of antibodies made against synthetic peptides, which may crossreact in immunofluorescence in a way not detected by other methods. This is frequently explainable by the nature of preservation of cell structures for immunofluorescence, in that fixation usually preserves molecules in their native conformations, molecular shapes that would not be preserved by some biochemical extraction methods. The observations relating to the effect of detergent treatments on preservation of membrane-associated antigens (6) also emphasize that some forms of fixation may not preserve an antigen in place sufficiently well for it to be detected by immunofluorescence.

8. Fixation methods play an important role in creating false-negative results in some cases. Formaldehyde fixation may crosslink cellular elements sufficiently to mask sites of antigen concentration. This is especially true in prolonged fixation of intact tissues, rather than the short incubation times for use with cultured cells. A similar problem exists in cultured cells with the use of glutaraldehyde as a primary fixative, in which many cellular sites are covered up by the tight crosslinking present in a glutaraldehyde-fixed cell. A uniquely accessible area of such cells is the region around microtubules that is accessible even after 2% glutaraldehyde fixation (4). The interior of the nucleus or mitochondria, on the other hand, are very easily rendered inaccessible to antibodies by tight fixation. These alterations are usually not related to unique chemical structural changes in the individual antigen, although that situation may theoretically exist in some amine-containing epitopes. Following glutaraldehyde primary fixation, for example, actin is accessible in surface ruffles, but not accessible in the microfilament bundles present in the same cell (4). This emphasizes a cardinal rule of immunocytochemistry in general: Lack of detection of an antigen does not necessarily imply that the antigen is not present in that site. That is, false negatives are frequent and can be caused by many things, especially by fixation.

9. Photography of fluorescent images in the past was most easily accomplished using black and white, high-speed film, such as Kodak Tri-X. When developed in Diafine, the relative ASA rating of this film is ~1,600. Historically and because of personal preference, many investigators in the past have used color films to record fluorescence images. There are several disadvantages to the use of color film:
   (a) The film sensitivity is usually lower, requiring longer exposure times;
   (b) The contrast and brightness of recorded images are usually less, and make presentation of projected 2 × 2 slides difficult because of their darkness; and
   (c) The processing of color materials for publication purposes is much more difficult, requires more elaborate darkroom facilities, and is much more expensive for journal presentation (~$1,000 for one color plate). However, digital imaging is rapidly reducing the cost of color reproductions.

   In addition, color film has an inherent artifact in areas of overexposure, in which the color of the film becomes yellow, no matter what the color of the exposing light. This produces apparent areas of enhanced concentration, which may or may not reflect the true intensity of label, especially in areas in which a low-level background image is added to the specific signal. This can lead to misinterpretations about selective areas of concentration of label. A similar artifact is also generated in digital imaging by using bright images that exceed the grayscale range of the digital image.

Color recording is important in some settings, especially in those in which either double exposures using labels of different color emission are desired or when filters that allow more than one fluorochrome signal through the camera are used. The advent of digital imaging has made color images easier to capture and to reproduce. Using black and white film or grayscale digital image capture, these double-label images can be recorded on two separate negatives or files using filters that separate both emissions discretely, and the images are then compared as individual panels. For various reasons, these grayscale images produce better clarity and greater flexibility in reproducing images on diffferent channels that often have different brightness or camera sensitivity profiles. Sometimes, however, the inherent clarity of points of reference in an image are enhanced by incorporating both label images in one color image (Fig. 3) (*see* Chapter 20). The recent availability of highly sensitive cooled CCD cameras that allow direct digital image capture has essentially made the use of film for image recording obsolete. The image in Fig. 3, for example, was recorded using a Zeiss Axiocam cooled CCD camera, and the individual channel images, captured in grayscale, were then assembled into a color overlay using Adobe Photoshop.

References

1. Willingham MC (1990) Immunocytochemical methods: useful and informative tools for screening hybridomas and evaluating antigen expression. Focus 12:62–67
2. Willingham MC, Pastan I (1985) An atlas of immunofluorescence in cultured cells. Academic, Orlando, FL
3. Willingham MC, Pastan I (1990) A reversible multi-well chamber for incubation of cultured cells with small volumes: application to screening of hybridoma fusions using immunofluorescence microscopy. Biotechniques 8:320–324
4. Willingham MC (1983) An alternative fixation-processing method for preembedding ultrastructural immunocytochemistry of cytoplasmic antigens: the GBS procedure. J Histochem Cytochem 31:791–798
5. Willingham MC (1980) Electron microscopic immunocytochemical localization of intracellular antigens in cultured cells: the EGS and ferritin bridge procedures. Histochem J 12: 419–434
6. Goldenthal KL, Hedman K, Chen JW, August JT, Willingham MC (1985) Postfixation detergent treatment for immunofluorescence suppresses localization of some integral membrane proteins. J Histochem Cytochem 33:813–820

Chapter 19

Fluorescent Visualization of Macromolecules in Drosophila Whole Mounts

Ricardo Guelerman Pinheiro Ramos, Luciana Claudia Herculano Machado, and Livia Maria Rosatto Moda

Abstract

The ability to determine the expression dynamics of individual genes "in situ" by visualizing the precise spatial and temporal distribution of their products in whole mounts by histochemical and immunocytochemical reactions has revolutionized our understanding of cellular processes. Drosophila developmental genetics was one of the fields that benefited most from these technologies, and a variety of fluorescent methods were specifically designed for investigating the localization of developmentally important proteins and cell markers during embryonic and post embryonic stages of this model organism. In this chapter we present detailed protocols for fluorescence immunocytochemistry of whole mount embryos, imaginal discs, pupal retinas, and salivary glands of *Drosophila melanogaster*, as well as methods for fluorescent visualization of specific subcellular structures in these tissues.

Key words: Drosophila, Immunocytochemistry, Fluorescent probes, DAPI, Phalloidin, Developmental cell biology, Whole mounts, Roughest protein, Gamma tubulin

1. Introduction

The ability to determine the expression dynamics of individual genes "in situ" by visualizing the precise spatial and temporal distribution of their RNA and protein products through histochemical and immunocytochemical reactions in whole mounts has revolutionized our understanding of cellular processes, especially during development (1–3). These methodologies, together with the advances in recombinant DNA manipulation and generation of transgenic organisms, have made it possible not only to correlate gene activity with specific morphological changes in cells and tissues but also to manipulate the level and distribution of their encoded proteins in vivo and directly observe their effects in

C. Oliver and M.C. Jamur (eds.), *Immunocytochemical Methods and Protocols*, Methods in Molecular Biology, Vol. 588, DOI 10.1007/978-1-59745-324-0_19,

the whole organism at single cell resolution (4–6). Drosophila developmental genetics was one of the fields that benefited most from these technologies, and a variety of fluorescent methods were specifically designed for investigating the localization of developmentally important proteins and cell markers during embryonic and post embryonic stages of this model organism (7–14). In this chapter we present detailed protocols for fluorescence immunocytochemistry of whole mount embryos, imaginal discs, pupal retinas, and salivary glands of *Drosophila melanogaster* as well as methods for fluorescent visualization of specific subcellular structures in these tissues.

2. Materials

2.1. General

2.1.1. Equipment

1. Stereomicroscopes.
2. Fluorescence, phase contrast and/or DIC microscopes.
3. Confocal microscope.
4. Digital imaging acquisition equipment.
5. Shaker.

2.1.2. Other

1. Mounting medium: glycerol/PBS 1:1.
2. Glass microscope slides 26×76 mm.
3. Coverslips 24×24 mm.
4. Eppendorf microcentrifuge tubes.

2.1.3. Solutions

1. 10× PBS: 13 mM NaCl, 70 mM Na_2HPO_4, 3 mM NH_2PO_4.
2. 4% Paraformaldehyde (Catalogue number T353-500, Fisher Scientific, Pittsburgh, PA) in phosphate buffer pH 6.8 (*see* Note 1).
3. N-Heptane (Merck): stored at room temperature.
4. Formaldehyde solution (Merck, Darmstadt, Germany; Catalogue number 1.04003.1000; 37% formaldehyde stabilized with about 10% methanol).

2.2. Embryo Collection and Dechorionation

1. Plastic Beakers (60 mm diameter) with small holes punched in their bottom with a hot needle.
2. Plastic Petri dishes 60×15 mm.
3. Double stick tape (Scotch 3 M).
4. Glass Petri dish.
5. Egg baskets (*see* Note 2 on how to construct them).
6. Pasteur pipettes.

7. Metal spatulas.
8. Yeast Paste.
9. 100% Bleach.
10. Grape juice agar medium for embryo collection: 227.5 mL grape juice, 43.5 g sucrose, 11 g Agar; 5 mL of an 1.25 N NaOH solution, 5.5 mL acid mix (418 mL propionic acid, 41.5 mL 85% phosphoric acid, distilled H_2O to make 1 L) (*see* Note 3).

2.3. Embryo Fixation and Devitellinization

2.3.1. Embryo Fixation Without Methanol (see "Fixation Without Methanol and Hand Devitellinization")

1. Fixation solution: heptane and 37% formaldehyde solution (Merk) 1:1 (*see* Note 4).
2. Small strips (approximately 5 × 2 cm) of Whatman 3MM blotting paper (Whatman Inc., Florham Park, New Jersey).
3. PBTA solution: 1× PBS, 0.05% BSA, 0.2% Triton X-100, 0.02% sodium azide.

2.3.2. Embryo Fixation with Methanol (see "Fixation with Methanol")

1. Fixation solution: 100 µL 10× PBS, 500 µL 4% freshly prepared formaldehyde (*see* Note 1), 400 µL distilled water. Always prepare it just before use!
2. Methanol (Merck) kept at –20°C – toxic!
3. 0.4% PBT: 1× PBS, 0.4% Triton X-100, Stored at 4°C.
4. BD Falcon™ plastic tubes.
5. Eppendorf® microcentrifuge tubes.

2.4. Phalloidin–DAPI Staining of Embryos

1. Phalloidin–Rhodamine or Phalloidin–Fluorescein (Invitrogen, Molecular Probes, Carlsbad, CA) 6.6 µM stock solution diluted 1:500 in PBTA (freshly diluted and kept in the dark).
2. DAPI (Molecular Probes) 100 µM stock solutions diluted 1:2,000 in PBTA (freshly diluted and kept in the dark).

2.5. Immunostaining of Embryos, Imaginal Discs and Pupae

1. 0.4% PBT: PBS + 0.4% Triton.
2. Ethanol (Merck) 30%, 50%, 80% and 100%.
3. Secondary antibody Cy™3 (1:300) (1.4 mg/mL, Jackson ImmunoResearch, West Grove, PA).

2.6. Salivary Gland Immunostaining

1. 0.1% PBT: PBS + 0.1% Triton.
2. PBSBT: PBS + 0.1% Triton X-100 + 1% BSA.

2.7. Dissection of Post-Embryonic Structures

1. No. 0 paintbrush.
2. Forceps (Dumont #5).
3. Odontologic needles (Senseus™ FlexoFile® endodontic instrument or similar).
4. Razor blades.
5. Kimwipes®.

3. Methods

3.1. Fluorescent Staining of Embryo Whole Mounts

Drosophila embryos are protected both by an outer layer called chorion and an impermeable and opaque vitelline membrane. Therefore preparation of whole mount *Drosophila* embryos for staining with antibodies and/or other fluorescent markers must go through the following steps: chorion removal, fixation, vitelline membrane removal, and membrane permeabilization. The next subsection introduces the basic procedures for embryo collection and chorion removal that are common to all protocols described here, as well as the two most common fixation methods: with or without methanol (the latter requiring hand devitellinization of embryos). The first one works well for immunostaining, while the second is ideal for F-actin staining with phalloidin.

3.1.1. Phalloidin and DAPI Staining (Fig. 1a)

DAPI (4′,6-Diamidine-2-phenylindole dihydrochloride), a fluorescent stain that specifically binds double stranded DNA, is widely used to specifically localize nuclei in developing embryos and as a counterstain. Phalloidin is a plant toxin that binds filamentous actin, thus allowing the visualization of cell borders by highlighting the F-actin network along cell membranes. Both are toxic and should be handled with care.

3.1.1.1. Embryo Collection and Dechorionation

1. Shake 200–400 flies from a culture vessel into a 250 mL plastic beaker and cover with a grape juice agar plate containing a small drop of yeast paste. Place it upside down so flies will lay their eggs on the grape juice (*see* Note 5).
2. Remove the plate from the beaker and add 100% bleach so as to completely cover the plate. Gently brush the embryos with a fine paintbrush to detach them from the plate.
3. Immediately pour the liquid from the collection plate containing the embryos into an egg basket, where they will be retained. Place the egg basket containing the embryos on an empty Petri dish and fill it with bleach so as to completely cover the embryos. Leave the embryos immersed in the bleach solution with constant agitation, for about 2 min (or until the dorsal appendages have dissolved in most embryos), then remove the egg basket. Rinse the embryos extensively in tap water to completely remove the bleach and yeast debris. Try to have as many of the collected embryos as possible in the center of the egg basket in order to minimize loss when transferring them out of the mesh.

3.1.1.2. Fixation without Methanol and Hand Devitellinization

1. Disassemble the egg basket and with a spatula carefully transfer the dechorionated embryos to a glass tube. Add 1 mL of the fixative solution (*see* Subheading 2.3.1) and fix for 45 min at room temperature.

2. Transfer the fixed embryos to a small strip of 3MM paper. Wait for about 15 s to allow the heptane to evaporate.
3. Put the 3MM paper strip (with embryos facing down) gently onto a strip of double-stick tape inside a plastic Petri dish and press very gently in the center and sides so that the embryos stick firmly to the tape. Remove the paper and immediately cover the embryos with about 200 μL of PBTA solution. The embryos are then ready to be dechorionated.
4. Remove the vitelline membrane by hand, individually, under a dissecting microscope using an odontological needle, by making a small hole in the vitelline membrane at one end of the embryo (*see* Note 6).
5. The devitellinized embryos will float on the PBTA solution. Use a pipette to transfer these embryos to a 0.5 mL microcentrifuge tube. At this point you can either store them at 4°C in PBTA for up to a week, or proceed immediately to the staining steps below.

3.1.1.3. Staining and Mounting on Slides

1. Wash the embryos two times with approximately 400 μL PBTA. Add phalloidin from the stock solution to a final dilution of 1:500 (*see* Subheading 2.4). Incubate for 20 min, in the dark, at room temperature. Then wash five times with PBTA, 5 min each wash.
2. Add DAPI from the stock solution to a final dilution of 1:2,000 (*see* Subheading 2.4). Incubate for 4 min in the dark at room temperature. Wash at least five times in PBTA, 5 min each, to remove excess dye. After removing as much of the PBTA as possible after the last wash, add 50% glycerol.
3. To mount the preparation, proceed as follows: First, to avoid flattening the embryos, take two coverslips and glue them with nail polish on each end of the slide. Then place the embryos in glycerol onto the middle of the slide and cover them with a coverslip so that it rests on the other two coverslips. Store the slides in the dark at 4°C.

3.1.2. Immunostaining of Drosophila Embryos (Fig. 1b)

This procedure works better with methanol fixation. Collection and chorion removal are performed as described in "Embryo Collection and Dechorionation" above.

3.1.2.1. Fixation with Methanol

1. Transfer the dechorionated embryos to a glass tube containing 1 mL heptane. Add the fixation solution with methanol (*see* Subheading 2.3.2) and wait until two phases form. The lower, aqueous, phase is formed by the fixative, with the heptane forming the upper phase. The embryos will be between the two layers. Leave the mixture for 20 min at room temperature.

2. Completely remove the lower (fixative) layer. Add 1 mL methanol and immediately mix it vigorously for about 15 s using a vortex mixer. As the phases reform, devitellinized embryos will sink and stay at the bottom of the tube. Remove the upper and lower layers (in this order), together with embryos that did not lose their vitelline membrane and remain floating between the two phases (*see* Note 7).
3. Transfer to a 0.5 mL microcentrifuge tube. Do a series of 5 min washes with about 400 μL of 80%, 50% and 30% methanol. After this do two more washes under the same conditions with 0.4% PBT.
4. Incubate with the primary antibody overnight, at 4°C, with gentle agitation. Shorter incubation times can be tried. The antibody concentration varies with each specific primary antibody. Then wash the embryos five times, 5 min each, with 0.4% PBT.
5. Incubate with the secondary antibody for 6 h, at 4°C, under constant agitation. Different dilutions should be tried to find out the ideal conditions. Then wash as described in the previous step.
6. Mount the slides as described in the previous section. Best results are obtained if the slides are mounted on the same day they will be analyzed microscopically.

3.2. Immunofluorescent Staining of Whole Mounts from Post-Embryonic Structures

In this section we will provide specific modifications from the previous protocols for immunostaining of whole mounts from post embryonic stages (Fig. 1c). An important difference between working with post embryonic structures as compared with embryos is that it is often necessary to dissect them out of the larval body or pupal case before fixing and performing the necessary incubations. Therefore, we have initially described in some detail, the dissection procedures used in our laboratory for obtaining the desired tissues. Also, although these protocols have been specifically optimized for eye imaginal discs and pupal retinas (*see* "Immunocytochemistry of Imaginal Discs and Pupal Retinas"), and salivary glands (*see* "Immunostaining of Salivary Glands") they should be applicable, with relatively few modifications, to imaginal discs other than eye-antennal structures, as well as additional structures such as Malpighian tubules.

3.2.1. Dissection Techniques

3.2.1.1. Larval Eye Imaginal Discs

1. We usually perform the procedure with L3 larvae, when the morphogenetic furrow is already formed and it is possible to recognize differentiating cell populations that will comprise the ommatidia.
2. Remove the larva from the wall of culture vial with a paintbrush (No. 0) (*see* Note 8).

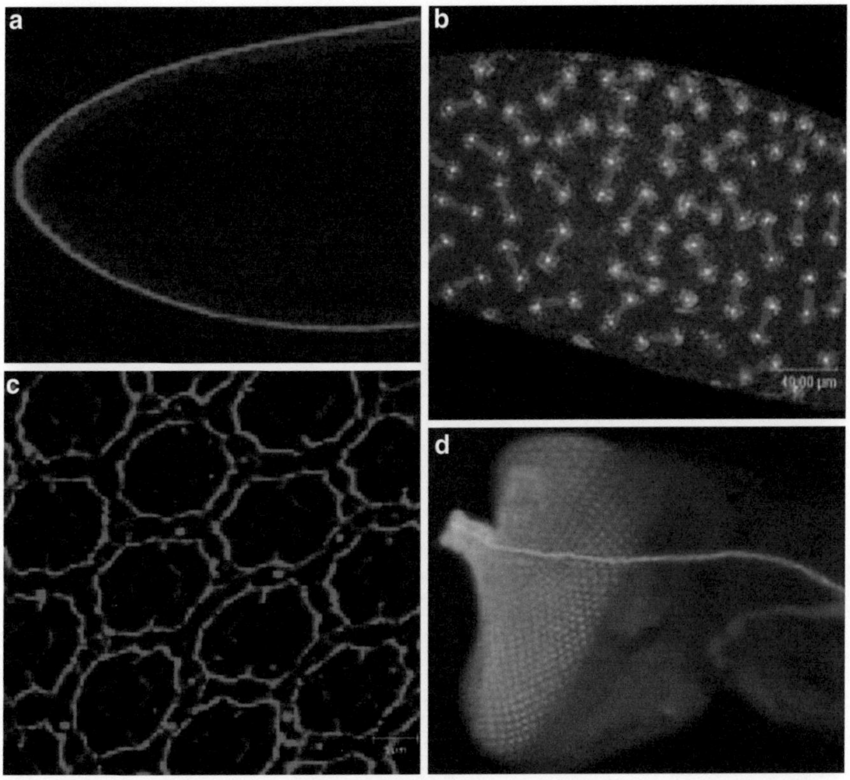

Fig. 1. Examples of fluorescence preparations of Drosophila whole mounts using the protocols is described in this chapter. All confocal images were obtained with a LeicaTCS4D confocal microscope. (**a**) Confocal optical section of a *D. melanogaster* embryo whole mount at blastoderm stage double stained with phalloidin–rhodamine (red) and DAPI (blue) to allow simultaneous visualization of nuclei and cortical actin around cell membranes. Anterior is to the *left*. (**b**). Confocal image of a syncytial stage *D. melanogaster* embryo whole mount with nuclei sincronously undergoing mitoses. The preparation was triple stained with phalloidin–rhodamine (red to visualize F-actin), DAPI (blue; DNA) and antigamma-tubulin antibody (yellow; centrosome, visualized with goat anti mouse Alexa 488 secondary antibody. (**c**) Confocal image of a Drosophila pupal retina, approximately 25% after puparium formation, immunostained with a mouse monoclonal antibody against the cell adhesion glycoprotein Roughest (Rst; *see* refs. (15) and (16)) and visualized with a Cy3 Goat antimouse secondary antibody. Note the strong immunoreactivity (*red*) at the borders between primary pigment cells and interomatidial cells, but not between the interomatidial cells themselves (For more details *see* refs. (17) and (18)). (**d**) Photomicrograph taken with a Zeiss Axiophot fluorescence microscope of a Drosophila eye-antennal imaginal disc whole mount stained with an antibody specific for sensory neurons (Mab22C10; *see* ref. (19)) and visualized with a FITC antimouse secondary antibody. Posterior is to the *left*. The ommatidial clusters containing the differentiating photoreceptors, behind the morphogenetic furrow, and the larval visual nerve, traversing the disc from the optic stalk are clearly stained (For details *see* ref. (20)).

3. Put the larva in a drop of PBS on a slide (*see* Note 9).
4. Under a stereomicroscope, hold the middle of larval body with a forceps and the mouth hooks with another (Fig. 2a). Firmly pull the mouth parts away from the rest of the body.
5. Look for the eye-antennal imaginal discs which will be attached to the mouth hooks and to the optic lobes and ventral nerve cord (Fig. 2b, c).

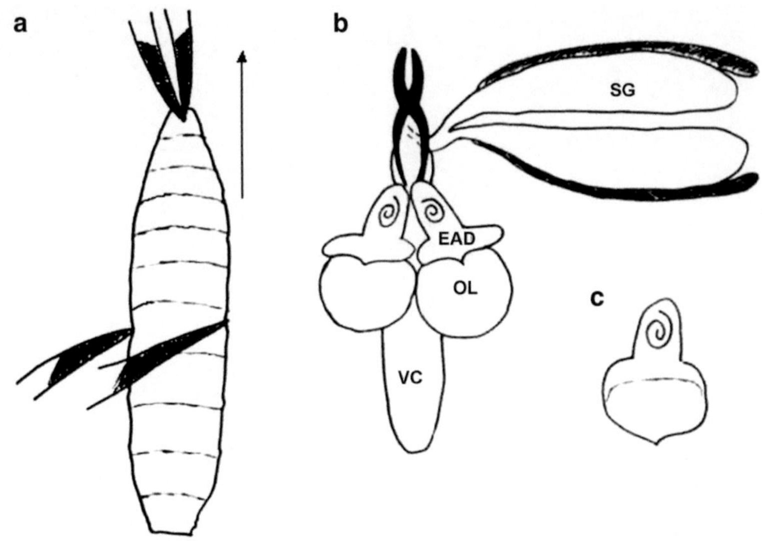

Fig. 2. (**a**) Schematic drawing illustrating the larval dissection procedure (For details *see* "Larval Eye Imaginal Discs" and "Salivary Glands"). (**b**) Drawing of eye-antennal imaginal discs (*EAD*) attached to the larval brain (comprising the optic lobes [*OL*] and the ventral cord [*VC*]. Salivary glands [*SG*], lined with fat bodies, (*in dark*) and attached to the larval mouth hooks are also shown. (**c**) Drawing of a single isolated eye-antennal imaginal disc.

6. Remove all the extra structures, such as salivary glands and fat body, and leave the discs attached to the mouth hooks and optic lobes (*see* Note 10).
7. After finishing step 6, quickly remove the discs from the PBS drop with a 200 μL micropipette with a cut tip and transfer them to a 200 μL microcentrifuge tube containing approximately 50 μL of PBS (*see* Note 11).
8. Clean the slide with a Kimwipe and start a new dissection (*see* Note 12).
9. After having put all dissected discs inside the microcentrifuge tube, close the lid and gently tap it on the bench so that they all go to the bottom of the tube (*see* Note 13).
10. Carefully, remove the PBS from the microcentrifuge tube and start the fixation procedure (*see* "Immunocytochemistry of Imaginal Discs and Pupal Retinas").

3.2.1.2. Pupal Retina

This protocol works well only for pupae with at least 12 h after puparium formation (at 25°C), when head eversion has already occurred. Also, retinas older than 50 h (25°C) are difficult to dissect because they strongly adhere to the cuticle.

1. Under a stereomicroscope, carefully hold the pupa with a forceps at the posterior end of the body. With another forceps remove the pupal case from the anterior end in order to expose the pupal head (Fig. 3a).

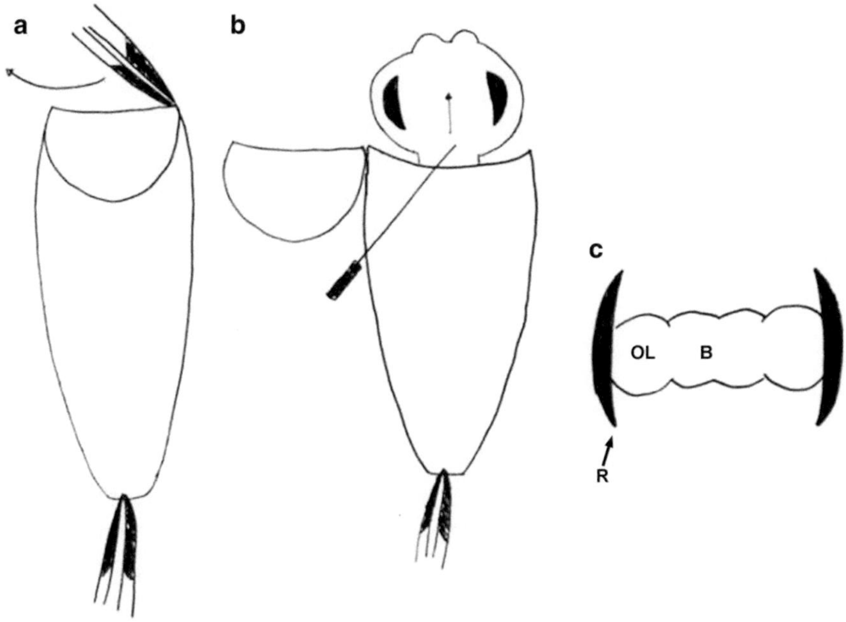

Fig. 3. Schematic drawings depicting the procedure for dissection of pupal retinas. (**a**) Opening of the pupal case. (**b**) Removal of the pupal head from the case. (**c**) The retinae (*R*) attached to the optic lobe (*OL*) and brain (*B*) (For a detailed description *see* "Pupal Retina").

2. Hold the pupa with a forceps at the posterior end and put the head inside a PBS drop onto a slide. Put a needle in the neck of the pupa and pull to the anterior end of the head (Fig. 3b).
3. Look for the pupal retinae attached to the optic lobe and brain inside the PBS drop (Fig. 3c) (*see* Note 14).
4. Clean the retina/optic lobe structures from the fat body and additional structures and proceed as described for eye imaginal discs in the previous section, steps 7–10.

3.2.1.3. Salivary Glands

1. Proceed the same way as described for eye imaginal discs (*see* "Larval Eye Imaginal Discs"), but instead of dissecting the eye-antenna discs and attached structures dissect only the salivary glands (Fig. 1a, b).
2. With two needles detach the fat body lining the outer rim of the salivary glands (Fig. 1b) taking care to do not disrupt the glands (*see* Note 15).

3.2.2. Immunocytochemistry of PostEmbryonic Structures Whole Mounts

3.2.2.1. Immunocytochemistry of Imaginal Discs and Pupal Retinas

The protocol for immunostaining imaginal discs and pupal retina is almost the same, but for imaginal discs, starting from step 2, use 0.1% PBT instead of PBS. Except where stated otherwise, all procedures are carried out at room temperature.

1. Fix the sample. This is an important step of any immunostaining technique and must be adequate for the antigen and specific

tissue, so when establishing a new protocol it is usually necessary to spend some time optimizing this step. In our experience, fixation for 30 min in 4% paraformaldehyde in PBS (Fisher Scientific) is suitable for membrane antigens (*see* Note 16).

2. Remove the fixation solution with a micropipette and add 2% glycine in PBS for 10 min (*see* Note 17).
3. Wash five times, 5 min each, with PBS under agitation. Note: the last wash can be longer if necessary (*see* Note 18).
4. Incubate with primary antibody at the recommended dilution for 1 h at room temperature or overnight at 4°C (12–16 h) (*see* Note 19).
5. Wash five times, 5 min each, with PBS. The last wash can last a bit longer, if necessary.
6. Incubate with the secondary antibody at the recommended dilution for 30 min to 2 h at room temperature or 4–6 h at 4°C.
7. Wash five times, 5 min with PBS (*see* Note 20).
8. Add glycerol: PBS (1:1) to the tube and immediately remove the samples with a cut tip (while they are floating) and place onto a slide. Dissect out the optic lobe with needles and mount the slide with only the eye disc, or retina, on it (*see* Note 21). Alternatively the slides with imaginal discs can be mounted as previously described for embryos (*see* "Staining and Mounting on Slides"). The samples can be circled with a nonfluorescent pen to facilitate viewing.
9. Controls: a basic control is to carry out the protocol without primary antibody. The times of fixation, washing and antibodies incubation must be the same as the sample. With Drosophila, good controls are null alleles for the gene that express the protein that is being labeled.
10. Visualize the immunostaining with a confocal microscope (*see* Note 22).

3.2.2.2. Immunostaining of Salivary Glands

1. Dissect as described above and transfer the salivary glands to a 1.5 mL microcentrifuge tube.
2. Fix with 500 μL of 4% paraformaldehyde (Fisher Scientific) and 500 μL of heptane for 20 min under agitation.
3. Carefully remove the lower phase (4% paraformaldehyde). Add 500 μL of methanol and leave for 1 min (*see* Note 23).
4. Remove upper phase (heptane) and the interphase.
5. Rinse three times with methanol.
6. Rinse with 500 μL methanol/500 μL PBT (PBS + 0.1% Triton).
7. Rinse three times with PBT, and then five times with PBSBT (PBS + 0.1% Triton + 1% BSA).

8. Block in PBSBT for 1 h at room temperature.
9. Add primary antibody at the appropriate concentration. Leave at 4°C overnight.
10. Wash six times in PBSBT, 10 min each.
11. Add secondary antibody. Leave at room temperature for 2 h.
12. Wash five times in PBSBT, 10 min each.
13. Transfer the glands to a microscope slide and mount them in 50% glycerol as described for embryos (*see* "Staining and Mounting on Slides"). Store at 4°C in dark for no longer than a week.

4. Notes

1. Protocol for the preparation of 4% paraformaldehyde, ready to use:
   (a) Dissolve 4 g paraformaldehyde in 35 mL of distilled water at 60°C. Stir 15 min.
   (b) Clear by adding a few drops of 1 N NaOH.
   (c) Add 40 mL of 0.06 M Na_2HPO4.
   (d) Adjust to pH 7.2 with 0.06 M KH_2PO4 (approx. 20 mL).
   (e) Freeze in 1 mL-aliquots. Do not freeze twice! Store thawed aliquots at 4°C for no longer than 2–3 days.
2. These baskets function as sieves, needed to hold the embryos during dechorionation and the washing steps following it. They can be made as follows: cut a plastic scintillation vial in half. Also cut off the top of the cap, so that it forms an open ring. Place a piece of fine synthetic mesh around the top of the vial and hold it in place by screwing the open top back on.
3. The order in which the reagents are mixed is important to ensure you get an homogeneous medium. You should first completely dissolve the sucrose in water and only then add the agar. Dissolve it by heating the solution in a microwave oven while preventing the mixture from boiling over. As soon as the agar is completely dissolved add the grape juice and wait for the mixture to cool down until you can hold it without burning your hands (about 55–60°C). Only then add the NaOH, the acid mix and pour onto 60 × 15 mm plastic Petri dishes. One recipe is enough to make about 80 plates. They can be stored at 4°C for up to a month.

4. In a 50 mL BD Falcon™ tube (BD Biosciences, San Jose, CA) (for 25–50 mL total volume) shake the mixture vigorously for 15 s. Let the solution settle in two phases. Repeat this mixing procedure several times during the day before using the solution. Make sure that the heptane becomes saturated with formaldehyde. The saturated heptane is the upper phase in the 1:1 formaldehyde:heptane stock. It is best to prepare the solution 1 day before it is to be used, shaking the tube periodically throughout the day. Wrap the tube in aluminum foil. This mixture is stored at room temperature and remains active for several months. If crystals form in the mixture upon addition of the formaldehyde, the solution will not work properly and should be discarded.
5. If you need embryos of roughly the same age you should discard the first two or three collections and change the collection plate every hour or less. In any case the yield will be significantly improved.
6. If the fixation was good, the embryo will come out easily, but with some embryos this method may not work well. In these cases, open up two holes, one at each end and push the embryo out.
7. At this point, if necessary, embryos can be stored at 4°C for 2–3 days, at least, by transfering them to a 0.5 mL microcentrifuge tube and washing twice, 5 min each, with 100% ethanol.
8. Usually L3 larvae will wander upwards on the vial wall for a while before they start the puparium formation.
9. If you find it difficult to hold the larva still in the PBS drop, it is possible to put the slide on a previously chilled metal block inside an ice box. This will dramatically slow down the larval movements.
10. Due to the penetration properties of a few antibodies, in some cases it is better to also remove the optic lobes before starting the fixation procedure.
11. Avoid bubbles or air formation inside the pipette tip that can lead to the discs sticking inside the tip. Optionally you can siliconize the tips to avoid the problem altogether.
12. Ideally you should start with at least 10 larvae from each group (control and experimental). The time of dissection of all larvae in a group should not exceed 30 min, after this time, degradation and differentiation can start occurring.
13. Look under the dissecting microscope to be sure that all the discs went to bottom of the tube. Sometimes the discs "float" at the surface of the PBS due the surface tension.
14. Sometimes the retina and optic lobe detach from the brain. In this case you will see retina-optic lobe as two separate structures.

15. The fat body usually is highly fluorescent in these preparations and must be removed.
16. The retinae or discs are fixed under lateral agitation inside a 250 μL microcentrifuge tube (when working with a small number of samples, tube and tips can be siliconized to prevent tissue adherence). The time of dissection should not exceed 30–40 min, to avoid degradation of tissue and mistakes in staging the period of development.
17. This procedure is optional, but as the glycine binds free aldehyde groups, it may reduce nonspecific binding of the primary antibody.
18. Optionally three washes of 10 min each can be performed instead.
19. When establishing a new protocol, the antibody dilution can start at 1:10 up to 1:100; usually more diluted antibodies result in less background. Also, sometimes there is a restriction in the quantity of antibody available in the laboratory, so it is best to find the optimal dilution. The time of incubation can be variable also, depending on thickness and permeability of the tissue and subcellular localization of the antigen. The maximum time for room temperature staining is usually 4–6 h and 18–20 h for overnight incubation at 4°C.
20. After this point it is possible, if desirable, to stain nuclei with DAPI. In these cases add DAPI diluted 1:2,000 during the last 5 min. Wash five times. For imaging DAPI, an UV excitation source and appropriate filter set are necessary.
21. Take care not to put an excessive quantity of mounting medium onto the slide. 50 μL is sufficient, otherwise the structures can float and be lost. If a larger volume is necessary because more than one sample collection is needed, the excess glycerol/PBS should be removed with a Kimwipe® twisted at one of the corners. Be careful that the discs do not get sucked up together with excess fluid. After this, place the coverslip over the sample. Do not press on the sample!! Drosophila tissues, especially retinae and imaginal discs, can be disrupted very easily and all your work will be lost!
22. The samples can be stored at 4°C for no longer than 1–2 weeks. Particularly for Drosophila whole mount preparations, imaging using a confocal microscope is always better than using an epifluorescence microscope, due the fact that imaginal discs, retinae, and embryos are not totally flat structures and in an epifluorescence microscope, the full staining of the structure may only visualized clearly by focusing on different focal planes.
23. Look under a stereomicroscope to be sure that the salivary glands where not removed with the fixative. During washes and staining the microcentrifuge tube must be kept under lateral agitation.

Acknowledgments

We would like to thank all past, present and visiting members of our laboratory, especially Drs. Bernard Bonengel and Martin Strünkelnberg, from the University of Freiburg, Germany, for their contribution in improving and streamlining the protocols described in this paper. We also thank Ms Marcia Graeff for her invaluable help with the operation of the confocal microscope, Ms Mara Silvia A. Costa for skilled technical assistance, Dr Enilza Espreafico (Ribeirão Preto, Brazil) for the gift of the antigamma-tubulin antibody, and Dr Karl Fischbach (Freiburg, Germany) for providing us with generous amounts of antiRst antibody.

References

1. Hashimoto H, Ishikawa H, Kusakabe M (1999) Preparation of whole mounts and thick sections for confocal microscopy. Methods Enzymol 307:84–107
2. Rosen B, Beddington R (1993) Whole-mount in situ hybridization in the mouse embryo: gene expression in three dimensions. Trends Genet 9:162–167
3. Stern CD (1998) Detection of multiple gene products simultaneously by in situ hybridization and immunohistochemistry in whole mounts of avian embryos. Curr Top Dev Biol 36:223–243
4. Chien R (1992) Signaling mechanisms for the activation of an embryonic gene program during the hypertrophy of cardiac ventricular muscle. Basic Res Cardiol 87(Suppl. 2):49–58
5. Brand AH, Manoukian AS, Perrimon N (1994) ctopic expression in Drosophila. Methods Cell Biol 44:445–487
6. Megason S, Amsterdam A, Hopkins N, Lin S (2006) Uses of GFP in transgenic vertebrates. Methods Biochem Anal 47:285–303
7. Zalokar M, Erk I (1977) Phase-partition fixation and staining of Drosophila eggs. Stain Technol 52:89–95
8. Mitchinson TJ, Sedat J (1983) Localization of antigen determinants in whole Drosophila embryos. Dev Biol 99:261–264
9. Patel N (1994) Imaging neuronal subsets and other cell types in whole-mount Drosophila embryos and larvae using antibody probes. Methods Cell Biol 44:445–487
10. Theurkauf W (1994) Immunofluorescence analysis of the cytoskeleton during oogenesis and early embryogenesis. Methods Cell Biol 44:507–532
11. Rothwell WF, Sullivan W (2000) Fluorescent analysis of Drosophila embryos. In: Sullivan W, Ashburner M, Hawley RS (eds) Drosophila protocols. Cold Spring Harbor Laboratory Press, Cold Spring Harbor, NY, pp 141–157
12. Blair SS (2000) Imaginal discs. In: Sullivan W, Ashburner M, Hawley RS (eds) Drosophila protocols. Cold Spring Harbor Laboratory Press, Cold Spring Harbor, NY, pp 159–173
13. Wolff T (2000) Histological techniques for the Drosophila eye. Part I: larva and pupa. In: Sullivan W, Ashburner M, Hawley RS (eds) Drosophila protocols. Cold Spring Harbor Laboratory Press, Cold Spring Harbor, NY, pp 159–173
14. Yin VP, Thummel CS (2004) A balance between the *diap1* death inhibitor and *reaper* and *hid* death inducers controls steroid-triggered cell death in *Drosophila*. Proc Natl Acad Sci U S A 101:8022–8027
15. Ramos RGP, Igloi GL, Baumann U, Maier D, Lichte B, Schneider T, Brandstätter H, Fröhlich A, Fischbach K-F (1993) The *irregular chiasm C-roughest* locus of Drosophila which affects axonal projections and programmed cell death encodes a novel immunoglobulin-like protein. Genes Dev 7:2533–2547
16. Schneider T, Reiter C, Eule E, Bader B, Lichte B, Nie Z, Schimansky T, Ramos RGP, Fischbach K-F (1995) Restricted expression of the cell adhesion molecule IrreC-rst is required for normal axonal projections of columnar visual neurons. Neuron 15: 259–271
17. Reiter C, Schimansky T, Nie Z, Fischbach K-F (1996) Reorganization of membrane contacts prior to apoptosis in the Drosophila retina: The role of the IrreC-rst protein. Development 122:1931–1940

18. Araujo H, Machado LCH, Mizutani CM, Silva MJF, Octacilio-Silva S, Ramos RGP (2003) Requirement of the *roughest* gene for differentiation and time of death of interommatidial cells during pupal stages of Drosophila compound eye development. Mech Dev 120:537–547
19. Zipursky SL, Venkatesh TR, Teplow DB, Benzer S (1984) Neuronal development in the Drosophila retina: monoclonal antibodies as molecular probes. Cell 36:15–26
20. Wolf T, Ready DF (1993) Pattern formation in the *Drosophila* retina. In: Bate M, Martinez-Arias A (eds) The development of Drosophila melanogaster. Cold Spring Harbor Laboratory Press, Cold Spring Harbor, NY, pp 1277–1325

Chapter 20

Overview of Conventional Fluorescence Photomicrography

J. Michael Mullins

Abstract

In an age of digital imaging, photographic film still provides a viable and effective means for recording fluorescence images by photomicrography. To maximize the quality of results that are obtained, a photographic emulsion with sufficient sensitivity for the low light level characteristic of Immunofluorescence must be selected, exposures adjusted for reciprocity failure, and modern, high numerical aperture objective lenses employed to produce the brightest possible image. Mounting media that reduce the effects of photobleaching on fluorochromes also help to maintain image brightness, and so reduce exposure times. Digital scanning of film-based micrographs provides the convenience of utilizing image processing software to adjust image density and contrast, and to produce quality prints.

Key words: Film, Photobleaching, Photographic emulsion, Photomicrography, Reciprocity failure

1. Introduction

The results of fluorescence labeling experiments are best photographed to produce a permanent record. Recent years have seen a major shift to digital imaging systems for photomicrography, but many laboratories still use, out of necessity or preference, conventional photographic emulsions for this purpose. Specific information is provided in the first two sections for those who intend to record fluorescence images on film.

2. Practical Effects of Reciprocity Failure

One of the major hurdles associated with fluorescence photography is that most commercially available films are designed to work best at exposure times in the range of 0.01–0.1 s. Because the

C. Oliver and M.C. Jamur (eds.), *Immunocytochemical Methods and Protocols*, Methods in Molecular Biology, Vol. 588,
DOI 10.1007/978-1-59745-324-0_20,

light levels emitted by antibody-tethered fluorochromes in a specimen are typically of low intensity, exposure times from one to several seconds are often necessary. A given quantity of light, delivered at low intensity over a longer period will have less effect on film than it will if delivered at high intensity over a correspondingly shorter period. This phenomenon, known as reciprocity failure, introduces some complications for photography.

Reciprocity failure of the film has two practical implications. The first is seen with the use of color films. Each of the three, color-sensitive layers of the film has a different reciprocity failure factor, resulting in incorrect color reproduction with long exposures. To correct this problem, color-compensation filters can be placed in the light path to the camera.

The second implication arises from the fact that all fluorochromes are susceptible to some degree of photobleaching as a result of exposure to the excitation light (*see* Subheading 20.2.3). Thus, long exposure time leads to bleaching, which in turn necessitates even longer exposure to insure an adequate image, etc. This is a vicious circle that is hard to avoid. The key is to reduce the exposure time by using a film as sensitive as possible, to optimize the intensity of the emitted fluorescence, and to take the photograph before bleaching has progressed much.

2.1. Film Selection

ISO 400 films such as Kodak Tri-X Pan or Ilford HP5 for black-and-white prints, or Ektachrome for color slides, are suitable for many applications. If needed, these films can typically be exposed using ISOs of 800 or 1600 and then push-processed to yield higher sensitivity. The alternative is obviously to employ films with higher standard ISO values when such sensitivity is necessary. A combination that has found favor in many laboratories is that of Kodak Tri-X film coupled with the Diafine two-bath developer (Acufine, Inc., Vernon Hills, IL) (1), which provides an ISO of 1600 and good grain structure. Higher ISO values correlate with a more conspicuous grain structure in the emulsion, which may be an issue if images are to be enlarged considerably. In general, black-and-white film has a finer grain than color slide or print films of the same ISO, and is less expensive to use. It is suitable for most situations, exceptions being multiple-labeling procedures in which emissions from two or more fluorochromes are to be photographed simultaneously, or when the visual appeal of color is desired for presentation.

2.2. Optimizing Fluorescence Intensity

Emitted fluorescence intensity may be optimized in two ways. To start with, high-intensity excitation light in the range of wavelengths at which the fluorochrome maximally absorbs should be used. Second, lenses of high numerical aperture (NA) are important, so the objective with the highest possible NA consistent with the desired magnification range should be selected.

With epifluorescence illumination, the objective of the microscope serves as both condenser and objective; therefore, fluorescence intensity is proportional to the fourth power of its NA. NA = n(sin α) where n is the refractive index of the medium between the objective lens and the coverslip and α is the ½ angle of the margins of the light cone captured by the lens. Theoretically, the largest ½ angle of light that a lens can gather approaches 90° (half of 180°), the sine of which is 1.0. Therefore, the maximum NA that can be obtained is dependent on the refractive index of the medium between the objective and the coverslip (2). The refractive index of air is 1.00, water is 1.33, glycerine is 1.47, and immersion oil is 1.52. Thus, the highest possible NA is approximately 1.5. Microscope manufacturers offer oil-immersion lenses with NAs approaching this theoretical maximum (e.g., 1.4), including planapochromatic objectives that provide excellent light transmission combined with good flatness of field and superb optical correction. The obvious drawback is that the price of such objectives is commensurate with their quality.

The use of efficient, multiple, antireflection coatings to reduce reflection of light by optical elements has greatly increased the intensity of fluorescence images compared to that obtained with previous optics that had less effective, single coatings. Thus, an older fluorescence microscope may not deliver as intense an image of a given specimen as will a system of more recent manufacture.

2.3. Reducing Exposure Times

Most microscopes are designed so that some or all of the light from the specimen may be directed either to the eyepieces for observation or to the camera for photography. To maximize the emitted fluorescence directed to the camera a 0–100% prism is necessary. This arrangement allows one to direct 100% of the light to the camera when taking a picture.

Dimming of the fluorescence image due to photobleaching of fluorochromes exposed to the intense, excitation light (3) produces further complications for observation and photography. The rate of photobleaching may be reduced by the addition of antifading (antibleaching) reagents to the mounting medium. These reagents are thought to work by scavenging free radicals, and so preventing them from damaging excited fluorochromes. Commonly used antifading reagents include 1,4-diazobicyclo-[2,2,2]-octane (DABCO) (4), *p*-phenylenediamine (PPD) (5, 6), *n*-propyl gallate (NPG) (7), and sodium azide (6). Bacallao et al. (9) obtained successful retardation of photobleaching with a combination of 100 mg/mL DABCO and 0.1% sodium azide in a mounting medium of 50% glycerol in PBS. They noted that in their hands *n*-propyl gallate produced a generally dimmer fluorescence image. Also, PPD has been reported to destroy stored samples over time (4). In addition to such "home brews," several commercial antifading agents of proprietary composition are available. For example,

Molecular Probes (Invitrogen, Molecular Probes, Carlsbad, CA) sells "Prolong," which reduces bleaching dramatically and also gels to provide the actual sealing of the coverslip to the slide. Comparative evaluations of the effectiveness of different antifading agents, including some commercial preparations, have been published (10–12). Of note from this work is the fact that in selecting an antifading agent, compromises may have to be made between higher initial fluorescence intensity vs. the slowest rates at which photobleaching is retarded. It should be noted that some antifading agents may be more useful than others for specialized purposes. Takizawa and Robinson (13), for example, found in work employing correlative fluorescence microscopy and immunogold labeling for electron microscopy in the same specimen, that DABCO dramatically reduced the signal from the silver-enhanced gold label, but that neither PPD nor NPG did so.

Automatic exposure systems often present difficulties in determining the correct exposure for fluorescence images. Since the background in a fluorescent specimen is ideally black, or nearly black, an exposure meter that determines exposure, based simply on the average intensity of the field will invariably produce overexposure. Metering systems that provide spot measurements of small areas of the image generally provide more accurate exposure, providing the spot area can be filled with regions of typical fluorescence intensity. Some photo systems (e.g., the Olympus PM30) provide metering modes in which the contribution of the dark, nonfluorescent background is discounted, allowing for accurate exposure assessment based only on fluorescence intensity. Expensive automatic exposure systems, however, are not a necessity. Exposure times can be determined manually by exposing a test roll of film to determine an appropriate exposure range for a given type of specimen. For the rare and exceptional specimen, manual or automatic bracketing of exposure times is a useful approaching for making certain of bagging a good image.

3. Counterstaining for Color Photography

When preparing color photographs or slides, a useful, general counter-stain for fluorescein-labeled specimens is Evan's blue. Under the 490 nm excitation light used for fluorescein, Evan's blue fluoresces red, providing a good contrast to the yellow–green emission of fluorescein. For sectioned material, 5–10 min in 0.1% Evan's blue in distilled water, followed by several rinses in distilled water before mounting is adequate. For whole mounts staining time should be reduced to 1 min. It should be noted that over-staining with Evan's blue can mask some specific fluorescence, especially if the signal is weak.

Counterstaining eliminates the problem that unlabeled regions of the specimen are not normally visible under epifluorescence. Without counterstaining, accurate localization of the antigen requires superposition or comparison of a fluorescence image with a phase or bright field image of the same specimen. With counterstaining, the entire specimen is present in the fluorescence image. Additionally, DAPI, which provides a nice DNA stain, can also be used for orientation of a fluorescence image. Vector Laboratories (Burlingame, CA) sells an antifading, mounting medium that includes DAPI, making counterstaining very easy.

4. Scanning Film Originals to Produce Digital Images

One of the great advantages of digital imaging is the use of the "desktop darkroom," consisting of a computer, an image processing program, and an ink-jet printer, to produce high quality prints. Ready availability of dedicated film scanners with resolutions of about 4,000 pixels per inch now allows workers who use film to enjoy the convenience of digital image processing. Image processing software, such as Photoshop (Adobe, Systems, Inc., San Jose, CA) can be easily used to adjust image contrast and density, and to selectively "burn in" or "dodge" portions of a digitized image. All such adjustments can then be retained for future printing, by simply saving them as part of a new file. Such adjustments were previously approachable only by those with skill in making conventional, black-and-white prints, and then only on a print-by-print basis. Additionally, individually photographed fluorochrome images from a multiples-labeled specimen can be readily merged into a single image in the computer; this obviates the problems of different fluorescence intensities that can obscure detail when single photographs, incorporating all emission wavelengths, are taken using a multipass filter set. Use of digital image processing, as with techniques used for image enhancement in the conventional black-and-white darkroom, must be used with care, so that the information in a specimen is not altered by the creation of artifacts.

References

1. Osborn M, Weber K (1982) Immunofluorescence and immunocytochemical procedures with affinity purified antibodies: tubulin-containing structures. Methods Cell Biol 24:97–132
2. Slayter EM (1970) Optical methods in biology. Wiley, New York, NY
3. Song L, van Gijlswijk RP, Young IT, Tanke HJ (1997) Influence of fluorochrome labeling density on the photobleaching kinetics of fluorescein in microscopy. Cytometry 27:213–223
4. Langanger D, DeMay J, Adam H (1983) 1, 4-Diazobizyklo-[2.2.2.] oktan (DABCO) verzogest das Ausbleichen von immunofluorenzpreparaten. Mikroskopie 40:237–241
5. Johnson GD, Nogueira Araujo GM de C (1981) A simple method of reducing the fading of

immunofluorescence during microscopy. J Immunol Methods 43: 349–350.

6. Johnson GD, Davidson RS, McNamee KC, Russell G, Goodwin D, Holborow EJ (1982) Fading of immunofluorescence during microscopy: a study of the phenomenon and its remedy. J Immunol Methods 55:231–242
7. Giloh H, Sedat JW (1982) Fluorescence microscopy: reduced photobleaching of rhodamine and fluorescein protein conjugates by n-propyl gallate. Science 217:1252–1255
8. Bock G, Hilchenbach M, Schauenstein K, Wick G (1985) Photometric analysis of antifading reagents for immunofluorescence with laser and conventional illumination sources. J Histochem Cytochem 33:699–705
9. Bacallao R, Bomsel M, Stelzer EHK, DeMay J (1989) Guiding principles of specimen preservation for confocal fluorescence microscopy. In: Pawley JB (ed) Handbook of biological confocal microscopy. Plenum, New York, pp 197–205
10. Krenik KD, Kephart GM, Offord KP, Dunnette SL, Gleich GJ (1989) Comparison of antifading agents used in immunofluorescence. J Immunol Methods 117:91–97
11. Longin A, Souchier C, Ffrench M, Bryon PA (1993) Comparison of anti-fading agents used in fluorescence microscopy: image analysis and laser confocal microscopy study. J Histochem Cytochem 41:1833–1840
12. Florijn RJ, Slats J, Tanke HJ, Raap AK (1995) Analysis of antifading reagents for fluorescence microscopy. Cytometry 19:177–182
13. Takizawa T, Robinson JM (2000) Analysis of antiphotobleaching reagents for use with FluoroNanogold in correlative microscopy. J Histochem Cytochem 48:433–436

Chapter 21

Overview of Confocal Microscopy

William D. Swaim

Abstract

Born out of the need to overcome an imaging problem in the 1950s, confocal microscopes today allow researchers to go beyond simple imaging and ask biochemical questions. This chapter provides background information on the development of modern confocal microscopes, their uses and applications. Sample preparation and observation are also discussed. Information is also provided about more advanced applications such as FRAP, FRET and 2-photon imaging. The requirements for setting up a confocal laboratory and the instrumentation needs are also discussed.

Key words: Confocal microscopy, Sample preparation, DAPI, FRAP, FRET, 2-Photon imaging

1. Introduction

The confocal microscope has moved from an elitist tool to a laboratory fixture in the past 15 years. What was once only found in well funded laboratories can now be seen in most college and research laboratories. Born out of the need to overcome an imaging problem in the 1950s, the systems of today have improved to the extent of allowing researchers to go beyond simple imaging and ask biochemical questions (1, 2).

Marvin Minsky designed the first confocal microscope in the mid-1950s in an effort to map neural connections. Later, a rediscovery of his designs and equipment launched a revolution in the science of imaging. His designs are still the basis for confocal microscopy today (Fig. 1). Having a confocal pinhole, the microscope is very efficient at rejecting out of focus fluorescent light. The practical effect of this is that the image comes from a thin section of the sample, and by scanning many thin sections through the sample, a very sharp three-dimensional image of the sample

C. Oliver and M.C. Jamur (eds.), *Immunocytochemical Methods and Protocols*, Methods in Molecular Biology, Vol. 588,
DOI 10.1007/978-1-59745-324-0_21, © Humana Press, a part of Springer Science+Business Media, LLC 1995, 1999, 2010

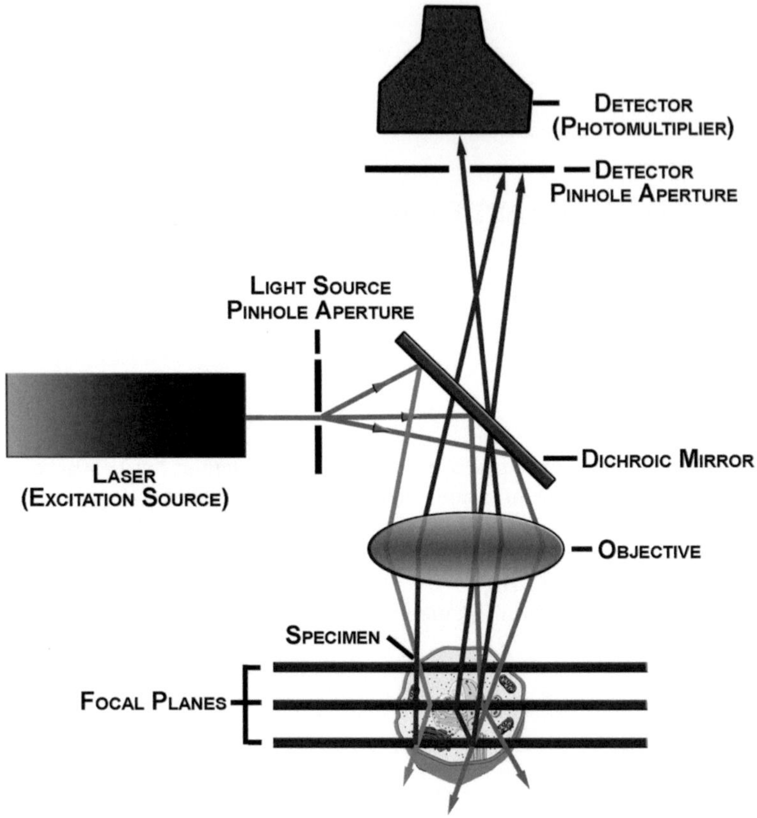

Fig. 1. Schematic diagram of a laser scanning confocal microscope.

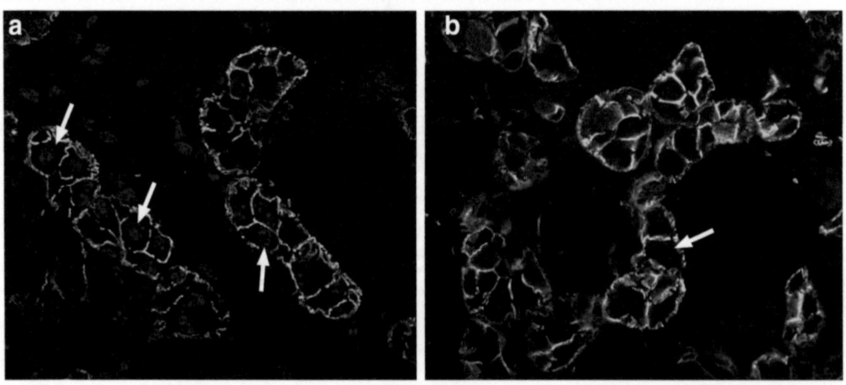

Fig. 2. Note in this comparison between a confocal image (**a**) and a standard fluorescence microscopy image (**b**), the increased sharpness of the confocal image. The plasma membranes and nuclei (*arrows*) of the individual cells are much easier to distinguish in the confocal image

can be built (Fig. 2). The modern confocal microscope, by allowing gigabytes of data, that are ready for analysis, to be available at your fingertips, the modern confocal microscope has greatly accelerated research involving imaging and morphometrics. Data acquisition and image analysis, once a laborious multistep process, has reaped the benefits of advances in desktop computer technology. In some cases today, the analysis can be performed during acquisition. In some software systems, wizards guide you through each step of the more advanced or specialized techniques and provide the analysis in raw data and report formats ready for presentation. While this seems fool-proof, it must be remembered that these systems are only as smart as the person sitting in front of the system.

2. Uses and Applications

Obviously, the first use of confocal microscopy is documentation of an experiment. Most facilities ask users to view their samples, if possible, on any of the available nonconfocal laser scanning fluorescent microscopes before using the system. If care is taken, this prescreening will not photobleach or damage the sample. However, prescreening can significantly eliminate wasting of time on assessing whether or not the sample is adequately prepared for analysis with the confocal microscope.

2.1. Sample Preparation

Preparation of samples for confocal imaging is one of the basic steps that can either make or break an experiment for imaging. The rule "Garbage In/Garbage Out" applies particularly well to imaging. For all the cost and technical advances that have gone into current confocal systems, there is one thing they cannot do: Make a bad sample look better! Failure at any step in the processing regimen negatively affects all subsequent steps. The images will only be as good as the WORST processing step!

2.1.1. Coverslips and Dishes

For fluorescence microscopy, 0.17 mm thick coverslips (#1½) are optimal. Round coverslips (12 mm diameter) will fit inside a 24-well plate, limiting the use of costly reagents. Although the fit is tight, with practice, one can easily master removing the coverslips without breaking them. When necessary, 35 mm diameter dishes with coverglass bottoms are an alternative. These dishes have the added benefit of allowing for live cell imaging with either an upright scope, using a dipping lens, or more commonly, an inverted microscope.

2.1.2. Fixation and processing

When it comes to fixation, less is more. Best results are obtained if one tries to just-adequately fix the sample to minimize problems in antibody binding (*see* Chapter 8). Typically, 2–4% formaldehyde is sufficient. In cases of aldehyde incompatibility with the antibody, ice cold methanol is an alternative. When using aldehydes, one must make sure that the fixative is freshly prepared (both working dilution and stock solutions) and that the osmolarity of all the fixative solutions is taken into account. Just enough for each experiment should be prepared so as not to carry over working dilutions from one experiment to the next. Samples may be immunolabeled using standard fluorescent immunolabeling methods (*see* Chapters 15–20). As in all immunolableling procedures, antibody solutions should be filtered (0.22 μm dia. filter) or centrifuged before use to remove any aggregates, and care must be taken to avoid specimen drying.

2.1.3. Mounting Medium

The mounting medium used for fluorescence, especially confocal microscopy can have a major impact on the success of the imaging. Fading is a major problem with this type of microscopy (3). The use of an antifade mounting medium is a critical part of specimen preparation. However, there are many excellent antifade mounting mediums commercially available and recipes exist for homemade mounting medium. There are incompatibility issues with some mounting media and certain types of fluorophores. For example, exposure to alcohol will cause GFP not to fluoresce When in doubt, ask the support personnel at the source of the fluorophore should be consulted. If an aqueous mounting medium is being used, it is advisable to seal the coverslip to the slide. Nail polish is probably the most commonly used sealant. However, colored nail polish should be avoided as the pigment in the polish is usually fluorescent. It is also advisable to use a nail polish that is labeled formaldehyde-free and usually sold as antiallergic. The formaldehyde, even in clear nail polish, may give a background fluorescence. Nail polish usually contains isopropyl alcohol as a solvent, and as mentioned above, that may interfere with some fluorophores. An alternative to nail polish is the use of a permanent mounting medium, diluted in an appropriate solvent such as xylene or toluene.

2.1.4. DAPI

Some mounting media come with DAPI or propidium iodide to label nuclei. As it is generally a good idea to have some sort of landmark in the image for the researcher to orient himself, DAPI is a great dye to use… except when the signal of interest happens to be nuclear. In this case, the DAPI signal MAY subdue the fluorophore one is trying to image or localize. The other issue with DAPI is that it has an extremely broad emission curve. This curve overlaps (think crosstalk) and bleeds into other channels (FITC, Alexa Fluor 488, and even as far as Texas Red). Other alternatives for nuclear labeling include Hoechst dye, the cell-impermeant TOTO, TO-PRO and SYTOX families of dyes and the cell-permeant SYTO family of dyes. Propidium iodide can also be used, but it unfortunately gives a broad emission peak in the red range, thus eliminating most red fluorescent fluorophores as choices for imaging. While trying to capture images simultaneously using both DAPI and FITC, we see that the UV lines that are being used to excite DAPI are also exciting FITC! If DAPI and FITC need to be imaged, then sequential imaging could be considered.

2.2. Sample Imaging Conditions

2.2.1. Environmental Chambers

Commercial or custom built environmental chambers are available to fit most microscopes. One custom built environmental chamber consists of a box of opaque dark plastic, with front and side ports for access to the objectives and for inserting the sample, mounted on a galvonometric stage. It is equipped with a port for CO_2 and heat, and provides a constant 5% CO_2 and a constant temperature environment. This allows for imaging times from minutes to hours with little change to the specimen.

2.2.2. Controls

Controls are absolute requirements for any procedure. Negative controls, i.e., no primary or secondary antibody or no primary antibody, allow the user to set the parameters to a baseline level. Any signal above this baseline is generally the signal of interest. When making single images from a sample, it is important to include a negative control first. This allows the user to set parameters that scale the intensity to between 0 and 255. By using a negative control, it is easy to avoid both oversaturation and undersaturation of the signal. When viewing the negative control laser power, AOTF (Acousto-optic tunable filter), gain, and offset controls should be adjusted to allow for detection on the lower end of the 0–255 scale. By setting the laser power and the AOTF at low and adjusting the gain higher one can minimize photobleaching of the sample. The settings in areas of the sample similar to those that will be imaged in the experimental samples must be focussed and adjusted. This will eliminate differences in the levels of autofluorescence. The control sample should be documented and the parameter settings saved. Parameter settings should not be changed for the remainder of the experiment, especially if samples under different treatments or conditions are being compared. If signal intensities and/or localizations are being compared, these settings must remain unchanged from the control slide.

2.2.3. Series and Stacks

When collecting a stack or series through the *z* axis (or top to bottom of the sample), the beginning and end points should be set accurately to cover the entire range of the area of interest. In most cases, this would be throughout the full thickness of the cells or tissues. But if one is only interested in a smaller subset of the sample, the top and bottom should be adjusted to include only the area of interest. There is nothing worse than to spend time in preparation only to cut off a region of the cell that makes the image complete. Also, it is advisable to start the stack just above the surface of the coverslip or slide. This will eliminate including labeled antibody that has nonspecifically bound to the substrate surface. With single photon imaging, the sample is bleached through the full thickness of the sample beneath the objective. Dwell time of the laser on the sample can cause bleaching of the fluorophores in the later sections of a series. Dwell time should be limited, especially during continuous scans while setting up the parameters for acquisition. Also, it should be borne in mind that Hg lamps will also fade signals. The area of the sample to be imaged should be found quickly and the light path blocked as soon as possible. Factors that affect the speed of imaging include format (512 × 512, 1,024 × 1,024, etc.), speed (200 Hz, 400 Hz, 1,000 Hz), averaging (2, 3, 4 … n), and the number of sections taken in the series. Again, the dummy-proof systems currently in use will help one determine not only the detector pinhole size to use, but also the number of optical sections to take for an "optimized" image. The user is the ultimate judge for these settings. In some cases, it is necessary to oversample in the axial plane. The imaging needs to determine this. If the image series is being reconstructed to be viewed laterally, it should be remembered that the axial direction is more ovoid than spherical and will appear "stretched" when viewed.

2.2.4. Timecourse Studies

Imaging studies performed for longer than a few minutes must be done under controlled conditions for temperature, CO_2, and humidity. Most cells grown at 37°C in 5% CO_2 and high humidity begin to change shape within minutes of being removed from this environment. If one is looking to localize or colocalize molecules within or on cells that are changing shape because of environmental changes, the analysis and results may be questionable at best. Shape changes may alter the results of a z-series or even shift the true top and bottom positions of a cell's basal or apical limits, resulting in only a partial series through the cell. Temperature control can be done either at the slide/dish level with a heating plate, by perfusing the system with the media at the required temperature, or by forced-air systems that heat the entire chamber. Each system has its advantages and disadvantages. In all of these, temperature gradients can exist, so that cells may actually be cooler than they are thought to be. Some researchers use objective heaters in order to minimize heat loss and dedicate these objectives to live; temperature-dependent imaging (constant heating/cooling with its concomitant expansion and contraction) takes a toll on objectives. Perfusion systems may cause movement as a result of the flow from inlet to outlet in the system, thereby causing the cells to shift. If the flow rate is too high, the cells can be seen moving in and out of focus in a pulsatile pattern with the pump. In these cases, hydrostatic systems may be a better choice. In the case of forced-air systems, dehydration is a constant battle to be fought.

2.3. Fluorescence Recovery After Photobleaching (FRAP)

FRAP has been used for more than 30 years to examine the mobility of lipids and proteins in cellular membranes (4–8). Today this method is being applied to virtually every cell compartment (5, 9–15). With FRAP, an attenuated laser beam is focused on a small area of a membrane that is uniformly labeled with a fluorescent lipid or protein, and the fluorescence intensity is monitored as a function of time. After a predetermined time, a small area is photobleached for a fraction of a second by a high intensity beam. This bleaching pulse reduces the fluorescence intensity of the bleached area. The bleached area subsequently recovers by the diffusion of unbleached molecules from the surrounding, unilluminated area. The mobile fraction or percentage recovery is determined by comparing the fluorescence intensity measured after bleaching with the intensity prior to bleaching. This calculation gives an indication of whether the molecule of interest is free to diffuse in the membrane or is bound and not able to do so (Fig. 3).

Although FRAP is a rather straightforward technique, care must be taken in the selection of the fluorophore. The fluorescent probe must be easily bleachable in a short period of time and at a laser intensity that will not damage or kill the cells of interest.

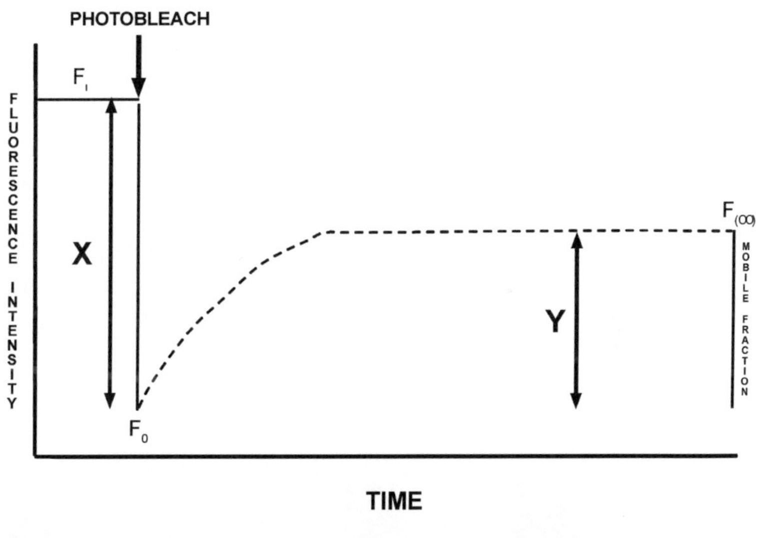

Fig. 3. Graph depicting data collected during a FRAP experiment. The initial fluorescence (F_i) of the sample is recorded before photobleaching (*arrow*). After photobleaching the amount of fluorescence is reduced significantly (F_0). Over time, the amount of fluorescence in the photobleached area increases as unbleached molecules diffuse into this area until there is a stabilization of the amount of fluorescence recovery and a plateau (F_{00}) is reached. The percent recovery can be calculated as follows: $(Y/X) \times 100 = \%$ recovery. In the diagram, the amount fluorescence lost because of photobleaching is X, and the amount of fluorescence that returned to the bleached area is Y. The percent recovery almost never reaches 100%. The slope of the curve shows the lateral mobility of the molecule of interest. The steeper the curve, the faster is the recovery indicating that the molecules are more mobile.

The most widely used probes today are green fluorescent protein and related fluorescent proteins. Antibodies conjugated to FITC or other easily bleached fluorophores may also be used. It is also important that the measurements be done under conditions ideal for the cell type studied. The use of an environmental chamber is recommended.

2.4. Fluorescence Resonance Energy Transfer (FRET)

Fluorescence Resonance Energy Transfer is not a new technique, but one that has seen a recent resurgence (16–19). First theorized by Förster (20), FRET gives relative information about the distance between molecules. Hence, Stryer (21) called it a "molecular ruler".It is a distance-dependent technique – useful between 10 and 100 Å. It is also orientation-dependent. Because of the dipole–dipole interaction, each molecule acts as a dipole antenna, capable of transferring energy (22, 23). It requires both a Donor and an Acceptor. The Donor must be fluorescent, but the Acceptor, while usually fluorescent, is not necessarily required to be so. The Donor and the Acceptor must be between 10 and 100 Å from each other. They must also be in the correct orientation for energy transfer. FRET and its orientation and proximity requirements could be considered to be like a handshake between two people – too close (i.e., nose-to-nose) and the handshake is improbable. If the two people are across the room from each other, the handshake is impossible. If the two people are within reach of each other, but one has his back turned to the other, again the handshake is impossible. Only when the two people are within reach of each other and facing one another (orientation dependence), is the handshake possible. The other requirement for FRET is that both parties should be willing to shake the hands with each other hand. Much in the same way, one molecule must be an acceptor of the donor. If any of these conditions are not met, FRET is unlikely (Fig. 4).

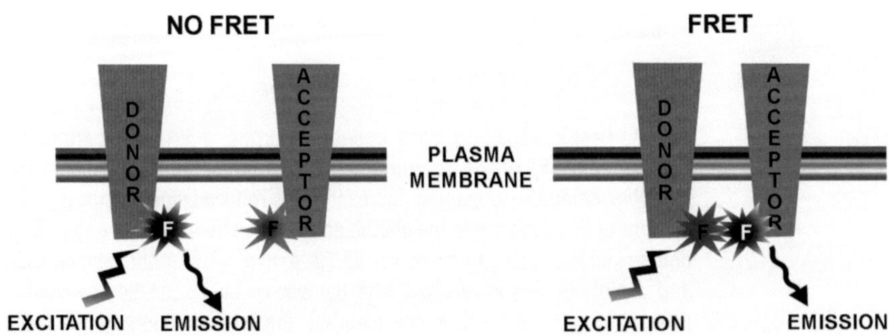

Fig. 4. An example of FRET between two different membrane associated molecules is shown. In the first example, the molecules are too far apart for any energy transfer to occur. Therefore there is no FRET. In the second example the molecules are in close proximity and when the fluorophore (F) on the donor molecule is excited, energy is transferred to the fluorophore on the acceptor molecule and the fluorescence characteristic of the second fluorophore is observed.

What happens during FRET? A fluorescent Donor molecule transfers nonradiative energy to an acceptor molecule via a dipole–dipole interaction. Upon transfer of energy, there is a concomitant decrease in the intensity and lifetime of the Donor emission. If there is a fluorescent Acceptor, the emission intensity of the Acceptor will increase via this transfer of energy from the Donor.

$$E = \frac{k_{ET}}{K_f + k_{et} + \sum_{ki}}$$

FRET Efficiency

The FRET efficiency (E) is the quantum yield of the energy transfer transition or the fraction of energy transfer event occurring per donor excitation event where k_{ET} is the rate of energy transfer, k_f the radiative decay rate, and the k_i are the rate constants of any other de-excitation pathway.

The FRET efficiency depends on various parameters such as the distance between the donor and the acceptor, the spectral overlap of the donor emission spectrum and the acceptor absorption spectrum as well as the relative orientation of the donor emission dipole moment and the acceptor absorption dipole moment. The efficiency of the energy transfer process varies in proportion to the inverse sixth power of the distance separating the donor and acceptor molecules. Therefore, FRET measurements can be utilized as molecular ruler to determine the distances between molecules labeled with an appropriate Donor and Acceptor fluorochrome if they are within 10 nm of each other.

What are the requirements for FRET imaging? The first and foremost requirement is an imaging system capable of exciting and detecting the two overlapping fluorescent probes (Table 1). There are a number of fluorescent combinations that are usable, some better than others (24, 25). FITC and TRITC were used originally as FRET pairs. The Cy dyes have been used as FRET pairs (Cy2-Cy3 or Cy3-Cy5). The Alexa Fluor Dyes can also act as FRET pairs (Alexa Fluor 488 – Alexa Fluor 546). More recently, Quantum Dots® (Invitrogen, Molecular Probes) have proven to be useful in FRET analysis (26). Fluorescent Proteins such as CFP-YFP, GFP-YFP and GFP-mRFP also act as FRET pairs (27). We use CFP-YFP as a FRET donor–acceptor pair in most live FRET imaging studies.

FRET may also be used to monitor protein conformational changes. In this case the target protein is labeled with a Donor and an Acceptor at two different loci. When a conformational change in the protein changes the distance or relative orientation of the Donor and the Acceptor, a FRET change is observed. FRET may also be used to investigate receptor–ligand binding by investigating the ligand-dependent conformational changes in the receptor following ligand binding.

Table 1
Donor–acceptor pairs for FRET

Laser	Donor	Acceptor	Donor Ex Acceptor Em
Violet	Alexa Fluor 405	Alexa Fluor 430	405/541
Violet	CFP	YFP	405/526
Violet	Cerulean FP	YFP	405/526
Argon	Cy2	Cy3	488/566
Argon	Cy3	Cy5	488/666
Argon	FITC	TRITC	488/577
Argon	PE	APC	488/660
Argon	Alexa Fluor 488	Alexa Fluor 514	488/541
Argon	Alexa Fluor 488	Alexa Fluor 532	488/553
Argon	Alexa Fluor 488	Alexa Fluor 546	488/572
Argon	Alexa Fluor 488	Alexa Fluor 610	488/626
Argon	GFP	YFP	488/526
Argon	GFP	mRFP	488/579
R-HeNe	Alexa Fluor 647	Alexa Fluor 680	633/700
R-HeNe	Alexa Fluor 647	Alexa Fluor 700	633/720
R-HeNe	Alexa Fluor 647	Alexa Fluor 750	633/780

We use two methods for measuring FRET. The first is the acceptor photobleaching method. In this method, the Donor emission is measured before and after the photobleaching of the Acceptor. After Acceptor photobleaching, the acceptor is incapable of receiving energy transferred from the Donor. In that case, the donor emission is increased. The inherent problem associated with sensitized emission is the crosstalk between channels. Therefore, images of donor-only and acceptor-only must be included in order to correct for bleed through from the Donor and Acceptor, both of which will impact on the FRET measurement. In the case of Acceptor photobleaching, measurement of the intensity and lifetime of the donor emission must also be made.

The second method for measuring FRET involves time-resolved fluorescence measurements. This method provides a way of obtaining average lifetimes without a precise knowledge of donor concentrations. The technique enables the quantitative determination of donor–acceptor separation distances, and is based on the measurements of the donor lifetime in the presence and absence of the acceptor. Measuring fluorescence intensity decay as a function of time elucidates the emission dynamics of the excited-state molecule, and consequently, more detailed information about the nature of the donor–acceptor interaction may be obtained. Fluorescence lifetime is based on the differences in the exponential decay rate of the fluorescence from a fluorescent sample. The primary advantage of time-resolved FRET in comparison to steady state FRET measurements is that Donor–Acceptor separation distances can be mapped with greater accuracy. This is due in part to the fact that fluorescent lifetimes do not depend upon local intensity or concentration. Fluorescent lifetimes are also largely unaffected by photobleaching. They are, however, highly sensitive to fluorophore environment, and even molecules with similar spectra may display distinct lifetimes under different conditions.

2.5. Two-Photon Imaging

Two-photon microscopy (also referred to as non-linear, multiphoton, or two-photon laser scanning microscopy) is an alternative to laser scanning confocal microscopy. Two-photon microscopy provides distinct advantages for three-dimensional imaging of living cells, especially within intact tissues such as brain slices, embryos, whole organs, and even whole animals, and in intravital microscopy Two-photon fluorescence microscopy was developed by Winfried Denk (28) in the laboratory of Watt W. Webb at Cornell University based on a concept first described by Maria Göppert-Mayer (29), and later patented by Winfried Denk, James Strickler and Watt Webb. In two-photon microscopy, a long wavelength excitation source is used so that the energy of a single excitation photon is not sufficient to excite a fluorescent molecule, but the combined energy of two excitation photons is. That is, two photons of low energy can excite a fluorophore in a quantum event, resulting in the emission of a fluorescence photon, usually at a higher energy than either of the two excitatory photons (Fig. 5). The probability that there will

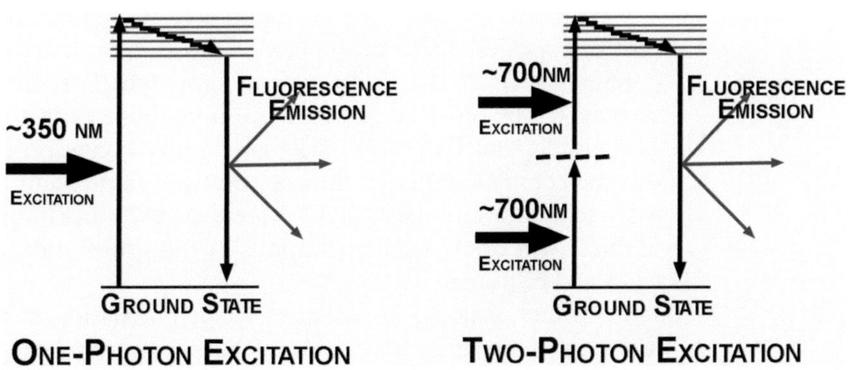

Fig. 5. In one photon excitation, a short wave length excitation, source is used so that the fluorophore is excited by a single photon. In two-photon excitation, a long wavelength excitation source is used and the energy of a single excitation photon is not sufficient to excite the fluorophore; but the combined energy of two excitation photons is capable of exciting the fluorophore.

be near-simultaneous absorption of two photons is extremely low, and a high flux of excitation photons is required. Therefore, a femtosecond laser, most commonly a Ti:Sapphire laser that emits IR light with a wavelength range from 700 to 1,000 nm in 100 fs pulses, is generally used. Because two photons must be absorbed in order to excite a fluorophore, the probability of fluorescent emission from the fluorophores increases quadratically with the excitation intensity. Much more two-photon fluorescence is generated where the laser beam is tightly focused than where it is diffuse. Two-photon imaging thus allows the user to excite only at the plane of focus, thereby limiting photobleaching to the focal plane and reducing tissue damage. Deeper penetration of the excitation wavelength into the sample with reduced light scattering can be accomplished with two-photon imaging than with single photon imaging. More extended live-cell imaging studies are also possible with two-photon imaging because of reduced phototoxicity and photobleaching (30).

3. Laboratory Requirements and Instrumentation Needs

Much of the time, fluorescence imaging is plagued by haze and light scattering. Even in single-cell imaging, these problems can appear and degrade imaging and subsequent analysis. In order to limit acquisition to mainly in-focus information, Minsky placed a pinhole in front of the detector. Pinholes today are generally adjustable to allow the user to choose the desired size. The basic requirements for confocal imaging are a microscope, a detector with pinhole, and an illumination source. Some laboratories have a particular need for upright or inverted platforms, while most core facilities plan for the need of either of the two microscopes and have both available, with the ability to switch from one to the other.

The choice of lasers for excitation is largely based on the current or expected needs of the laboratory. Although it is easier to configure a system with all the possibilities when ordering, some systems can be retro-fitted with add-on modules, postinstallation. UV, visible, and IR (or near-IR) lasers offer excitation throughout the complete range of fluorophores and fluorescent proteins. UV excitation is used for DAPI more than any other fluorophore. HeNe lasers offer excellent options in the green and red range (543 and 633 nm).

Another major consideration when purchasing a system is service and service contracts. Good, fair, or poor service can make or break a laboratory. The points to consider include (1) the availability of a dedicated service engineer in the area/region, (2) the average down time for the system of choice, (3) the company's policy when calling in a service request, (4) the terms of the service contract, (5) the services covered and those not covered with the contract, (6) the company's expectation of the laboratory's role in the troubleshooting, maintenance, and minor repair and (7)coverage for/need for all components third-party sources for certain parts (lasers, microscope, chillers/heat exchangers)?

Room design is a necessary forethought when considering buying a system. Will the system be installed in a dedicated space, or will it be a curtained-off area of the general lab space? Will the system fit into the space available for it? Certain systems have installation constraints. Some systems are required (because of the components themselves) to be installed in a linear or an L-shape with length requirements. This does not permit the system to be installed piece-meal into a small closet or room. Adequate space must also be afforded for access by service personnel as well as building maintenance. Is there a fire sprinkler directly above the most electronically sensitive parts of the system, or can it be relocated elsewhere? Where will the user(s) sit? Is it convenient to move from the computer desk to the microscope to the laser control? Does the room have adequate cooling and ventilation? Will the heat exchangers/chillers be located outside the room to limit noise, airflow, and heat production? Room lighting is also a consideration. Rheostat-controlled incandesent lighting is a good addition to the room to limit fluorophore bleaching as long as there is no direct illumination of the microscope area. Some components require an air table to limit building vibration. The building air should be adequate to lift the slab or an air compressor may be necessary. Are there potential water leaks in the room selected for installation? Will this affect the area where the components will be placed? Are the leaks frequent? These are important aspects to be considered. Access to the confocal microscope is critical for multiuser facilities. An electronic entrance will provide security and convenience. Every trained user and service personnel should have his/her own PIN to use to gain access into the room. Only after successful training should users receive their PIN. The entry history can be downloaded to determine who entered the room last, in case there is a problem.

Training may be done on an as-needed basis with the maximum number of trainees limited to four, because of time and room constraints. A training session for four people should be of about 2 days duration. This will give each potential user adequate hands-on experience in all aspects of use under supervision prior to unlimited access. Usage can be controlled through an on-line calendar. E-mail requests can be sent to the facility manager via a web page sign up system. Only trained users should have access to solo appointment requests. Individuals who are not trained must schedule use with the facility manager. E-mail requests should be time-stamped and added to the calendar by the facility manager on receipt.

No one should be allowed to simply show up to use the system. This will afford the further advantage of making usage tracking easier to when it is time for annual or semi-annual reports (oversight committees, funding requests, etc).

References

1. Pawley JB (ed) (2006) Handbook of biological confocal microscopy. Springer Science + Business Media, LLC, New York
2. Hibbs AR (2004) Confocal microscopy for biologists. Springer Science + Business Media, Inc, New York
3. Ono M, Murakami T, Kudo A, Isshiki M, Sawada H, Segawa A (2001) Quantitative comparison of anti-fading mounting media for confocal laser scanning microscopy. J Histochem Cytochem 49:305–311
4. Axelrod D, Koppel DE, Schlessinger J, Elson E, Webb WW (1976) Mobility measurement by analysis of fluorescence photobleaching recovery kinetics. Biophys J 16:1055–1089
5. Chen Y, Lagerholm BC, Yang B, Jacobson K (2006) Methods to measure the lateral diffusion of membrane lipids and proteins. Methods 39:147–153
6. Edidin M, Zagyansky Y, Lardner TJ (1976) Measurement of membrane protein lateral diffusion in single cells. Science 191:466–468
7. Jacobson K, Dersko Z, Wu ES, Hou Y, Poste G (1976) Measurement of the lateral mobility of cell surface components in single living cells by fluorescence recovery after photobleaching. J Supramol Struct 5:565–576
8. Peters RJ, Peters J, Tews KH, Bahr W (1974) A microfluorimetric study of translational diffusion in erythrocyte membrane. Biochim Biophys Acta 367:282–294
9. Henis YI, Rotblat B, Kloog Y (2006) FRAP beam-size analysis to measure palmitoylation-dependent membrane association dynamics and microdomain partitioning of Ras proteins. Methods 40:183–190
10. Hernandez-Verdun D (2006) Nucleolus: from structure to dynamics. Histochem Cell Biol 125:127–137
11. Howell BJ, Hoffman DB, Fang G, Murray AW, Salmon ED (2000) Visualization of Mad2 dynamics at kinetochores, along spindle fibers, and at spindle poles in living cells. J Cell Biol 150:1233–1250
12. Houtsmuller AB (2005) Fluorescence recovery after photobleaching: application to nuclear proteins. Adv Biochem Eng Biotechnol 95:177–199
13. Kenworthy AK (2006) Fluorescence-based methods to image palmitoylated proteins. Methods 40:198–205
14. Kimura H (2005) Histone dynamics in living cells revealed by photobleaching. DNA Repair 4:939–950
15. Lele TP, Thodeti CK, Ingber DE (2006) Force meets chemistry: analysis of mechanochemical conversion in focal adhesions using fluorescence recovery after photobleaching. J Cell Biochem 97:1175–1183
16. Jares-Erijman EA, Jovin TM (2006) Imaging molecular interactions in living cells by FRET microscopy. Curr Opin Chem Biol 10: 409–416
17. Piston DW, Kremers GJ (2007) Fluorescent protein FRET: the good, the bad and the ugly. Trends Biochem Sci 32:407–414
18. Schmid JA, Birbach A (2007) Fluorescent proteins and fluorescence resonance energy transfer (FRET) as tools in signaling research. Thromb Haemost 97:378–384
19. Vogel SS, Thaler C, Koushik SV (2006) Fanciful FRET. Sci STKE 331:re2.
20. Förster T (1948) Intermolecular energy migration and fluorescence. Annalen der Physik (Leipzig) 2:55–75
21. Stryer L (1978) Fluorescence energy transfer as a spectroscopic ruler. Ann Rev Biochem 47:819–846
22. Selvin PR (1995) Fluorescence resonance energy transfer. Meth Enzymol 246:300–334
23. Selvin PR (2000) The renaissance of fluorescence resonance energy transfer. Nature Struct Biol 7:730–734
24. Chapman S, Oparka KJ, Roberts AG (2005) New tools for in vivo fluorescence tagging. Curr Opin Plant Biol 8:565–573
25. Sapsford KE, Berti L, Medintz IL (2006) Materials for fluorescence resonance energy transfer analysis: beyond traditional donor–acceptor combinations. Angew Chem Int Ed Engl 45:4562–4589
26. Clapp AR, Medintz IL, Mattoussi H (2006) Förster resonance energy transfer investigations using quantum-dot fluorophores. Chemphyschem 7:47–57

27. Takanishi CL, Bykova EA, Cheng W, Zheng J (2006) GFP-based FRET analysis in live cells. Brain Res 1091:132–139

28. Denk W, Strickler J, Webb W (1990) Two-photon laser scanning fluorescence microscopy. Science 248:73–76

29. Göppert-Mayer M (1931) Über Elementarakte mit zwei Quantensprüngen. Ann Phys 9:273–295

30. Helmchen F, Denk W (2005) Deep tissue two-photon microscopy. Nat Methods 2:932–940

Chapter 22

Overview of Laser Microbeam Applications as Related to Antibody Targeting

P. Scott Pine

Abstract

This chapter reviews several techniques which combine the use of laser microbeams with antibodies to study molecular and cellular biology. An overview of the basic properties of lasers and their integration with microscopes and computers is provided. Biophysical applications, such as fluorescence recovery after photobleaching to measure molecular mobility and fluorescence resonance energy transfer to measure molecular distances, as well as ablative applications for the selective inactivation of proteins or the selective killing of cells are described. Other techniques, such as optical trapping, that do not rely on the interaction of the laser with the targeting antibody, are also discussed.

Key words: Laser, Microbeam, Antibody, Fluorescence, FRAP, FRET, Ablation, Photobleaching

1. Introduction

Laser-based microscopic systems (laser microbeams) are becoming popular tools for investigating various aspects of molecular and cellular biology (1). Depending on the wavelength, energy and beam geometry employed, laser microbeams can be used for fluorescence excitation, microsurgery, cellular ablation, or micromanipulation of cells and organelles. The use of antibodies permits the targeting of specific antigens or cell types for analysis or treatment. Integrating a laser, microscope, and detection system (camera or photomultiplier tube) with a personal computer creates a workstation capable of controlling data acquisition parameters and performing subsequent data analysis. An example of one such workstation is shown in Fig. 1.

Several properties of lasers make them an ideal source of photons. For example, laser light is monochromatic, available in wavelengths ranging from the UV to the infrared depending on

C. Oliver and M.C. Jamur (eds.), *Immunocytochemical Methods and Protocols*, Methods in Molecular Biology, Vol. 588, DOI 10.1007/978-1-59745-324-0_22, © Humana Press, a part of Springer Science+Business Media, LLC 1995, 1999, 2010

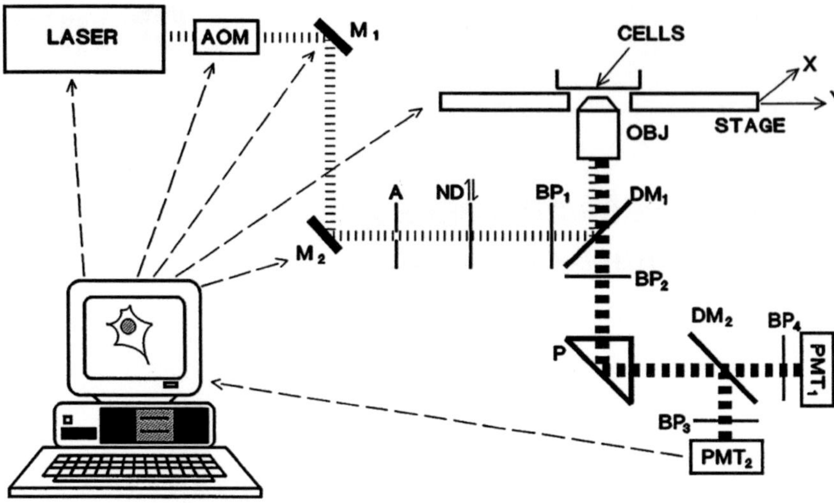

Fig. 1. Schematic diagram of the epi-illumination optical path in the inverted microscope and the computer input and output used to control laser excitation and fluorescence emission detection. The output wavelength is determined by the type of laser. The intensity of the laser output can be controlled by varying the current to the laser, varying the frequency of an acousto-optic modulator (AOM) and selecting the modulated beam with an aperture (A), and/or placing neutral density filters (ND) in the optical path. Fluorescence excitation and emission detection can be achieved using the combination of filters (excitation bandpass (BP_1), dichroic mirror (DM_1), and emission bandpass (BP_2)) found in the conventional filter cubes available for fluorescence microscopes. The emission's signal is passed to a photomultiplier housing by a prism (P) that distributes the light to the eyepiece lenses (not shown) and accessory ports. Dual emission signals can be monitored by two photomultiplier tubes (PMT_1 and PMT_2) using a combination of bandpass filters (BP_3 and BP_4) and a dichroic mirror (DM_2). The computer can generate two-dimensional images by correlating the PMT signal with the *x*, *y* coordinates of the cell relative to the laser beam. This can be achieved by changing the sample position relative to a fixed laser beam using a motorized stage or by changing the position of the spot illuminated by the laser beam using a combination of galvanometric mirrors (M_1 and M_2).

the medium stimulated to emit light. It has directionality. For all practical purposes, the light emitted by a laser can be considered parallel, making it possible to achieve microscopically focused spot sizes with diameters on the order of one wavelength of light ($\approx 0.5\ \mu m$ for lasers emitting in the visible region of the spectrum). Laser light maintains its brightness. The wave fronts of laser light are in phase, a phenomenon known as coherence, and they do not destructively interfere with each other. This property allows the beam to retain its intensity over greater distances than the light produced by conventional thermal sources.

The laser beam can be directed along one of several optical paths available in either the upright or inverted microscope configurations. For fluorescence applications, it is often convenient to make use of the standard epi-illumination pathway by simply replacing the arc lamp with a laser.

However, some systems use the accessory camera ports, which are usually used for collecting the emitted light. In this case, the laser beam is directed back toward the objective in order to achieve epi-illumination. For applications such as microsurgery or optical trapping, even the transillumination pathway can be used. Precise positioning of the microbeam can be achieved with a combination of mirrors (for the *x–y*, specimen plane) and lenses (for *z*-axis, focal-point distance).

The following discussion provides an overview of several applications selected for their use of (or potential use of) antibodies in combination with a laser microbeam to investigate some aspect of molecular or cellular biology.

2. Biophysical Applications

2.1. Introduction

Laser microbeams offer several advantages over other fluorescence excitation techniques. In spectrofluorometry, observations are often made on a population of cells in a cuvette, resulting in a combined signal that lacks information about individual cellular responses. In flow cytometry, many individual cells are measured, but there is no temporal resolution as each cell is observed only once, and there is no spatial resolution because the entire cell is illuminated as it passes through the laser beam (*see* Chapter 31). In conventional fluorescence microscopy, individual cells can be monitored over time, and information about the two-dimensional spatial distribution of fluorescence can be obtained. However, some samples may be more susceptible to photobleaching by the arc lamps used for excitation, and the temporal resolution may be limited to video-rate data acquisition (30 frames/s) (*see* Chapter 15).

Fluorescence excitation with a laser microbeam allows for a smaller region to be illuminated. Monitoring fluorescence with a sensitive photomultiplier tube also permits the use of lower intensities of irradiation for shorter periods of time. Therefore, unwanted photobleaching can be significantly reduced. If the spot size is adjusted to illuminate an entire cell, information analogous to spectrofluorometry or flow cytometry can be obtained on an individual cell basis with a high degree of temporal resolution. If the spot size is smaller than the cell, similar information can be obtained from a particular location within the cell.

By varying the location of the laser spot in the *x–y* plane using galvanometric mirrors for positioning (laser scanning) or moving the specimen relative to a fixed laser beam (stage scanning), a two-dimensional array of data points can be generated. This produces an image with a spatial resolution corresponding to the spot size. Laser scanning has the advantage of collecting two-dimensional images at up to video rates, whereas stage scanning permits areas larger than the objective's field of view to be imaged. In addition, laser microbeams provide a point source of illumination with sufficient intensity for use in confocal microscopy, which allows for the construction of three-dimensional images by optical sectioning along the *z*-axis (*see* Chapter 21).

2.2. Epitope-to-Epitope Distance Measurements

Fluorescence resonance energy transfer (FRET) is a technique that has been used to measure distances between pairs of proximal fluorochromes. A suitable pair consists of a donor fluorochrome, which has an emission spectrum that significantly overlaps with the absorption spectrum of an acceptor fluorochrome (2). With the availability of monoclonal antibodies to many cell-surface determinants, intramolecular distances between nearby epitopes and intermolecular distances between adjacent cell-surface macromolecules can be investigated to analyze molecular interactions influencing important cellular events. Such monoclonal antibodies can be conjugated to fluorescein-isothiocyanate (FITC) as the donor, and either tetramethyl-rhodamine-isothiocyanate (TRITC) or phycoerythrin (PE) as the acceptor.

Two important factors determine the efficiency with which energy is transferred from the donor to the acceptor: the extent of spectral overlap and the distance that separates the donor–acceptor pair (Fig. 2a). The spectral overlap for any particular pair (e.g., FITC-TRITC or FITC-PE) is constant. However, the rate of energy transfer is extremely sensitive to changes in distance because it is inversely proportional to the sixth power of the distance separating the two fluorochromes. By using the same donor–acceptor pair, FRET is useful for studying relative changes in either molecular conformation or intermolecular interactions.

The energy-transfer efficiency can be measured in several ways. In the absence of an energy acceptor, a donor fluorochrome in the excited state will return to the ground state with energy being lost in the form of emitted photons (i.e., fluorescence). However, if a suitable acceptor fluorochrome is nearby, the energy will be transferred in a nonradiative manner, and the fluorescence intensity of the donor will be reduced (i.e., quenched) (Fig. 2b). In addition, the acceptor fluorochrome will become excited, resulting in the emission of fluorescence with the characteristic spectrum of the acceptor. By measuring the fluorescence intensities of the donor fluorochrome (both quenched and unquenched) and the acceptor fluorochrome (both enhanced and nonenhanced), determinations of energy-transfer efficiencies have been made using spectrofluorometry (3), flow cytometry (4), and fluorescence microscopy (5).

In the microscopic technique, photobleaching FRET (5), the intensity of fluorescence excitation is increased to cause photobleaching of the donor fluorochrome, and the decay kinetics are measured in the absence or presence of an acceptor fluorochrome. If the acceptor is in close proximity to the donor, then the availability of excited-state donors for photobleaching is reduced, thus making the photobleaching process slower.

The photobleaching method has been adapted for use with a laser microbeam system (6). The advantage of this system is that it allows for the selection of individual cells to be analyzed.

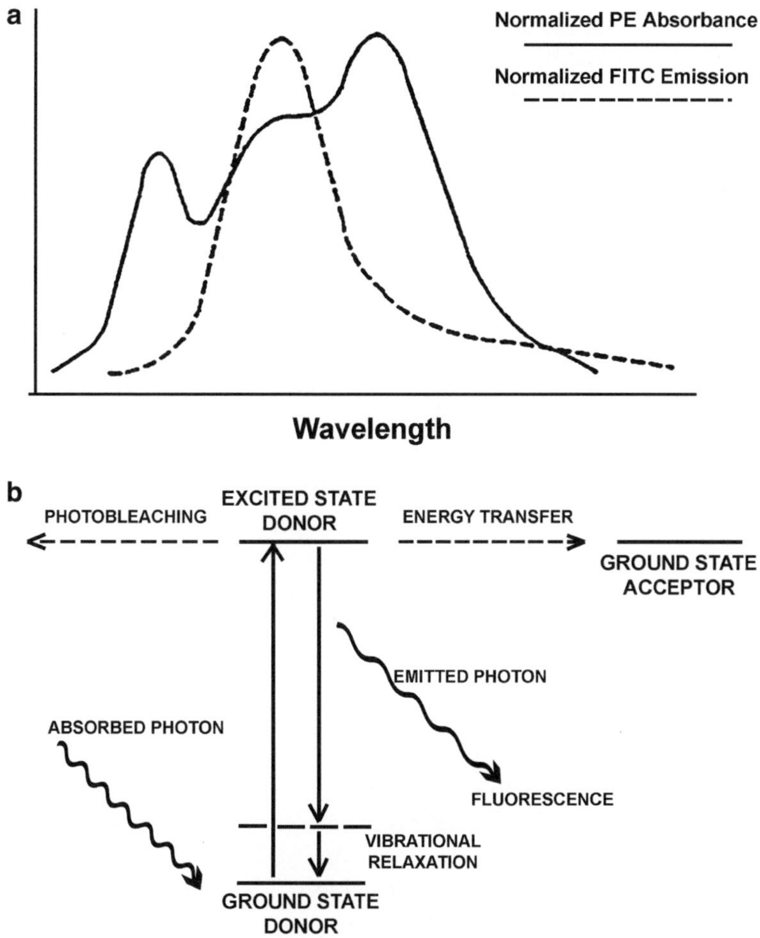

Fig. 2. Parameters affecting the efficiency of energy transfer. (**a**) Overlay of FITC emission spectrum and PE absorbance spectrum normalized to maximum fluorescence intensity and maximum optical density, respectively. FITC fluorescence intensity was measured as a function of the emission's wavelength using a fluorimeter with an excitation wavelength of 488 nm. PE optical density was measured as a function of wavelength using a spectrophotometer. (**b**) Schematic representation of energy absorption and the possible pathways for the subsequent energy release (abbreviations as in the text).

The laser beam can be tuned to the wavelength closest to the excitation maximum of the donor (the 488-nm line of an argon ion laser is used for FITC excitation), and the beam can be optically expanded to irradiate an entire cell. A cell density which permits the irradiation of one cell without any signal contribution from neighboring cells, should be used. The intensity of the laser beam can be adjusted to bleach a cell completely in a brief amount of time (<1 s). The photomultiplier tube can resolve thousands of time-points during the photobleaching, permitting an accurate computer fitting of the decay curves.

By comparing the kinetic parameters of a donor-only sample to a donor-plus acceptor sample (≈50 cells/sample), statistically significant shifts can be determined for donor–acceptor pairs that have an average separation of <17 nm. This technique has been used to measure conformational changes in the CD4 antigen of human peripheral blood T cells (7), as well as the relationships between various CD3 antigens and nearby accessory molecules (8).

2.3. Measurement of Protein Mobility Within Cell Membranes

Photobleaching may also be used to induce spatial gradients of fluorescence intensity by introducing localized regions of bleached (nonfluorescing) probes. Various parameters can be measured depending on the initial distribution of the probe and the geometry of the laser beam used for bleaching and monitoring. Fluorescence redistribution after photobleaching (FRAP) is a technique most commonly used for measuring the ability of cell-surface proteins and lipids to diffuse laterally within the plane of cellular membranes (9). Variations on this technique have been used to look at gap junctional communication using total cell photobleaching (GAP-FRAP) (10), rotational mobility using polarization photobleaching (pFRAP) (11), and receptor–ligand binding kinetics using total internal reflectance microscopy (TIR-FRAP) (12).

In one FRAP configuration (13), the laser is focused to illuminate a small (≈1 μm) spot on the surface of a cell labeled with a monoclonal antibody conjugated to a fluorochrome (Fig. 3). Initially, the laser power is set at a level low enough to monitor the fluorescent signal emitted from the spot with a minimum amount of photobleaching. Then the laser is pulsed at a higher power to bleach a large proportion of the fluorochromes present within the measured spot. Immediately after the spot is bleached, the power is returned to the lower monitoring level, and the fluorescence within that spot is measured over time. If the protein is free to move within the plane of the membrane, then random diffusion will allow unbleached fluorochrome molecules to diffuse into the spot, and the fluorescent signal will increase. The diffusion coefficient can then be calculated from the rate of recovery, and the proportion of molecules free to diffuse (the mobile fraction) can be determined from the magnitude of the recovery. Some of the molecules may be free to diffuse only a short distance. Changing the spot size may provide some information regarding limitations to the distance a molecule may diffuse. For an additional approach to studying boundary limitations, *see* Subheading 4.3.

Another variation of the FRAP technique scans the laser in one dimension across the cell producing a "line-scan" profile of fluorescence intensity (14). For a round cell whose surface is evenly labeled with a fluorescently conjugated antibody, a line scan typically produces a profile with two peaks of fluorescence, as the laser beam is illuminating more fluorophores at the edges of

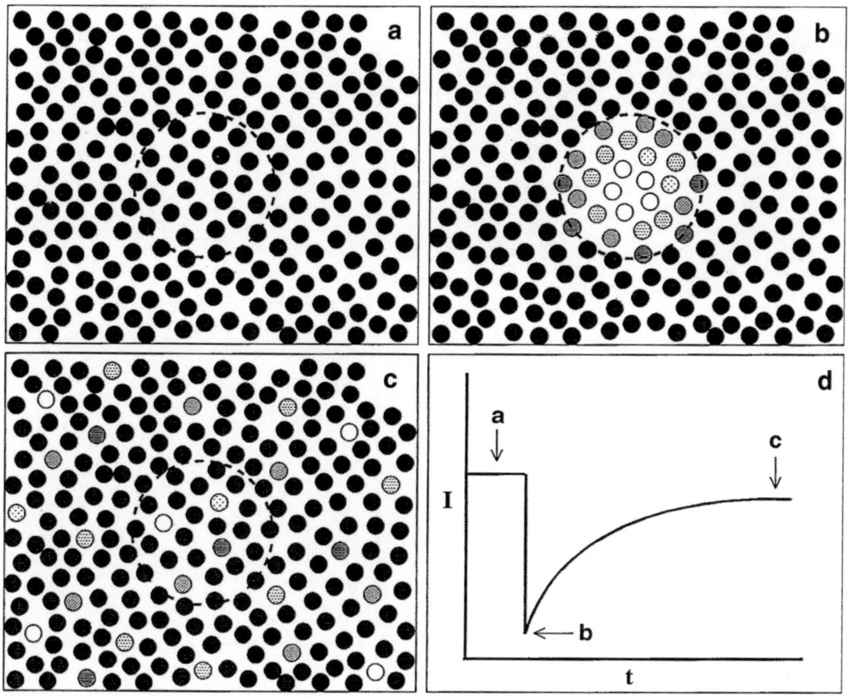

Fig. 3. Schematic diagram of the "spot" photobleaching method of FRAP. (**a**) The *darkened circles* represent fluorescently labeled molecules evenly distributed over a two-dimensional surface (assumed to be an infinite plane). (**b**) The *white* and *light gray circles* represent the initial postbleach distribution of photobleached molecules within a 1-μm diameter spot. (**c**) Redistribution of photobleached and unbleached molecules as a consequence of random diffusion over time. (**d**) *Curve* representing the fluorescence intensity within the 1-μm diameter spot monitored over time; *arrows* a, b, and c indicate the time-points that correspond to their respective panels. The rate of recovery from point b to point c is used to determine the diffusion constant. The magnitude of the recovery is determined by comparing the fluorescence intensity at point c with the initial intensity at point a, and is used to determine the mobile fraction.

the cell (Fig. 4). In this approach, one of the two edge peaks is bleached, and then line scans are repeatedly recorded as a function of time. The coefficient of diffusion is calculated from the rate of recovery of the bleached peak, and the mobile fraction is determined from the extent of recovery. In addition, changes in the integrated area under the curve can be used to correct for any minor photobleaching caused by the laser during the postbleach phase of the measurements.

3. Ablative Applications

3.1. Introduction

In addition to being used as sources of fluorescence excitation, lasers can provide a high power source of irradiation for microsurgery and for inducing cellular injury and/or death (1).

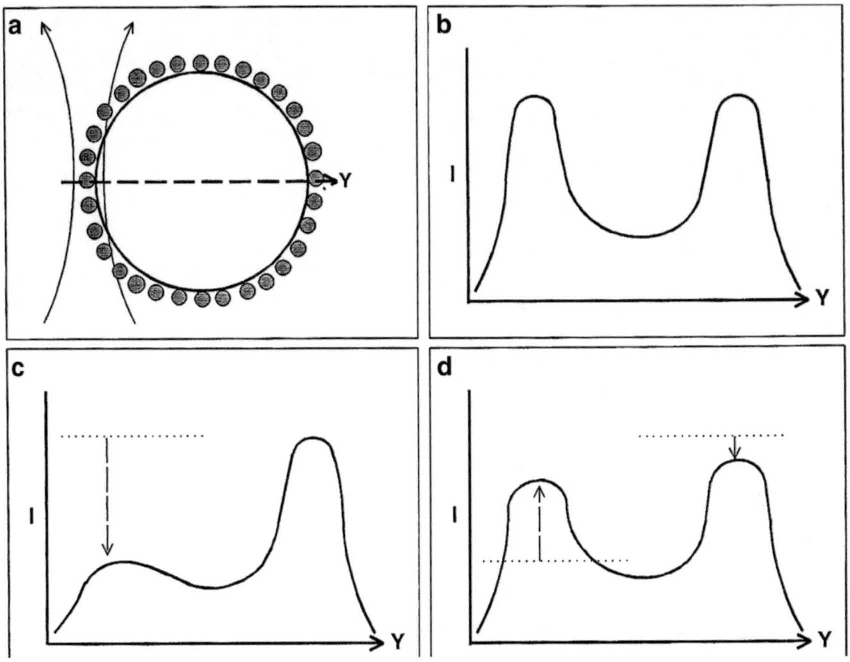

Fig. 4. Schematic diagram of the "line-scan" photobleaching method of FRAP. (**a**) *Darkened circles* represent fluorescently labeled molecules distributed along the surface of a 1-μm-wide "slice" through a round cell as viewed from the side. The laser beam waist is represented by the two *arrows curving upward*, which point in the direction of light propagation. The *dashed line arrow* represents the scanning direction, *y*, with a fixed position *x* in the specimen plane. The movement of the cell relative to the laser beam results in a line-scan profile of fluorescence intensity as a function of *y*. (**b**) The prebleach profile appears bimodal with the two peaks corresponding to the edges of the cell because the laser excites more fluorescent molecules when illuminating the cell tangentially. (**c**) The postbleach profile after one of the edges has been photobleached. The *dashed arrow* indicates decrease in fluorescence intensity owing to photobleaching. (**d**) The redistribution of fluorescent molecules results in an increase of fluorescence intensity at the bleach edge and a decrease at the opposite edge. Note: The redistribution is not limited to the slice illustrated in panel (**a**), but actually occurs across the entire surface of the cell, i.e., the surface of a sphere. Recovery curves analogous to those of the spot photobleaching method can be made by monitoring the change in fluorescence intensity at the bleach position of the line-scan profiles.

UV wavelengths (200–400 nm) are absorbed by many of the proteins within cells. In addition, some proteins, such as hemoglobin and melanin, absorb strongly in the visible region of the spectrum (400–700 nm). As a result of this absorption, the photon energy is converted to heat, and the proteins become thermally denatured leading to photocoagulation. The extent of photocoagulation can be controlled by varying both the power of the laser and the duration of irradiation. When an extremely short pulse of very high power is used, the temperature rise becomes exceptionally large because there is insufficient time for thermal diffusion to occur. This can result in vaporization at the point of irradiation (i.e., photoablation).

3.2. Specific Damage

Chromophore-assisted laser inactivation (CALI) is a technique that has been used to destroy the function of antibody-targeted proteins selectively (15). In this application, the antibody (or some other protein-specific ligand) is conjugated to a chromophore that has an absorption maximum at a wavelength that is not absorbed by any of the endogenous biomolecules. Irradiation of the cell with laser light of this wavelength results in the thermal denaturation of the proteins in close proximity to the chromophore. The effectiveness of this heat transfer decreases substantially with distance so that only the targeted proteins are significantly inactivated (16).

In one application, CALI was used to investigate the function of fascilin I, a cellular adhesion molecule (17). An antibody to fascilin I was conjugated to malachite green, a chromophore with an absorption maximum at 620 nm, a wavelength that is not strongly absorbed by cellular components. The chromophore-labeled antibodies were introduced into grasshopper eggs by microinjection. The embryos were irradiated with a neodymium: yttrium-aluminum-garnet (Nd:YAG) pumped tunable dye laser to achieve the necessary high power laser light at a wavelength of 620 nm. During axonal outgrowth, sister axons normally form a single fascicle, but laser irradiation resulted in defasciculation of those neurons that normally express fascilin I on their surface during differentiation. From these experiments, the investigators were able to show that fascilin I performs a function in axon adhesion during limb bud development.

3.3. Specific Killing

Fluorescence-activated cell sorters (FACS) have been used to separate subpopulations of cells for subsequent treatment or analysis (*see* Chapter 31). However, this approach requires that the cells be in suspension. In the case of adherent cells, some cannot be easily suspended, or the treatments used to suspend them may interfere with subsequent analysis. In these situations, a laser microbeam system capable of fluorescence imaging can serve two purposes. At low power, the laser can excite fluorescence to produce an image, and at a higher power, the laser can be used to kill the undesired cells.

For the same laser beam to be used for fluorescence excitation and killing, the identifying fluorochrome must be excitable by a wavelength of light that can also be absorbed by the cell and converted to thermal energy. However, for cells that do not contain endogenous biomolecules with the requisite absorption spectrum, it is necessary to provide some other method of absorbing the photons from lasers that emit visible light. For this purpose, photoabsorptive dyes have been introduced into cells to make them susceptible to high-intensity irradiation (18), and special substrates have been employed that can absorb light and convert it to thermal energy for transfer to adjacent cells (19, 20).

Based on the qualitative and quantitative analyses of a two-dimensional fluorescent image scan using a low laser power, areas within the field can be chosen for rescanning at a higher "killing" laser power. This results in the selective cell death of those cells that meet a specific fluorescence-labeling criteria, i.e., selecting for those cells that are either above or below a certain fluorescence-intensity threshold value (*see* Fig. 5).

3.4. Cookie Cutter

This technique is based on the use of a proprietary substrate from Meridian Instruments (Okemos, MI) consisting of a special film coating on 35-mm Petri dishes (19, 20). This film can be welded to the surface of the dish with high-power visible laser light. This application is particularly useful for rare-event cell selection (21). If a small percentage of a mixed-cell population can be identified fluorescently, then the low-power laser setting and the stage scanning feature of the laser microbeam system can be used to locate

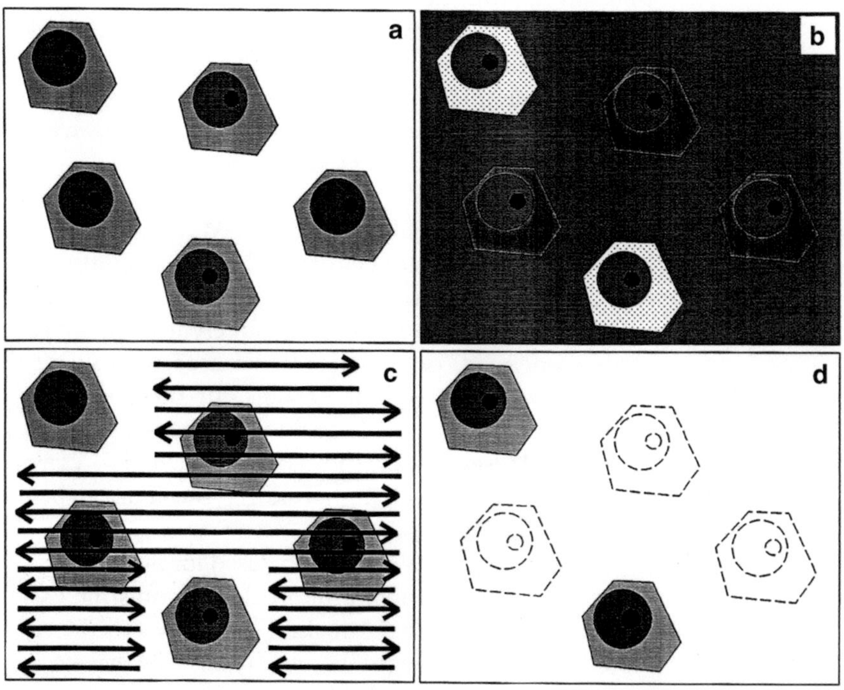

Fig. 5. Schematic diagram of the steps involved in ablative sorting on the basis of fluorescence-intensity criteria. In this case, a positive sort is made for cells above a threshold fluorescence-intensity value. (**a**) Field of view representing a light microscope image of undistinguishable cells. (**b**) Two-dimensional image reconstruction based on fluorescence intensity as measured by a stage-scanning laser microscope. (**c**) Using fluorescence intensity criteria, cells are selected for "saving" from subsequent rescanning at the higher "killing" power, which will be activated only in the areas represented by the *arrows* (*arrows* point in the direction of stage movement during scanning). (**d**) *Dotted outlines* represent ablated cells, which usually appear disrupted, blebbed, or shriveled.

those cells. When the cells of interest are found, a high-power laser setting is used to create octagonal welds around the cells (Fig. 6). The film is then peeled away from the dish, leaving "cookies" containing the specific cells on the dish. If there are any contaminating cells within the cookies, they can be killed using the technique described in Subheading 3.3.

4. Optical Trapping Applications

4.1. Introduction

Recently, infrared laser microbeams (wavelengths >700 nm) have been used to produce electromagnetic fields capable of exerting a sufficient force on cells or organelles to hold them within the path of the laser beam near the focal point, a process referred to as optical trapping (22). Laser light can exert a force on a particle in the optical path as a result of refraction and reflection of the light. This force, known as radiation pressure, results from the exchange of momentum between the photons and the particle. In the case of an inverted microscope with an epi-illuminating optical trap, this force would "lift" the particle as the objective was raised toward the stage, whereas in the case of a transilluminating optical trap, this force would "push" the particle toward the substrate (*see* Fig. 7). In both cases, the lateral trapping force (i.e., the force perpendicular to the optical axis) is directed toward the center of the laser beam and "pulls" the particle into the optical trap. This

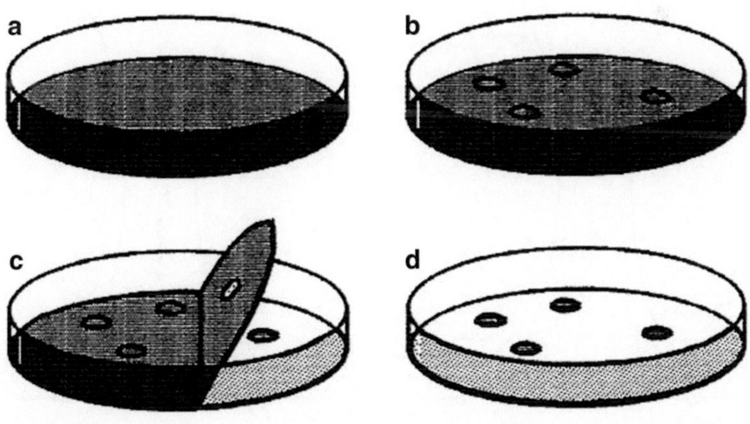

Fig. 6. Schematic diagram of the steps involved in the "cookie cutter" method of cell selection. (**a**) Cells are grown on plastic Petri dishes covered with a darkened nylon film. (**b**) Based on fluorescence-intensity image scans using a stage-scanning laser microscope, rare event cells are identified and octagonal welds are made around those cells to fuse the film to the dish. (**c**) The film is then peeled away from the dish. (**d**) The "cookies" containing the desired cells remain on the dish so that the cells may be analyzed further or subsequently cloned.

approach provides a sterile, gentle, noninvasive means for the micromanipulation of cells and organelles. Several practical applications of optical trapping (also referred to as optical tweezers) have been demonstrated (23–29), and those making use of antibodies are discussed in Subheadings 4.2. and 4.3.

4.2. Micromanipulation of Cells for Sorting Purposes

In one application, an epi-illuminated optical trap was used in conjunction with an inverted fluorescence microscope so that individual cells could be identified with FITC-conjugated antibodies, and subsequently trapped for further micromanipulation (24). In the first part of the experiment, as a demonstration of a sorting technique, the trapped cells were transferred into a capillary tube that was located in the Petri dish along with the cells. The optical trap was used to lift the fluorescently tagged cells to a height greater than the thickness of the capillary tube wall. Then the stage was translated so that the capillary tube "slid" over the trapped cell. The capillary tube containing the selected cells could then be removed from the dish to transport the cells for further treatment. In the second part of the experiment, fluorescently tagged natural killer (NK) cells were optically trapped and then placed in contact with target cells to observe the subsequent interaction. Using optical traps to place cells in close proximity has also been used in combination with a UV laser microbeam for laser-induced cell fusion (25).

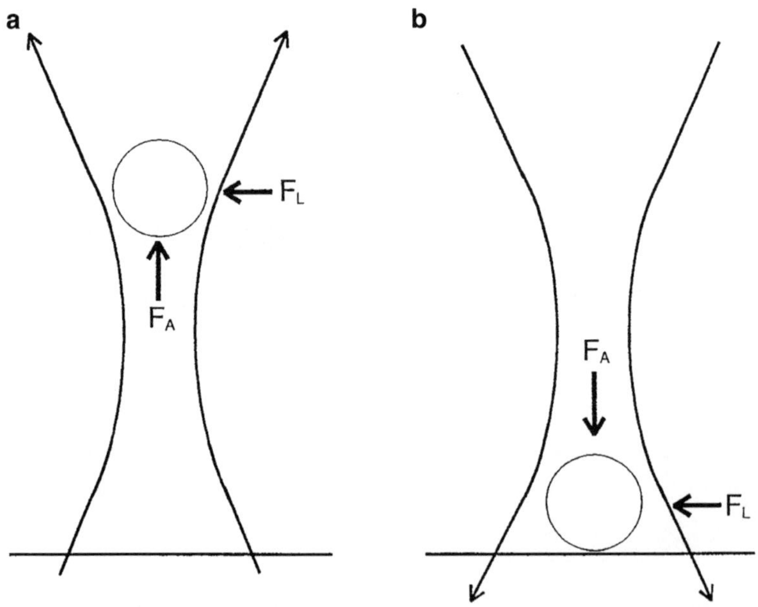

Fig. 7. Schematic diagram of forces exerted on a cell when using an inverted microscope with (**a**) epi-illumination (i.e., laser focused through the objective) or (**b**) transillumination (i.e., laser focused through the condenser). F_A is the axial force and F_L is the lateral trapping force. *Curved arrows* represent the laser beam waist and point in the direction of light propagation.

Because optical trapping does not require physical contact, cells can be manipulated in a completely enclosed environment in which physical and chemical parameters can be maintained over time. Specially designed chambers have been used that contain multiple compartments into which cells can be sorted automatically on the basis of optical characteristics not recognizable by conventional flow-sorting techniques (26, 27).

4.3. Micromanipulation of Cell-Surface Proteins

In another application, an optical trap was used to manipulate cell-surface proteins (29). First, colloidal gold particles conjugated to monoclonal antibodies were bound to the cells. Then an optical trap was used to drag the particle across the surface of the cell and thereby, drag the cell-surface protein through the membrane. When the cell-surface protein encountered a "boundary," the lateral force of the optical trap was overcome, and the particle was released. This approach was used to compare boundary limitations experienced by two different major histocompatability complex (MHC) class I glycoproteins. One was an integral membrane protein with a transmembrane region and cytoplasmic tail (H-2D^b), and the other (Qa2) was a cell-surface protein anchored by a glycosylphosphatidylinosital (GPI) linkage.

5. Concluding Remarks

The techniques discussed in this chapter are intended as an overview of how laser microbeams might be used in conjunction with antibodies to address various aspects of molecular and cellular biology. There may be other applications that were not covered, and there will likely be the development of additional approaches as laser microbeams become increasingly available. Although microscopes are already a common tool of biological research, lasers are increasingly becoming as widely used. With decreases in their size, complexity, and cost, lasers may become a standard accessory to the research microscope.

Acknowledgments

My thanks to Dr. Juanita Anders of the Uniformed Services University of the Health Sciences, Bethesda, MD, for two careful readings of the manuscript, which resulted in numerous clarifications and improvements. This chapter was written in my private capacity. No official support or endorsement by the Food and Drug Administration is intended or should be inferred.

References

1. Berns MW, Wright WH, Wiegand Steubing R (1991) Laser microbeam as a tool in cell biology. Int Rev Cytol 129:1–44
2. Matyus L (1992) Fluorescence resonance energy transfer measurements on cell surfaces. A spectroscopic tool for determining protein interactions. J Photochem Photobiol B Biol 12:323–337
3. Szollosi J, Damjanovich S, Mulhern SA, Tron L (1987) Fluorescence energy transfer and membrane potential measurements monitor dynamic properties of cell membranes: a critical review. Prog Biophys Mol Biol 49:65–87
4. Szollosi J, Matyus L, Tron L, Balazs M, Ember L, Fulwyler MJ, Damjanovich S (1987) Flow cytometric measurements of fluorescence energy transfer using single laser excitation. Cytometry 8:120–128
5. Jovin TM, Arndt-Jovin DJ (1989) FRET microscopy: Digital imaging of fluorescence resonance energy transfer. Application in cell biology. In: Kohen E, Ploem JS, Hirschberg JG (eds) Microspectrofuorometry of single living cells. Academic, Orlando, FL, pp 99–117
6. Szabo G Jr, Pine PS, Weaver JL, Kasari M, Aszalos A (1992) Epitope mapping by photobleaching fluorescence resonance energy transfer measurements using a laser scanning microscope system. Biophys J 61:661–670
7. Szabo G Jr, Pine PS, Weaver JL, Rao PE, Aszalos A (1992) CD4 changes conformation upon ligand binding. J Immunol 149:3596–3604
8. Szabo G Jr, Pine PS, Weaver JL, Rao PE, Aszalos A (1994) The L-selectin (Leu8) molecule is associated with the TcR/CD3 receptor; fluorescence energy transfer measurements on live cells. Immunol Cell Biol 72:319–325
9. Wolf DE, Edidin M (1981) Diffusion and mobility in surface membranes. In: Baker P (ed) Techniques in cellular physiology. EIsevier, North Holland, pp 1–14
10. Anders JJ, Woolery S (1992) Microbeam laser-injured neurons increase in vitro astrocytic gap junctional communication as measured by fluorescence recovery after photobleaching. Lasers Surg Med 12:51–62
11. Velez M, Barald KF, Axelrod D (1990) Rotational diffusion of acetylcholine receptors on cultured rat myotubes. J Cell Biol 110:2049–2059
12. Hellen EH, Axelrod D (1991) Kinetics of epidermal growth factor/receptor binding on cells measured by total internal reflection/fluorescence recovery after photobleaching. J Fluorescence 1:113–128
13. Edidin M, Zagyansky Y, Lardner TJ (1976) Measurements of membrane protein lateral diffusion in single cells. Science 191:466–468
14. Koppel DE (1980) Lateral diffusion in biological membranes: a normal mode analysis of diffusion on a spherical surface. Biophys J 30:187–192
15. Jay DG (1988) Selective destruction of protein function by chromophore assisted laser inactivation. Biochemistry 85:5454–5458
16. Linden KG, Liao JC, Jay DG (1992) Spatial specificity of chromophore assisted laser inactivation of protein function. Biophys J 61:956–962
17. Jay DG, Keshishian H (1990) Laser inactivation of fascilin I disrupts axon adhesion of grasshopper pioneer neurons. Nature 348:548–550
18. Miller JP, Selverston AI (1979) Rapid killing of single neurons by irradiation of intracellularly injected dye. Science 206:702–704
19. Schindler M, Allen ML, Olinger MR, Holland JF (1985) Automated analysis and survival selection of anchorage-dependent cells under normal growth conditions. Cytometry 6:368–374
20. Schindler M, Jiang L-W, Swaisgood M, Wade MH (1989) Analysis, selection, and sorting of anchorage dependent cells under growth conditions. Methods Cell Biol 32:423–446
21. Jiwa AH, Wilson JM (1991) Selection of rare event cells expressing (beta)-galactosidase. Methods 2:272–280
22. Weber G, Greulich KO (1992) Manipulation of cells, organelles, and genomes by laser microbeam and optical trap. Int Rev Cytol 133:1–41
23. Ashkin A, Dziedzic IM, Yamane T (1987) Optical trapping and manipulation of single cells using infrared laser beams. Nature 330:769–771
24. Seeger S, Monajembashi S, Hutter K-J, Futterman G, Wolfrum J, Greulich KO (1991) Application of laser optical tweezers in immunology and molecular genetics. Cytometry 12:497–504
25. Wiegand Steubing R, Cheng S, Wright WH, Numajiri Y, Berns MW (1991) Laser induced cell fusion in combination with optical tweezers: The laser cell fusion trap. Cytometry 12:505–510
26. Buican TN, Smyth MJ, Crissman HA, Salzman GC, Stewart CC, Martin JC (1987) Automated single-cell manipulation and sorting by light trapping. Appl Opt 26:5311–5316

27. Buican TN, Neagley DL, Morrison WC, Upham BD (1989) Optical trapping, cell manipulation, and robotics. SPIE Proc 1063:190–197
28. Berns MW, Aist JR, Wright WH, Liang H (1992) Optical trapping in animal and fungal cells using a tunable, near-infrared titanium–sapphire laser. Exp Cell Res 198:375–378
29. Edidin M, Kuo SC, Sheetz MP (1991) Lateral movements of membrane glycoproteins restricted by dynamic cytoplasmic barriers. Science 254:1379–1382

Chapter 23

Immuno-Laser Capture Microdissection of Rat Brain Neurons for Real Time Quantitative PCR

Denis G. Baskin and L. Scot Bastian

Abstract

Laser capture microdissection (LCM) is a technical approach for obtaining microscopic samples as small as individual cells from tissues for molecular analysis. While the principles and details of the operation of LCM instruments, the technical requirements for obtaining identified cells for LCM "picking", all share the common feature of using a laser in combination with a microscope to microdissect and remove cells from tissue slices (or cultured cells) mounted on a glass slide. The use of LCM is becoming widespread in pathology laboratories and is increasingly being used for gene expression studies in cell biology. The approach is particularly powerful when used in conjunction with immunostaining techniques to obtain enriched RNA samples from cells that have been collected by picking and gathering phenotypically similar cells from anatomically complex organs such as the brain. In the present chapter, we describe an approach for combining immunocytochemistry with LCM to obtain RNA for real time quantitative PCR.

Key words: Laser capture microdissection, Immunocytochemistry, Immunohistochemistry, Fixation, PCR, Brain, Neuron, Gene expression

1. Introduction

A major challenge in molecular microscopy is to identify and isolate specific cells of interest that are located within the architecture of complex tissue and organs. For cells in suspension, this separation can be achieved by the application of fluorescence activated cell sorting. However, the separation of an organ or tissue into its constituent cells for molecular analysis is not practical or feasible, for many solid organs and tumors. Therefore, it is a challenge to obtain identified cells that express specific markers of function from within complex organs such as the brain, for analysis of the expression of specific genes by techniques such as polymerase chain reaction (PCR). Despite the powerful analytic

C. Oliver and M.C. Jamur (eds.), *Immunocytochemical Methods and Protocols*, Methods in Molecular Biology, Vol. 588,
DOI 10.1007/978-1-59745-324-0_23, © Humana Press, a part of Springer Science+Business Media, LLC 1995, 1999, 2010

capabilities of in situ hybridization techniques for detecting gene expression in tissue sections at the transcriptional level, in situ hybridization has the drawbacks of being technically demanding and rarely permits the detection of more than a few mRNA species from cells within a section of a solid tissue. The development of laser capture microscopy (LCM) has facilitated our ability to overcome the limitations of in situ hybridization for molecular analysis of DNA and RNA in tissue sections. With LCM, small anatomic regions can be excised from an organ or tumor and subjected to biochemical and molecular analysis. Moreover, relatively pure populations of cells can be picked from sections of a complex organ such as the brain and subjected to multiplex analysis (including microarray analysis) for the expression of many genes simultaneously (1, 2).

In the present chapter, we focus on the problem of using LCM to recover specific mRNA for real-time quantitative PCR (here referred to as PCR) from rat brain neurons. We describe the principles and approach for the microdissection of small regions such as hypothalamic nuclei and also for picking cells that have been identified by immunocytochemistry. This technique, referred to as Immuno-LCM (3, 4), has been applied to the analysis of pathological tissues for several years (1, 5, 6), and more recently has been finding increased application in characterizing gene expression in specific brain neurons identified by immunocytochemistry (1, 7–13). Our approach here is to discuss general guidelines for investigators who wish to apply this technique to rodent brain tissue, but the methods have general applicability to other organs and tissues as well (*see* Note 1.)

2. Materials

1. Brain tissue.
2. Isopentane (2-methylbutane).
3. Dry ice.
4. Cryostat.
5. Ethanol.
6. Xylene.
7. Staining jars (Coplin jars).
8. Plastic gloves.
9. Uncoated microscope slides.
10. Primary antibodies.
11. Fluorescent labeled second antibodies.
12. phosphate buffered saline (PBS).

13. Diethylpyrocarbonate (DEPC).
14. Laser capture microdissection instrument.
15. Substrates ("caps") for collecting picked cells.
16. –80°C freezer.
17. Primers for real time quantitative PCR (QPCR).
18. Reagents for extraction of RNA for PCR.

3. Methods

3.1. Fixation and Tissue Preparation for Immuno-LCM

The challenge of immuno-LCM is to obtain the tissue and process it for immunocytochemistry and LCM in such a way as to minimize the loss and degradation of RNA. The use of formaldehyde-fixed, paraffin-embedded tissues for immuno-LCM may have merit for the analysis of DNA, but it has severe drawbacks for the analysis of mRNA. While effective methods for obtaining specific RNA from formaldehyde-fixed, paraffin-embedded or cryostat-sectioned tissues have been published (4), and commercial kits are available for this purpose, the quantity and quality of usable mRNA for PCR analysis of gene expression would appear to be compromised. While this approach may be suitable for LCM of large numbers of cells that express certain gene products at high concentrations, such as those from tumors, it would seem to be less useful for immuno-LCM of small numbers of cells in which the expression of genes may be relatively low. The procedure of perfusion of rodent brain with formaldehyde based fixatives, while customary for immunocytochemistry, has severe drawbacks for the analysis of neuronal mRNA by PCR as much of the RNA is fragmented and degraded by formalin. The use of ethanol fixation is reportedly superior to formaldehyde for retention of RNA in tissues and has been adopted for LCM analysis of fresh-frozen tissues (14–17). Moreover, a common strategy to preserve mRNA is the use of brief immunostaining protocols (3, 7, 13, 18) (*see* Note 2).

We have found that using cryostat sections of frozen rat brain in combination with rapid immunostaining protocols after alcohol fixation works well for immuno-LCM, and real time QPCR for mRNA. Our goal has been to isolate mRNA from immunocytochemically identified populations of hypothalamic and brain stem neurons that express genes involved in the regulation of food intake and body weight (19, 20). These cells are located in regions that are very small and the analyses often involve relatively few cells, requiring the picking of cells from several sections to obtain adequate material for analysis. Most of our studies are done on pools of 100–300 cells that have been picked by LCM after immunofluorescent staining (19, 20).

This chapter summarizes our experience with this approach and describes some of the critical parameters involved in the preparation of rat neural tissue for LCM, with particular emphasis on protocols applied to the Arcturus Autopix LCM. This instrument has been superceded by more recent models, which are now marketed and distributed by MDS Analytical Technologies (http://www.moleculardevices.com). The principles described here, however, are applicable to tissue preparation for most LCM instruments. We describe two basic protocols for the isolation of samples of rat brain, first from unstained microdissected regions, and second, from brain cells that express specific antigens identified by immunostaining. In addition, we compare the effects of different fixation conditions on tissue recovery and RNA content using real-time QPCR.

3.2. Tissue Treatment and Sample Slide Preparation

To isolate RNA from cells or tissues, it is recommended that fresh, unperfused samples be snap-frozen in dry icecooled iso-pentane prior to storage at –80°C. The tissue should be cryosectioned at a thickness between 7 and 12 μm and thaw-mounted on clean slides. In our hands, 10 μm sections work well. If the goal is to measure RNA content, appropriate measures, such as wearing gloves and using a fresh box of slides should be undertaken to avoid RNA degradation. If untouched slides are used, they need not be specially treated prior to use. Slides with special coatings are not recommended, as the coatings could interfere with the removal of the cells. This potential problem should be evaluated prior to using the slides for LCM. To minimize RNA degradation, the slides should not be heat-dried after contact with the section. After sectioning, the slide-mounted tissues are transferred to an –80°C freezer where they can be stored for several weeks prior to LCM. It is not clear how long various RNA species are stable under these conditions, so caution should be exercised when using archived frozen sections. In our hands, there appears to be modest reduction of mRNA yield in sections stored at –80°C for several months. To minimize RNA degradation by ribonucleases and extraction from the picked cells, aqueous steps should be performed rapidly. We prepare aqueous solutions with 0.1% DEPC that has been allowed to stand overnight at room temperature followed by autoclaving to remove the DEPC.

3.3. Fixation of Slide-Mounted Tissue Sections

To allow efficient extraction of intact mRNA, it is recommended that alcohol fixatives be used in lieu of cross-linking agents such as paraformaldehyde. In our experience protocols that have been developed for studying paraformaldehyde-fixed paraffin-embedded archival specimens in tandem with RNA amplifications produce low yields of RNA from microdissected brain regions and picked cells. Fixation of tissue with methanol or ethanol preserves immunoreactivity and mRNA in many cases. Accordingly, we immerse slide-mounted tissue sections in ice-cold methanol or ethanol for 3 min prior to immunostaining (*see* Note 4). We have found that alcohol fixation produces immunocytochemical staining equivalent to that resulting from formaldehyde fixation, at least with antibodies for oxytocin, tyrosine hydroxylase, and Fos protein (*see* Notes 5 and 6).

3.4. Dehydration

The purpose of dehydration is to extract traces of water that interfere with cell removal by the laser. Although staining is optional for LCM specimens, if immunostaining has been performed, the samples must be thoroughly dehydrated to allow for an efficient removal of cells from the slide. Dehydration of the samples is accomplished through a gradual replacement of the aqueous solvents with ethanol, using a graded series of ethanol. This is followed by replacement of the ethanol with a clearing agent, such as xylene, followed by a final air drying step. The drying step is extremely critical for picking cells with the AutoPix LCM. We have had excellent success at removing cells with the AutoPix when we closely adhere to the drying procedure. After the PBS rinses (in the case of sections that have been immunostained), the slides are dipped in 75% ethanol (1 min), 95% ethanol (1 min), and 100% ethanol (twice for 1 min each). These steps are followed by several changes of xylene over 5 min and air drying. The 100% ethanol should be absolutely dry. We obtain absolute ethanol in 500 ml bottles and use molecular sieves. The slides are not cover-slipped. They should be examined in the LCM instrument immediately after drying, and the cells of interest should be picked as soon as possible to obtain the best results (*see* Note 7).

3.5. Immunocytochemical Staining of Cells for LCM Picking

Immunocytochemical staining of sections prior to LCM is not required for the isolation of a targeted cell population if the cells can be identified by morphological criteria (such as hippocampal pyramidal neurons), but it is essential if specific cells cannot otherwise be recognized, as is the case, for example, of catecholamine neurons in the hindbrain (*see* Note 3). The latter neurons must be immunostained with antibodies to a catecholamine synthetic enzyme such as tyrosine hydroxylase, to be differentiated from the adjacent non-catecholaminergic cells. As immunostaining introduces the potential for RNA extraction and degradation, it should be processed rapidly. We recommend the following general procedure as a starting point for investigations that involve immunostaining neurons prior to picking by LCM. Investigators can modify the protocols to suit the particular requirements of their studies (*see* Note 8).

After fixation in ice-cold methanol, the slides are dipped in PBS twice for 15 s each; then, primary antibody is added and the slides are incubated at room temperature for 3 min. Because of the very brief incubation, the antibody needs to be used at a much higher concentration than is customary for longer incubations. For example, an antiserum that we would normally dilute to 1:2000 for an overnight incubation in the refrigerator would be diluted to only 1:50 or 1:25 for the Immuno-LCM protocol. Following the primary antibody step, the slides are treated with four 15-s rinses in ice-cold PBS and then exposed to a drop of fluorescent second antibody (e.g., goat anti-rabbit IgG-Cy3) diluted 1:50 for 3 min, followed by four 15 s rinses in ice-cold PBS. Because of the very rapid protocol, the timing is critical and only a few slides can be handled efficiently at one time. The procedure does not lend itself to batch processing. We usually perform this protocol on only one or two slides at a time. The slides are viewed without coverslips.

4. Notes

1. Successful identification and picking of neurons for immuno-LCM requires careful optimization of sample preparation protocols and instrument settings to ensure efficient sample recovery. For example, the tissue collected should be cryosectioned at less than 12 μM thickness and mounted on uncoated slides. Thicker sections interfere with cell removal. If the goal is to recover RNA, then normal precautions should be taken to minimize the activity of endogenous RNAses and prevent the introduction of exogenous RNAse: Gloves should be worn, staining jars should be washed with RNAse decontaminating solutions, aqueous solutions should be treated with DEPC, and warming of slides when in aqueous solutions should be minimized.
2. We find that it is useful to conduct preliminary PCR studies on cell populations in the region of interest prior to picking by immuno-LCM. This allows us to determine if the PCR probes can detect the RNA transcripts of interest in unfixed tissue samples and gives a baseline for evaluating the efficacy of immuno-LCM for the same transcripts. Figure 1 shows a typical example of a regional microdissection. In this example, the tissue was not stained and thus was only subjected to the dehydration, clearing and drying steps. Figure 1a shows the SCN after cells were picked by gross LCM. The tissue was viewed with bright field optics; the areas where cells were removed appear as light areas in the image. The picked cells are missing in the image, as they were transferred to the plastic substrate ("cap"), which is seen in Fig. 1b. After collection, the cells on the cap can be lysed, the RNA extracted and column-purified, and analyzed for content of specific templates.

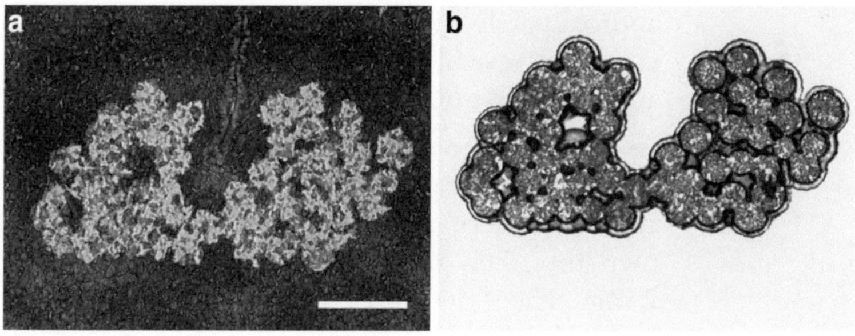

Fig. 1. Laser capture of neurons from a coronal cryostat slice of rat suprachiasmatic nucleus (SCN). **(a)** Image of SCN after cells had been removed from the section. **(b).** Image of the clear transparent LCM plastic cap showing cells that were picked from the slice in **a**. Scale bar = 100 μm.

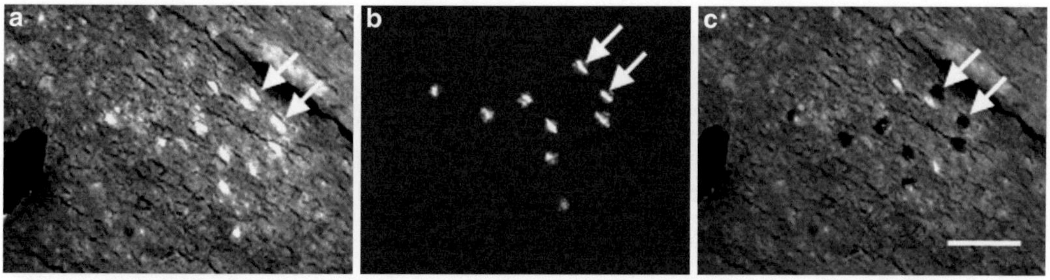

Fig. 2. Immuno-Laser capture of neurons from a coronal cryostat slice of the nucleus of the solitary tract (NTS) in the rat caudal brainstem. **(a)** A slice of the NTS that was immunostained for tyrosine hydroxylase (TH) using fluorescent CY3 second antibodies. TH-positive neurons show bright fluorescence (two indicated by arrows). **(b)** Image of the collection cap showing TH-positive neurons picked from the slice shown in **a** (*arrows* indicate the same two cells that are indicated by *arrows* in **a**). **(c)** Image of the same slice shown in **a** after removal of the cells by LCM. Cells visible in **a** are missing in **c** (*arrows* point to same two neurons indicated by *arrows* in **a**). Scale bar = 50 μm.

3. To identify and collect a subpopulation of rat brain cells that express a specific phenotype, we utilize this fast immunostaining protocol that marks the population of interest with a fluorescent tag while preserving the integrity of the RNA. We have found that this method easily reveals the hindbrain catecholamine neurons that have been immunostained with antibodies to tyrosine hydroxylase (TH). Figure 2a shows neurons from the rat nucleus tractis solitarius (NTS) in the hindbrain that were rapidly immunostained for TH using a mouse anti-TH monoclonal antibody (Cat# 318, Chemicon International, Millipore Corpo-ration, Billerica, MA) diluted 1:25 in PBS followed by a secondary goat anti-mouse-Cy3 antibody (Jackson ImmunoResearch, Fort Washington, PA; Cat# 115-165-068) that was diluted 1:50 in PBS. Figure 2b shows an image of the plastic collection cap after the targeted cells have been removed and transferred. Figure 2c shows the same region as seen in Fig. 2a after the cells were removed; the blank areas represent the hole left by the picked cells that are seen on the plastic cap in Fig. 2b. Using this method, we pick

approximately 100–200 TH-positive cells onto one substrate cap from several brainstem sections. This procedure provides adequate TH mRNA for real time QPCR (20).

4. As a first step toward optimizing Immuno-LCM with alcohol fixation, we compared four different alcohol treatments. Serial cryosections of rat hindbrain were fixed in ice-cold 100% methanol, 70% methanol, 100% ethanol, or 70% ethanol for 2 min. The slides were treated for 1 min in cold PBS followed by dehydration as described above. A comparison of the amount of tissue removed by the AutoPix after these different conditions suggests that the different fixations resulted in visibly different amounts of tissue removed from the sections. All, however, produce samples that are suitable for efficient cell picking (Fig. 3). It appears, though, that fixation in 70% alcohol produced better tissue recovery in this experiment.

5. To determine optimum alcohol fixation conditions for the integrity and recovery of the RNA from the tissue, the extracts from each fixation were column-purified on RNA Arcturus Picopure RNA Isolation Kit™, and residual DNA was degraded

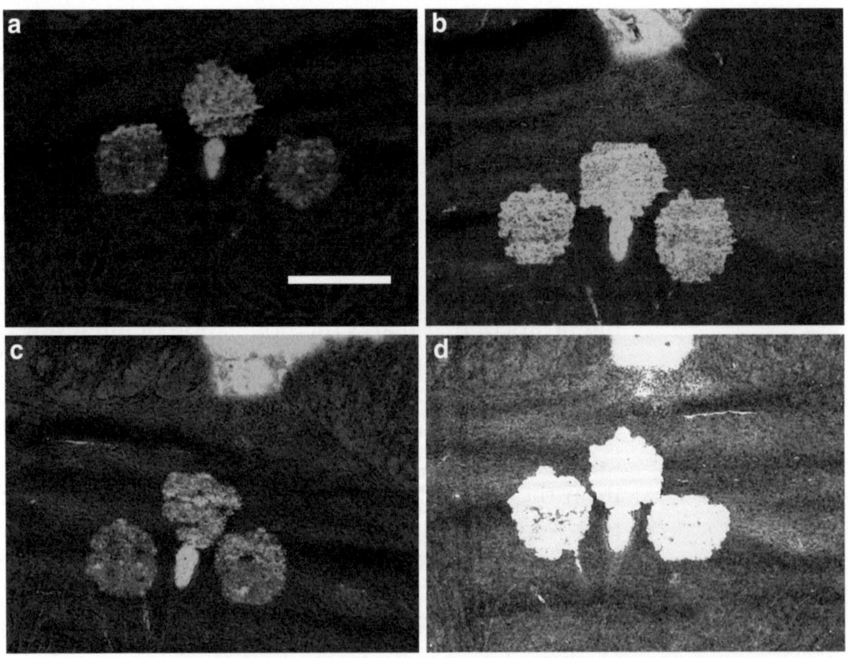

Fig. 3. Images of adjacent cryostat slices of unfixed caudal brainstem at the level of the area postrema after LCM removal of area-equivalent tissue. The areas sampled by LCM are seen as circular light patches, one in the center above the central canal and two laterally (hypoglossal nucleus). Prior to LCM, each slice (mounted on a slide) was fixed for 2 min in a different concentration of ethanol or methanol. **(a)** 100% methanol. **(b)** 70% methanol. **(c)** 100% ethanol. **(d)** 70% ethanol. The tissue from pooled replicates by each fixation was processed for GAPDH mRNA levels by real time quantitative PCR. The differences in background intensity reflect the actual differences in background brightness from the different treatments. Scale bar = 200 μm.

by treating the columns with the RNAse-Free DNAse (cat# 79254, Qiagen USA , Valencia, CA). Equal portions of each eluate were reverse-transcribed into cDNA using the Applied Biosystems (Applied Biosystems, Foster City, CA) High Capacity cDNA Archive Kit™ (Cat# 4322171). Equal portions of the resulting template were analyzed for content of GAPDH using QPCR. The probe and primers were designed with the aid of Primer Express™ version 2.0.0 software (Applied Biosystems). Briefly, according to the manufacturer's instruction GAPDH was measured using 1 μM upstream (5′-GCCAGC-CTCGTCTCATAGACA-3′) and 1 μM downstream primers (5′-GTCCGATACGGCCAAATCC-3′) in conjunction with 0.4 μM probe primer (VIC-5′-ATGGTGAAGGTCGGT-GTG-3′) in a reaction containing Applied Biosystems Taqman Universal PCR Master Mix. GAPDH content, as a measure of overall mRNA yield, was measured in triplicate on ABI Prism 7000 Sequence Detection System (Applied Biosystems). The samples were incubated at 50°C for 2 min followed by 95°C for 10 min, then at 95°C for 10 min, and then run through 40 cycles of 95°C for 15 s followed by 60°C for 1 min.

6. A comparison of the relative content of the GAPDH template in the samples obtained from each fixation condition is shown in Fig. 4. The highest yield of GAPDH mRNA was obtained with 70% ethanol fixation. By comparison, 100% methanol fixation produced 40% less yield of GAPDH mRNA. The 100% ethanol and 70% methanol fixations yielded more GAPDG mRNA than from 100% methanol but less than with 70% ethanol.

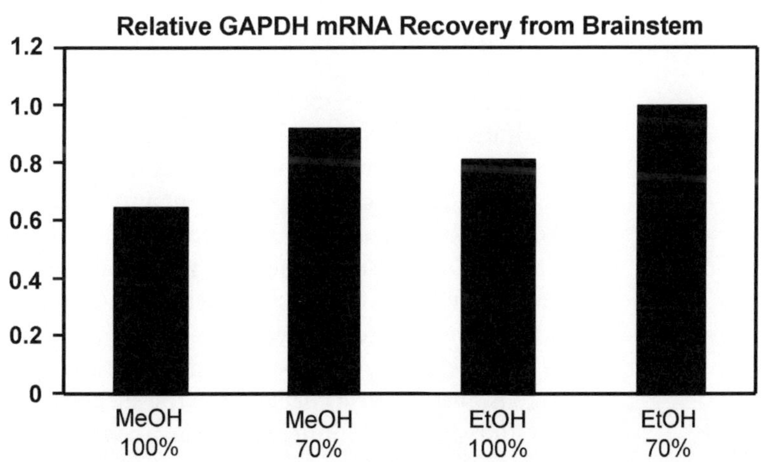

Fig. 4. Histogram comparing relative recovery of GAPDH mRNA from brainstem LCM samples fixed with four different conditions shown in Fig. 3 and analyzed by real time quantitative PCR. The highest yield resulted from fixation in 70% ethanol (bar on *right*). The bars represent the relative amounts of GAPDH PCR signal from the four conditions relative to 70% ethanol. It can be seen that the highest yields resulted from 70% alcohol concentrations. The absolute alcohols produced as much as 40% less GAPDH mRNA yield.

Interestingly, the relative yields of GAPDH mRNA appeared to parallel the amounts of tissue removed by the AutoPix, as seen in Fig. 3 This observation is anecdotal, but suggests that the different alcohol concentrations tested, produced variable recovery of RNA (e.g., cells) from the tissue sections and did not compromise the integrity of the RNA. Taken together, these data indicate that, at least with rat brain tissue, the use of 70% ethanol might be optimal for RNA recovery from tissue picked by LCM.

7. Dehydration and drying are critical steps in tissue processing. It is important to use a fresh bottle of 100% ethanol in the dehydration protocol. Absolute ethanol is hygroscopic, and an open bottle will draw water from the atmosphere leading to inadequate dehydration and difficulty in removing the cells from the surface of the slide. Alternatively, molecular sieves might be employed to absorb water from the ethanol, but we have not tested this. In our experience, air-drying for 10 min was adequate, but a humid atmosphere may necessitate drying in the presence of a desiccant.
8. The parameters for the rapid immunofluorescence staining protocol must be determined by trial and error before LCM. The objective is to obtain the brightest possible specific immunofluorescence so that the cells of interest can be visualized with the AutoPix. High background fluorescence is sometimes tolerated to achieve this goal. The concentrations, incubation, and wash times of primary and secondary antibodies described above have worked well for a variety of antibodies in our experience, but it is likely that different antibodies will require different incubation times and/or concentrations depending on the avidity of the antibody and the concentration of the antigen. The fixation, antibody incubations and PBS washes were carried out using ice-cold solutions and a cold block. The dehydration, clearing and drying steps were done at room temperature. It is recommended that candidate antibodies be pre-tested using standard overnight immuno-staining protocols prior to the application of the fast immunostain protocol. In our limited observations, the rapid stain protocol requires an approximately 100-fold higher concentration of antibody than the optimal titer for overnight immunostaining. Extremely low titer, relatively nonspecific antibodies, or low-abundance antigens, may prove a challenge to the successful application of the rapid-stain technique, but adjustments in staining times, incubation temperatures, or more sensitive fluorochromes, may increase the specificity to acceptable levels. We have also successfully used Biotin-linked primary antibodies in conjunction with fluorochrome-conjugated streptavidin to amplify low level signal and reduce background.

Acknowledgments

This material is based upon work supported in part by the Office of Research and Development Medical Research Service, US Department of Veterans Affairs, and by the facilities at the Department of Veterans Affairs Puget Sound Health Care System, Seattle, Washington, and in part by NIH grant DK17046 to the Diabetes Endocrinology Research Center, University of Washington. Dr. Baskin is Senior Research Career Scientist in the Research and Development Service, Department of Veterans Affairs Puget Sound Health Care System, Seattle, WA.

References

1. Fend F, Kremer M, Quintanilla-Martinez L (2000) Laser capture microdissection: methodical aspects and applications with emphasis on immuno-laser capture microdissection. Pathobiol 68:209–214
2. Taatjes DJ, Palmer CJ, Pantano C, Hoffmann SB, Cummins A, Mossman BT (2001) Laser-based microscopic approaches: application to cell signaling in environmental lung disease. Biotechniques 31:880–882, 884, 886–888, 890, 892–894.
3. Fink L, Kinfe T, Stein MM, Ermert L, Hanze J, Kummer W, Seeger W, Bohle RM (2000) Immunostaining and laser-assisted cell picking for mRNA analysis. Lab Invest 80: 327–333
4. Fassunke J, Majores M, Ullmann C, Elger C, Schramm J, Wiestler OD, Becker AJ (2004) In situ-RT and immunolaser microdissection for mRNA analysis of individual cells isolated from epilepsy-associated glioneuronal tumors. Lab Invest 84:1520–1525
5. Fend F, Raffeld M (2000) Laser capture microdissection in pathology. J Clin Pathol 53:666–672
6. Fend F, Emmert-Buck MR, Chuaqui R, Cole K, Liotta LA, Raffeld M (1999) Immuno-LCM: Laser capture microdissection of immunostained frozen sections for mRNA analysis. Am J Pathol 154:61–66
7. Uz T, Arslan AD, Kurtuncu M, Imbesi M, Akhisaroglu M, Dwivedi Y, Pandey GN, Manev H (2005) The regional and cellular expression profile of the melatonin receptor MT1 in the central dopaminergic system. Brain Res Mol Brain Res 136:45–53
8. Xiang CC, Mezey E, Chen M, Key S, Ma L, Brownstein MJ (2004) Using DSP, a reversible cross-linker, to fix tissue sections for immunostaining, microdissection and expression profiling. Nucleic Acids Res 32:e185
9. Meguro R, Lu J, Gavrilovici C, Poulter MO (2004) Static, transient and permanent organization of GABA receptor expression in calbindin-positive interneurons in response to amygdala kindled seizures. J Neurochem 91:144–154
10. Ginsberg SD, Che S (2004) Combined histochemical staining, RNA amplification, regional, and single cell cDNA analysis within the hippocampus. Lab Invest 84:952–962
11. Vincent VA, DeVoss JJ, Ryan HS, Murphy GM Jr (2002) Analysis of neuronal gene expression with laser capture microdissection. J Neurosci Res 69:578–586
12. Greene JG, Dingledine R, Greenamyre JT (2005) Gene expression profiling of rat midbrain dopamine neurons: implications for selective vulnerability in parkinsonism. Neurobiol Dis 18:19–31
13. Bi WL, Keller-McGandy C, Standaert DG, Augood SJ (2002) Identification of nitric oxide synthase neurons for laser capture microdissection and mRNA quantification. Biotechniques 33:1274–1283
14. Soukup J, Krskova L, Hilska I, Kodet R (2003) Ethanol fixation of lymphoma samples as an alternative approach for preservation of the nucleic acids. Neoplasma 50:300–304
15. Su JM, Perlaky L, Li XN, Leung HC, Antalffy B, Armstrong D, Lau CC (2004) Comparison of ethanol versus formalin fixation on preservation of histology and RNA in laser capture microdissected brain tissues. Brain Pathol 14:175–182
16. Hu SP, Yang JS, Wu MY, Shen ZY, Zhang KH, Liu JW, Guan B (2005) Effect of one-step 100% ethanol fixation and modified manual

microdissection on high-quality RNA recovery from esophageal carcinoma specimen. Dis Esophagus 18:190–198

17. Gillespie JW, Best CJ, Bichsel VE, Cole KA, Greenhut SF, Hewitt SM, Ahram M, Gathright YB, Merino MJ, Strausberg RL, Epstein JL, Hamilton SR, Gannot G, Baibakova GV, Calvert VS, Flaig MJ, Chuaqui RF, Herring JC, Pfeifer J, Petricoin EF, Linehan WM, Duray PH, Bova GS, Emmert-Buck MR (2002) Evaluation of non-formalin tissue fixation for molecular profiling studies. Am J Pathol 160:449–457
18. Fink L, Kinfe T, Seeger W, Ermert L, Kummer W, Bohle RM (2000) Immunostaining for cell picking and real-time mRNA quantitation. Am J Pathol 157:1459–1466
19. Blevins JE, Morton GJ, Williams DL, Caldwell DE, Schwartz ML, Bastian LS, Baskin DG (2005) Third and fourth ventricular administration of MTII enhances the satiety response to CCK-8. Program No. 580.5. 2005 Abstract Viewer/Itinerary Planner. Society for Neuroscience, Washington, DC, 2005. Online.
20. Williams DL, Schwartz ML, Bastian LS, Blevins JE, Baskin DG (2008) Immunocytochemistry and laser capture microdissection for real-time quantitative PCR identify hindbrain neurons activated by interaction between leptin and cholecystokinin. J Histochem Cytochem 56:285–293

Chapter 24

Overview of Antigen Detection Through Enzymatic Activity

Gary L. Bratthauer

Abstract

The identification of antigenic substances with antibodies can only occur through the use of a reporter molecule. One way of doing this is through the use of enzymes. Enzymes act upon a substrate and that substrate, or a molecule affected by that substrate, in turn becomes detectable by a variety of methods. There are many enzymes available for this purpose. The most common is peroxidase. Another widely used enzyme is alkaline phosphatase. Each enzyme has a few chromogenic substrate solutions with which it can react to change a color visualized through the use of selected instruments, including the microscope. Antibodies can be labeled with an enzyme directly, or secondary antibodies can be labeled with the enzyme and employed in an indirect technique. Also, immunoglobulin labeled polymers labeled with enzyme can be used and the enzymes themselves can serve as antigens in immunoenzyme complex procedures. Finally, avidin or biotin can be labeled with enzyme, and used either singly or in complexes, and peroxidase mediated biotin amplification can be used to increase the sensitivity in some procedures.

Key words: Enzyme, Peroxidase, Alkaline phosphatase, Primary antibody, Secondary antibody, Avidin, Biotin, Substrate, Immunepolymer, Immune complex

1. Introduction

The use of enzymes together with immunoglobulins to identify specific substances emerged with the work by Nakane and Pierce who labeled an immunoglobulin with the peroxidase enzyme rather than with a fluorescent compound (1). The difficulty with this approach lies in attaching a relatively large molecule like an enzyme to another large molecule like an immunoglobulin without compromising either molecule's ability to function. In this case, labeling can occur without appreciable functional loss. The labeled antibody is still able to bind the antigen and the attached enzyme is still able to catalyze the oxidative reaction. This direct

C. Oliver and M.C. Jamur (eds.), *Immunocytochemical Methods and Protocols*, Methods in Molecular Biology, Vol. 588, DOI 10.1007/978-1-59745-324-0_24, © Humana Press, a part of Springer Science+Business Media, LLC 1995, 1999, 2010

labeled technique was the forerunner of numerous other methods which bring enzymes and antibodies together to allow the enzyme action to identify the location of the antigen through the antibody intermediary.

Along with the direct labeled methods, the indirect labeled methods were developed providing amplification and universality. By using a labeled secondary antibody, any number of primary antibodies can be used (to which the secondary antibody binds) (2). This allows great freedom in selecting antigens to study and the antibodies to study them. All that is needed is a secondary "anti-antibody" reagent with an enzyme attached: a far less costly means of antigen detection. This makes the technique much more universal in application than the direct techniques.

The other overriding and perhaps more important aspect of this technique is the increased amplification of the signal obtained. By allowing multiple secondary antibodies, each with several enzyme molecules attached to bind to the primary antibody, the amount of enzyme at the site of the primary antibody–antigen interaction can be increased along with the resultant signal. This makes the reaction easier to observe, but also increases the visibility of weak reactions, thereby increasing the overall sensitivity of the method. In addition, the background is reduced and the primary antibodies can be diluted even further with little loss in detectability. This produces a technique that is not only more cost effective but also more specific because of a decrease in the concentration of any non-specific antibodies in the primary antiserum.

Increased amplification yielding more sensitivity and more specificity, along with a universal methodology providing ease of use and applicability, are the essential principles governing all further modifications of this technology as shall be shown in Chapters 25–27.

2. Enzymes Used for Antigen Detection

There are a few common enzymes that have been employed in these types of assay systems over the years, but chief among them has been the peroxidase enzyme (3). Peroxidase has an oxidative function when transferring electrons, in conjunction with a source of oxygen, to a molecule that becomes oxidized. The peroxidase enzyme found in the horseradish plant has been used for its ability to carry out this function, the fact that it is easily obtained, and for the antigenic differences from most mammalian forms of the enzyme. The oxidative function of this enzyme allows for the use of chromogens that, when oxidized, not only change color but precipitate in such a manner as to render a permanent preparation.

Another common enzyme used in these procedures is alkaline phosphatase. Alkaline phosphatase will cleave phosphates off a donor molecule, which in turn acts as a mediator of a color change involving a third molecule. This system is often used because alkaline phosphatase can create more of the color producing molecules per enzyme molecule than can peroxidase, resulting in better sensitivity. Alkaline phosphatase systems are especially sensitive for examining protein or nucleic acid blots with enzyme labels. The problem when examining tissue is the presence of the endogenous enzyme in the tissues being examined. Quenching the endogenous alkaline phosphatase activity can be difficult. The standard treatment is to use levamisole in a blocking step incubation, but the exact conditions for successful inactivation are often varied depending on the tissue, and the endogenous activity can persist (4).

Other minor enzyme systems, such as beta-galactosidase, can be used. (5). This system works well; however, it can lead to some false positive problems resulting from endogenous enzymes having a similar reactivity (6). Another enzyme not commonly used is glucose oxidase. A glucose oxidase system can provide a sensitive and specific assay, if other endogenous enzyme activity is a problem.

3. Chromogenic Substrates

In addition to the many enzyme systems available, there are with each, a series of chromogenic substrate solutions that can be used to create different colors and locations of reaction products. For the peroxidase system, there are numerous oxidizable compounds that precipitate as a permanent color. The most common and still widely used is 3,3′diaminobenzidine tetrahydrochloride (DAB). This compound precipitates to a golden brown color when in solution with peroxidase and hydrogen peroxide. This brown color has many subtleties and readily stands out in a tissue section. With practice, it is possible to differentiate specific from non-specific staining patterns merely by examining the characteristics of the precipitated pigment. This material is also insoluble in alcohol and xylene, and therefore the tissue may be routinely dehydrated and cleared without loss of chromogen.

A drawback of the use of this chromogen is its close resemblance to some endogenous pigments like melanin. Most of the time the characteristics and color subtleties of this compound are enough to distinguish it from melanin, lipofuchsin, hemosiderin, or formalin pigments. However, on occasion, depending on the tissue, the endogenous pigment may be startlingly close in appearance to DAB. In these situations, it may be necessary to try a different molecule that precipitates as an alternate color. One such molecule is 3-amino-9-ethylcarbazole (AEC).

AEC precipitates as an insoluble color substance when subjected to peroxidase and hydrogen peroxide. The color is a bright red and is often more intense than that achieved with DAB. It does not conflict with any endogenous pigments. The drawback of the use of this chromogen is that it is soluble in alcohol. This means that the tissue sections cannot be dehydrated and cleared as is commonly done. An aqueous mounting medium has to be used and the sections often appear thickened under the microscope. Sometimes there is a loss of resolution when using high magnification. One mounting medium used with some success is Crystal/Mount (Biomeda Corp., Foster City, CA). It is baked to an insoluble plastic. While the plastic coat protects the specimen and removes the refractility associated with wet mounts, the surface of the plastic is quite fragile and may be easily scratched. However, once the compound has dried and hardened the section can be coverslipped using an organic mounting medium such as Permount, and the slide can be made more permanent. The resolution (Fisher scientific, pittsbargh, PA), though, may not be as good as with an alcohol- dehydrated, xylene-cleared, specimen.

There are other chromogens that can be employed when using peroxidase enzymes. The compound 4-chloro-1-naphthol is one that is often used in immunoblotting, and occasionally, for tissue examination (7). The signal achieved with this material is thought to be superior to that obtained with other chromogens. The blue color, though, which is the precipitant product, is harder to visualize under the microscope as blue has traditionally been the color of histology counterstains like hematoxylin. Many peroxidase chromogens used in other assays like o-phenylenediamine change color when oxidized but are soluble in aqueous solutions and will not precipitate as a permanent pigment. They are thus, unsuitable for tissue analysis. Most of these oxidizable substrates are potential carcinogens and should be handled appropriately. There is, though, a compound which is thought to be safer for handling, called tetramethylbenzidene (TMB) (8). TMB precipitates to a dark blue-black and is insoluble in alcohol. Now, numerous commercially available chromogens that are insoluble in alcohol and precipitate red, blue, or purple in the presence of peroxidase and hydrogen peroxide, are produced by a number of immunohistology companies (Vector Laboratories, Burlingame CA; Biocare Medical, Concord, CA).

These compounds can be used in place of DAB or along with DAB when two color assays are desired. Two color assays can also be accomplished by altering the enzyme system used for one of the assays. Another method is to alter the color product of the DAB chromogen for one of the assays. This can be done by adding a heavy metal compound such as cobalt or nickel to the dilute solution (9). The resultant precipitate will be blue to black, not brown. It is helpful in this circumstance to use a Methyl Green counterstain that will enhance the black precipitate and avoid the confusion of color seen with some other counterstains.

Alkaline phosphatase acts on many substrates as well, each precipitating as a different color. For example, a combination of 5-bromo-4-chloro-3-indolyl phosphate (BCIP) and nitro blue tetrazolium (NBT) results in permanent blue precipitates at the site of the alkaline phosphatase localization. There are other compounds that can also be tried, such as Fast Red TR/Naphthol AS-MX (Sigma Chemical Co., St. Louis, MO) which precipitates as a red color.

The use of multiple chromogens and multiple enzymes has emerged as a process whereby numerous antigens can be identified with increased sensitivity. The sensitivity is increased through more substrate precipitation or greater color resolution. Sometimes, though, it is better to keep to simple methods when starting to work with these systems. The peroxidase and alkaline phosphatase enzymes are most widely used because they are easily controlled, the assays work, and experience creates many avenues for problem solving. The peroxidase enzyme system is highlighted in Chapters 25–27 because it is easy to consume the endogenous enzyme activity, the substrates are varied and obtainable, and the products are familiar and recognizable.

4. Enzyme Conjugation to Immunoglobulins

4.1. Direct Label Technique

Using an enzyme labeled primary antibody, a very quick direct assay is obtained. This assay may not be as sensitive as others, and may involve more background, but a labeled antibody can still be used if detection by other means is problematic. One example would be using a human-derived antibody to analyze a human sample. With a directly labeled antibody, a simple antibody incubation step followed by the enzyme–substrate combination, is all that is required. Labeling an immunoglobulin with an enzyme can be difficult. There can be problems with free enzyme sticking to the section, unlabeled antibody decreasing the sensitivity, and denaturation occurring, which creates labeled fragments that can interfere with the test.

In this technique, once the specimens have been prepared (*see* Chapters 8–14), the antibody solution at the appropriate dilution is applied. Following 30 min of incubation, extensive washing is performed before incubation with the chromogen. The washes should total 30 min. The antigen is then detected by incubation in the chromogenic substrate solution.

4.2. Indirect Label Technique

With this technique, the often numerous primary antibodies used do not all have to be labeled with enzyme, provided they are all of the same species to which a secondary antibody raised against immunoglobulin, will bind. The secondary antibody, labeled with enzyme, provides for the detection of all the primary antibodies without the need for them to be individually conjugated with enzyme. The problems of background and denaturation associated with conjugation are still present and can be troublesome. However, an increment of sensitivity, greater than that obtained by the previous method, can be achieved.

This method is about 50 min longer than the direct label technique as the primary antibody incubation is performed for 30 min with an unlabeled antibody directed against the antigen of interest. Following the washing steps, the labeled antibody must then be applied for 30 additional minutes followed by a slightly reduced, 20 min wash. The antigen is once again detected with substrate incubation. This process only works if the secondary antibody is reactive against the species from which the primary antibody was obtained and recognizes the primary antibody immunoglobulin type.

Amplification can be attained with this type of method by employing two indirect techniques simultaneously. After the specimen is thoroughly rinsed following the labeled secondary antibody incubation, a third antibody, which is enzyme labeled and reactive against the species of immunoglobulin responsible for the secondary antibody, may be used.

5. Enzyme Incorporation into Antibody-Rich Polymers

Immunepolymers have been utilized to avoid problems with endogenous biotin and still maintain a high sensitivity of detection. Now sold as biopolymers of varying sizes by a number of companies (Dako Inc. Carpinteria CA, Biocare Medical, Vector Laboratories), this immunoenzyme technique achieves both sensitivity and speed in a universal reagent. The secondary antibodies are attached to an inert polymer molecule labeled with horseradish peroxidase. These antibodies can be directed against both rabbit and mouse immunoglobulins. This technique requires only two steps and often does not require a protein blocking reagent. If needed, though, a universal non-serum blocking solution may be used. By allowing any monoclonal or polyclonal reagent to be detected with this one compound, and by achieving high levels of sensitivity with numerous incorporated enzyme molecules, this type of system becomes ideal for rapid turn-around situations while maintaining the sensitivity developed with the longer, more involved, techniques. This system is available as a kit, or as a single reagent, and the polymer/enzyme/antibody solution is ready to use.

6. Enzyme Incorporation in Immune Complexes

Other sandwich type techniques are entirely immunologic. The peroxidase-anti-peroxidase (PAP) technique (*see* Chapter 25) was developed to alleviate the problems of antibody conjugation with enzyme and also to amplify the number of enzyme molecules that can be directed to a given site. By making use of the proteinaceous antigenicity of the peroxidase enzyme, Sternberger developed an immune complex of enzyme and anti-enzyme (10). This complex in solution in a 3:2, enzyme:antibody molar ratio, allows enzyme incorporation through a linking antibody intermediate. The linking secondary antibody, produced in an alternate species, binds the primary antibody and the PAP complex provided they are from the same species used as the immunoglobulin antigen introduced to the species providing the secondary antibody.

The advantage of this technique over the indirect techniques is an increase in sensitivity. A slight disadvantage comes with the increased time taken for the three step procedure and a possible increase in background due to the increase in sensitivity. Time factors are not really an issue, though, because good reproducible results are desired regardless of the perceived inconvenience. The main problem with this type of assay is the need for PAP made from many species as quality primary antibodies are generated in rabbits, mice, guinea pigs, goats, rats, and sheep. Also, there are other methods that may provide more sensitivity than this method.

In addition to peroxidase mediated immunologic assays, there are also alkaline phosphatase-anti-alkaline phosphatase (APAAP) reagents available (11). The general overall principle governing these immunologic assays remains the same.

7. Enzyme Conjugation to High Affinity Molecules

The overriding problems seen with the direct and indirect techniques are the conjugation of a large enzyme to a large immunoglobulin while preventing denaturation, removing unconjugated species of both reagents, and preserving the normal function of both reagents. The more widespread means of labeling currently in use involves the vitamin biotin and the protein avidin. By biotinylating a compound, it can be linked to any other compound virtually irreversibly through an avidin intermediate. The use of the avidin D-biotin systems in the newer detection methods alleviates some of the problems cited above. These molecules are sufficiently small to prevent the problem of inactivation that is so common with large and cumbersome enzyme conjugations. Biotinylation is not a difficult process (*see* Chapter 7). There are numerous biotin labeling kits available commercially and many procedures adapted for coupling (12). Some allow for labeling to amino groups, and others to the sulfhydryl groups available on the immunoglobulin molecule. Initially, biotin conjugation to antibody was detected by enzyme conjugation to avidin, or avidin was used as an intermediary in a bridged avidin-biotin technique. The Avidin-Biotin Complex (ABC) molecule (*see* Chapter 26) was developed by Hsu and associates to increase the number of enzyme molecules available near any one antibody (13). Essentially, by biotinylating an enzyme and reacting that enzyme-labeled biotin with avidin, a complex consisting of four molecules of biotin for every avidin and two molecules of avidin for every biotin, builds. This complex, then, is able to bind the biotin attached to a secondary antibody.

Variations on this biotin binding sandwich technique involve the use of enzyme labeled streptavidin which is a compound with a lower isoelectric point than avidin D. The lower isoelectric point helps to prevent some charge mediated non-specific binding. Also, long-arm spacer biotinylated secondary antibodies, which help alleviate the steric hinderance of these giant complexes so near to the antibody, can be used. Labeled avidin techniques were developed that reduced the potential for steric hinderance. The notion that the more enzyme available at the antigen site, the more amplification, and the better the result, is generally true. With the ABC technique, though, the complex can get too large for proper localization. It is sometimes better to make the complex smaller and allow more of them to reach the biotin molecules on the antibody. This is the theory of the labeled avidin type systems. It is true that in some cases a smaller enzyme complex can provide an increased signal through greater resolution in detection.

This material represents the past and present of the most common enzyme mediated methods of antigen detection. There are alternate procedures available involving such methods as anti-biotin antibody steps that combine the avidin-biotin systems with a further anti-biotin/anti-enzyme sandwich for still greater increased sensitivity. Also, there are methods that follow a PAP procedure with a biotinylated antibody to the PAP immunoglobulin followed by ABC detection (14). The obvious problem created with this approach is the tremendous increase in the steps involved and the ever increasing difficulty associated with troubleshooting and quality control in such a system. But, for an individual assay in a research setting where utmost amplification is required, there are many combinations of methods and reagents which may be appropriate.

8. Detection of Precipitated Marker Molecules

In the ongoing quest for signal amplification, a catalyzed reporter molecule process was developed for immunoassays (15). This method was developed to accentuate the signal seen using an avidin-biotin type of detection. This process had application in formalin-fixed, paraffin-embedded tissue to increase the sensitivity to the point where, in combination with antigen recovery methods, compounds that were previously negative could be identified (16). The method uses a biotinylated tyramine which, when exposed to the oxidative effects of peroxidase on hydrogen peroxide, becomes radicalized and attaches covalently to electron rich amino acids in the vicinity of the peroxidase enzyme. The amount of biotin deposited at this site is tremendously enhanced as the enzyme action progresses. After a marker enzyme labeled avidin molecule is used to bind to the numerous biotin molecules present, the chromogenic substrate can be employed. By first using a detection molecule substrate, followed by the indicator molecule substrate, up to a 10,000-fold increase in sensitivity may be obtained with some tests. These types of detection substrate chemicals are available from DuPont NEN (TSA) and from the Dako Inc. Corporation (CSA) in kit form.

9. Conclusions

There are inherent problems associated with enzyme mediated methods, regardless of the method used. The right conditions must be met, of course, for the enzyme action to take place. Unlike fluorochromes or gold particles, (two other labeling compounds) enzymes need to act chemically for the assay to work. Also, the enzyme action must only represent the identified molecule. Endogenous enzyme or enzyme-like activity can create problems only realized in systems that use enzymes. Also, the use of enzymes demands more attention to detail because of the increase in sensitivity often obtained. The problem of unwanted reactivity is enhanced in enzyme-mediated reactions more so than in others, due, in part, to the additional level of sensitivity brought about by the continuous action on a substrate. There are certain specimen preparations, which create problems for some of the sandwich methods. Frozen or fresh cell preparations may have inherent avidin-binding properties as can some fixed preparations. While this should not preclude the use of these methods, one should be aware of the potential limitations and have alternate methodologies available for confirmatory testing.

Each enzyme method offers a unique feature that, under the right conditions, is the ideal choice. The direct method is advantageous in situations in which an anti-antibody step would be prohibitive. In this case, owing to the problems of directly-labeled enzyme, a better choice would perhaps be biotinylating the primary antibody and using labeled avidin or ABC for detection. If this is not possible because of the tissue being used, direct enzyme labels might be needed.

To quickly screen antibodies under consideration for use, an indirect method would be fine. However, once a reagent has been shown to be promising, a more powerful PAP or ABC system should be used to decrease potential background problems and boost sensitivity.

Among the sandwich techniques, the ABC is the most universal, with the PAP the least prone to non-specific staining. More sensitivity can be had with labeled avidin methods or the newer more inventive amplified amplifications. A universally applied method with an alternate technique available, like the PAP or labeled polymer methods for occasional problem specimens, will most often suffice for most laboratory situations.

Once a system is chosen, each facet of that system should be analyzed for potential problems. If the technology is understood, problem solving becomes easier. The simpler the system utilized, from the buffers and antibodies, to the enzyme and chromogen, the easier it is to investigate when things go awry, which unfortunately is always a possibility. When selecting a method, a system which has familiar technology should be chosen, performance tested on several known positive specimens, and positive and negative controls should always be performed with every assay to monitor performance.

References

1. Nakane P, Pierce G (1966) Enzyme-labeled antibodies: Preparation and application for the localization of antigens. J Histochem Cytochem 14:929–931
2. Farr A, Nakane P (1981) Immunohistochemistry with enzyme labeled antibodies: A brief review. J Immunol Meth 47:129–144
3. Swanson P (1988) Foundations of immunohistochemistry. Am J Clin Pathol 90:333–339
4. Ayala E, Martinez E, Enghardt M, Kim S, Murray R (1993) An improved cytomegalovirus immunostaining method. Lab Med 24:39–43
5. Sakanaka M, Magari S, Shibasaki T, Shinoda K, Kohno J (1988) A reliable method combining horseradish peroxidase histochemistry with immuno-β-Galactosidase staining. J Histochem Cytochem 36:1091–1096
6. Flugelman M, Jakitsch M, Newman K, Casscells S, Bratthauer G, Dichek D (1992) In vivo gene transfer into the arterial wall through a perforated balloon catheter. Circulation 85:1110–1117
7. Musiani M, Zerbini M, Plazzi M, Gentilomi G, LaPlaca M (1988) Immunocytochemical detection of antibodies to Epstein-Barr virus nuclear antigen by a streptavidin-biotin-complex assay. J Clin Microbiol 26: 1005–1008
8. Bos E, van der Doelan A, van Rooy N, Schuurs A (1981) 3,3',5,5'-tetramethylbenzidine as an Ames test negative chromogen for horseradish peroxidase in enzyme-immunoassay. J Immunoassay 2:187–204
9. Hsu S, Soban E (1982) Color modification of diaminobenzidine (DAB) precipitation by metallic ions and its application for double

immunohistochemistry. J Histochem Cytochem 30:1079–1082

10. Sternberger L (1979) Immunocytochemistry. Wiley, New York, NY
11. Hinglais N, Kazatchkine M, Mandet C, Appay M, Bariety J (1989) Human liver Kupffer cells express CR1, CR3, and CR4 complement receptor antigens. Lab Invest 61:509–513
12. Tse J, Goldfarb S (1988) Immunohistochemical demonstration of estrophilin in mouse tissues using a biotinylated monoclonal antibody. J Histochem Cytochem 36:1527–1531
13. Hsu S, Raine L, Fanger H (1981) Use of avidin-biotin-peroxidase complex (ABC) in immunoperoxidase techniques: A comparison between ABC and unlabeled antibody (PAP) procedures. J Histochem Cytochem 29: 577–580
14. Swanson P, Hagen K, Wick M (1987) Avidin-biotin-peroxidase-antiperoxidase (ABPAP) complex. Am J Clin Path 88:162–176
15. Bobrow MN, Litt GJ, Shaughnessy KJ, Mayer PC, Conlon J (1992) The use of catalyzed reporter deposition as a means of signal amplification in a variety of formats. J Immunol Meth 150:145–149
16. Merz H, Malisius R, Mannweiler S, Zhou R, Hartmann W, Orscheschek K, Moubayed P, Feller AC (1995) A maximized immunohistochemical method for the retrieval and enhancement of hidden antigens. Lab Invest 73:149–156

Chapter 25

The Peroxidase–Antiperoxidase (PAP) Method and Other All-Immunologic Detection Methods

Gary L. Bratthauer

Abstract

Immunoenzyme procedures take on many forms, including, simply, antibody coupled to enzyme. These direct techniques require the labeling of all the primary antibodies and can produce more background. A more economical method uses a secondary antibody or one that has the primary antibody as its antigen. Labeling this secondary antibody with enzyme provides detection for many primary antibodies directed against different antigens of interest. A more sensitive approach involves the use of antibodies directed against enzyme connected to same-species primary antibodies by a secondary linking antibody. This "all immunologic" technique is more sensitive and can result in less background than the covalently labeled methods. Finally, an immune polymer consisting of several secondary antibodies along with many enzyme molecules embedded on one long chain carbon polymer, can be used. This can provide a faster, more universal detection procedure with adequate sensitivity and specificity.

Key words: Direct assay, Indirect assay, Peroxidase–antiperoxidase method, Immune polymer, DAB chromagen, PBS buffer, TBS buffer

1. Introduction

These methods have, as an underlying unification, the sole use of antibody-antigen interaction to provide the binding of reagents, ultimately leading to the localization of enzyme at the site of cellular antigen. The earlier direct and indirect techniques, while still in use today, were found to be less sensitive than the later peroxidase–antiperoxidase (PAP) techniques. The newer immune complex polymer type of detection system increases the amplification with an indirect style of reaction, still keeping the binding entirely immunologic. Some of these techniques have been supplanted by the avidin-biotin binding methods which will follow in a later chapter. However, there are still times when a nonavidin/biotin

C. Oliver and M.C. Jamur (eds.), *Immunocytochemical Methods and Protocols*, Methods in Molecular Biology, Vol. 588, DOI 10.1007/978-1-59745-324-0_25, © Humana Press, a part of Springer Science+Business Media, LLC 1995, 1999, 2010

system is preferred. The following procedure highlights the PAP type of reaction, it being the most commonly used immunologic reaction method, and additional versions such as direct, indirect, and polymer types of procedures are discussed at the end of the chapter.

The PAP method was pioneered by Sternberger in 1979 *(1)*. The method uses an immunological sandwich amplification and the enzyme peroxidase to effect a signal. The unique feature of this procedure is the enzyme/antibody solution: the PAP immune complex. The horseradish peroxidase (HRP) enzyme, itself an immunogenic protein, is used to inoculate a given species, and a polyclonal immune response is generated against the enzyme. This antiserum is harvested and placed in solution with the enzyme so that immune complexes, which remain soluble, are formed. These complexes form with a molar ratio of two molecules of IgG to three molecules of enzyme. Furthermore, not only does this complex remain soluble, but the enzymatic activity of the peroxidase is not affected by the attached immunoglobulins. The antiperoxidase antibodies are from the same species as that which has produced a primary antibody raised against a tissue antigen. These two antibodies, one directed against the tissue antigen and the other directed against the peroxidase enzyme, can be linked by another antibody raised in an alternate species against the immunoglobulin from the first species (Fig. 1).

The peroxidase enzyme most often used is that found in the horseradish plant. HRP is a 40 kDa enzyme capable of stimulating an immune response. The principle of the technique is the same as in other immunolocalization techniques that provide a means of getting a marker molecule (the enzyme) in close proximity to an antigen through the use of antibodies. The difference in this technique is that the three step approach provides a further step in amplification, and this reaction is entirely based on

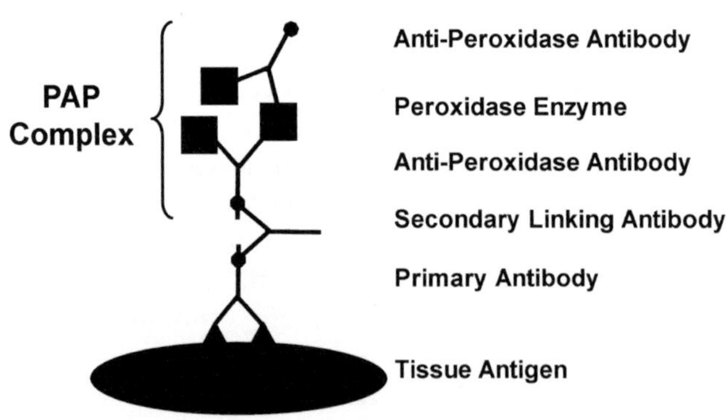

Fig. 1. Diagram illustrating the molecular interactions of the PAP procedure. The PAP complex is comprised of HRP bound to an antiperoxidase antibody generated in the same animal species as the primary antibody, which recognized the tissue antigen of interest. The primary antibody and the PAP complex are linked via a secondary antibody generated in a second animal species against immunoglobulin of the primary animal species (immunoglobulin; peroxidase enzyme).

immunologic binding. Without the need for the conjugation of a marker molecule to an antibody, reactivity can be achieved with less background and more sensitivity *(2)*. The only background problems occur as a result of the antibody binding nonspecifically; this can sometimes be corrected with the use of detergents and by more extensive washing steps. In cases where endogenous biotin binding capabilities preclude the use of the popular avidin–biotin complex (ABC) procedure (*see* Chapter 26), the PAP technique is a convenient alternative.

One disadvantage of the PAP method is that the primary antibody and the PAP complex must be from the same species. To have readymade PAP complexes from multiple species to accommodate the vast library of primary antibodies available is costly and unwieldy. In fact, a particular PAP complex may not be available for all primary antibody species although many exist for the most common ones. Also, the sensitivity is slightly less than that obtained by other technologies. However, for reducing background and for ease in problem solving, this technique is still quite effective.

Finally, a PAP assay system is nice to have available for detecting more than one antibody on an individual specimen. In double labeling experiments, having two completely different assay systems reduces the chances of cross-over reactivity. The first antigen can be detected using the standard ABC procedure (*see* Chapt. 26), and the second antigen can be detected using the PAP system. This way, no harsh acid treatments need to be performed to remove the first series of reagents in preparation for the second. By using PAP instead of ABC for the second antigen detection, there is no danger of binding to the biotin present on the secondary antibody used for the first antigen detection.

2. Materials

1. Gloves, gowns and masks.
2. Ultra low freezer (–70°C).
3. 45 L carboy.
4. Vortex.
5. Adjustable pipetman pipets with tips.
6. 4 mL glass Wheaton vials (Wheaton Science Products., Millville, NJ)
7. Humid chamber leveling tray with lid for horizontal antibody application.
8. Absorbent paper towels.

9. Staining racks and dishes for solution incubation.
10. Stirring block with stir bars.
11. Light microscope.
12. Coverslips.
13. Phosphate-buffered saline (PBS): 0.01 M sodium phosphate, 0.89% sodium chloride, pH 7.40 ± 0.05, or Tris-buffered saline (TBS plus, Biocare Medical Corporation, Concord, CA) (*see* Note 1).
14. 10 N sodium hydroxide and concentrated hydrochloric acid for adjusting pH.
15. PAP immune complex reagent (DakoCytomation Corporation, Carpinteria, CA).
16. Primary antibody reactive against the desired antigen from the same species as that used for the PAP immune complex (*see* Note 2).
17. A secondary linking antibody solution reactive against the immunoglobulin of the species responsible for the other two reagents.
18. 10% normal serum from the species from which the secondary antibody was generated in TBS or PBS.
19. Chromogen-substrate solution: 3,3'diaminobenzidine tetrahydrochloride (DAB) (Sigma-Aldrich, St. Louis, MO), 5 g bottle; 30% hydrogen peroxide (H_2O_2) (*see* Note 3).
20. 30% bleach in water.
21. Counterstain (e.g., Mayer's Hematoxylin).
22. 6 M ammonium hydroxide diluted 1:50 in deionized water.
23. 100% ethanol.
24. Xylene.
25. Permount mounting medium (Fisher Scientific, Pittsburgh, PA).

3. Methods

3.1. The Peroxidase–Antiperoxidase Method

Depending on the starting material, preantibody incubation steps may vary, and these are outlined in Chapters 8–14. The following assay begins with the removal of the slides from the overnight 10% normal serum incubation step. As the PAP is generally produced from rabbits, a good secondary antibody to use is an anti-rabbit antibody produced from swine. Therefore, the overnight serum incubation in this case would have been with 10% normal swine serum in PBS or TBS.

1. Align a humid staining chamber, leveling the slide bars, and adding water to the chamber (*see* Note 4).
2. Remove the slides from the dish of serum, and place them on the bars in the chamber. Cover the specimens with 10% normal swine serum in PBS or TBS, and replace the chamber cover.
3. Prepare the antibody solutions in PBS or TBS. If thawing out fresh frozen reagent, allow plenty of time for the aggregates to disperse; and likewise for any reconstitution of lyophilized material (*see* Note 2).
4. Blot off the 10% swine serum from each slide by placing the end of the slide on absorbent paper towels.
5. Add the primary rabbit antibody directed against the antigen desired to the slide, making sure to cover the entire specimen. Work quickly to avoid any drying. Cover the chamber and incubate for 30 min (*see* Note 5).
6. Rinse the specimens using PBS or TBS with wash bottle force or a siphon stream. Rinse for several seconds allowing the buffer to freely flow off the end of the slides sitting on the racks in the chamber. Repeat three times, allowing a min or two between subsequent washings to enable any nonspecifically adherent immunoglobulins to slowly diffuse away (*see* Note 6).
7. Blot off the excess buffer from each slide by placing the end of the slide on absorbent paper towels.
8. Add more 10% normal swine serum, covering the specimens to further guard against nonimmunologic binding. Cover the chamber and incubate for 10 min (*see* Note 7).
9. Rinse with buffer briefly, then add more 10% normal swine serum and cover the chamber for 10 min incubation.
10. Blot off the 10% swine serum from each slide by placing the end of the slide on absorbent paper towels.
11. Add the swine anti-rabbit IgG secondary antibody to the slide making sure to cover the entire specimen. Work quickly to avoid any drying. Cover the chamber and incubate for 30 min (*see* Note 8).
12. Rinse the specimens using PBS or TBS with wash bottle force or a siphon stream. Rinse for several seconds, allowing the buffer to freely flow off the end of the slides sitting on the racks in the chamber. Repeat three times, allowing a min or two between subsequent washings to enable any nonspecifically adherent immunoglobulins to slowly diffuse away.
13. Blot off the excess buffer from each slide by placing the end of the slide on absorbent paper towels.

14. Add the PAP complex to the slide making sure to cover the entire specimen. Work quickly to avoid any drying. Cover the chamber and incubate for 30 min.
15. Rinse the specimens using PBS or TBS with wash bottle force or a siphon stream. Rinse for several seconds, allowing the buffer to freely flow off the end of the slides sitting on the racks in the chamber. Repeat three times allowing a minute or two between subsequent washings to enable any nonspecifically adherent immunoglobulins to slowly diffuse away.
16. Place the slides in a staining slide rack and incubate for 10 min in a dish of PBS or TBS. Do not allow specimens to dry.
17. Prepare the chromogen solution (*see* Notes 3, 10).
18. Place the rack of slides into the chromogen solution, cover, and incubate for 15 min.
19. Remove the slide rack and wash in a dish with three changes of deionized water, for 2 min each time.
20. Counterstain with Mayer's hematoxylin for 1–5 min depending on the concentration and color intensity desired (*see* Note 9).
21. Rinse with deionized water, three changes, 2 min each time.
22. Develop the nuclei blue with a 10 s incubation in ammonium hydroxide in water.
23. Rinse with deionized water, three changes, 2 min each time.
24. Dehydrate the specimens with 100% ethanol, four changes, 2 min each time.
25. Clear the specimens with xylene, 4 changes, 2 min each time.
26. Coverslip with Permount, dry and observe. A positive reaction should be visible as a brown precipitate. The nuclei should be light blue (*see* Notes 10–11).

3.2. Additional Methods

3.2.1. Direct Assay

This test requires an antibody, which is labeled with enzyme directed against the compound of interest. Though expensive, less sensitive, and occasionally plagued with background problems, this type of assay is still used, especially in cases where, for example, a particular patient has an antibody reactive with a virus or endogenous protein; this antibody is then conjugated with enzyme from the patient's serum in order to be used on a cellular substrate. Also, these types of tests are performed as strictly detection methods. A popular marker molecule in use today is digoxigenin. Nucleic acid probes labeled with digoxigenin are often detected in situ or in vitro, using antibody enzyme conjugates directed against digoxigenin.*(3)* In performing these types of assays, the blocking serum or protein solution could be either the normal serum of the species providing the antibody or one of the many universal blocking solutions available commercially.

For the procedure, the conjugated antibody reagent in Subheading 3.1, step 5 should be used followed by step 7 to step 16. The time of incubation in DAB or other substrate should be closely monitored as this type of test can lead to false positive results if there is heavy background present.

3.2.2. Indirect Assay

This test requires that an antibody be directed against another species immunoglobulin, conjugated with a marker molecule such as HRP. These techniques are also not used very often, but some newer technologies use affinity purified reagents, which decrease the problems associated with free antibody or enzyme. Moreover, these reagents can be designed for detecting more than one antibody species. In this manner, a universal type of secondary detection system can be employed. One must be cautious of the synergistic effects of pooled immunoglobulin; but overall, these reagents can provide a rapid, very effective, nonbiotin type of reactivity using a universal antibody solution. In performing these kinds of assays, a species specific (if sole species antibody solutions are used) or universal (if antibodies from multiple species are used) blocking solution is utilized.

For the procedure, the conjugated anti-immunoglobulin reagent in Subheading 3.1, step 11 is used, followed directly by step 13 to step 16. Again, monitoring the DAB or other substrate development can be critical to a successful result.

3.2.3. Immune Polymer Assay

This newer type of indirect detection attaches the various immunoglobulins (reactive against the immunoglobulins of the most popular species used in these types of techniques) to a large inert polymer substance *(4)*. This polymer substance has HRP molecules embedded within it (Fig. 2). In this way, this compound can react with any primary antibody and provide a large amount of enzyme molecules to act towards signal production. One problem with the large size of the complex is resolution. However, for antigens in small amounts, the amplification achieved is worth the loss in resolution, especially if the antigen is not large enough in quantity to create the problem of over-reactive localization. A recent alternative to the use of large polymers is the use of antibodies conjugated to enzyme-laden small micropolymers (Vector Laboratories, Burlingame, CA). The use of smaller molecules allows for better resolution and increased sensitivity, according to the manufacturer.

These tests are also relatively fast, omitting the final immunoglobulin reagent, and are at least as sensitive as the three step procedures. In these assays a universal blocking solution may be required as some of the antibodies used for detection may be from multiple species. In some cases, a blocking step may not be

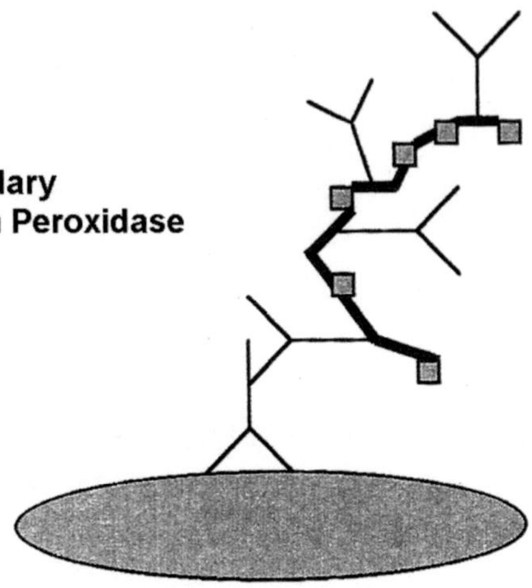

Fig. 2. Diagram illustrating the immune polymer method, Dako's Envision™. This is a two step, fast method, which allows the use of a more dilute primary antibody. The enzyme-containing polymer reagent is "universal" in that it contains anti-rabbit/mouse immunoglobulins and will bind to rabbit or mouse primary antibodies (immunoglobulin; □ peroxidase enzyme).

necessary because of the charge of the polymer. These types of tests are beneficial when time is an important factor.

For the procedure, use a polymer reagent in Subheading 3.1, step 11 is used, followed directly by step 13 to step 16. It should be remembered that it may not be necessary to block for nonspecific binding with this reagent. Therefore, following Subheading 3.1, step 7, one could go directly to step 11. Also, as this reagent is a commercially prepared one, no further dilution is required.

4. Notes

1. If large volumes of PBS are required, 45 L of a simple buffer with low ionic strength may be prepared as follows:
   (a) Weigh 50 g of sodium phosphate and 150 g of sodium chloride and dissolve in a 4 L flask, filled to within 100 mL of the 4 L mark.
   (b) Bring the pH of the solution to 6.8 with 10 N sodium hydroxide (about 20 mL).
   (c) Fill the remainder of the flask to 4 L and check the pH.
   (d) Dilute the flask to 45 L in carboy.
   (e) Mix well by shaking/rotating the carboy.
   (f) Remove a beaker of solution and check the pH; it should be close to 7.4. If it is not, adjust with appropriate volumes

vof hydrochloric acid or sodium hydroxide. The final pH of the 0.01 M PBS should be 7.40 ± 0.05.

Alternatively, for smaller volumes and convenience, PBS or TBS buffers may be commercially obtained.

2. Antibody solutions are made with PBS or TBS to a predefined dilution. These are experimentally determined on a known positive specimen. Usually, working antibody concentrations are in the range of 10–20 μg/mL. However, depending on the individual reagent, this concentration could vary considerably. For a beginning titration, start at 1:10, and do serial 1:10 dilutions resulting in 10, 100, 1,000, and 10,000-fold dilutions of concentrated or "neat" antibody. Assay a known positive specimen following the procedure, and examine the sections. Optimum results will occur within a range of the dilutions. Once a range is established, another titration can be performed within that range of 1:2 serial dilutions to better optimize the final dilution. The antibodies can be stored concentrated in aliquots in an ultra-low freezer at –70 to –80°C. However, it is unwise to store the PAP reagent in the freezer as the freeze/thaw process disrupts the immune complex and the enzyme. The other antibodies are stable in the freezer indefinitely but should be thawed once and used, not refrozen. If desired, antibodies can be thawed and diluted to a concentrated stock solution from which more dilute working solutions can be prepared. These stock solutions can be kept at 4 to 8°C for 1 week.
3. The chromogen, DAB, is a potential carcinogen and should be handled accordingly. For small operations, commercially available tablets or prediluted concentrates exist, designed to provide about 100 mL of reagent. These are preferred in those situations where there are few slides because of the reduced contact this type of prepared chromogen offers. However, for large volumes, or in case alterations to the procedure are desired, the following is one method of preparing the DAB chromogen:
   (a) Purchase DAB in 5 g bottles and store desiccated in a –20°C freezer;
   (b) Working in a fume hood and wearing the appropriate gloves, gown and mask, add PBS to the 5 g bottle, and mix until dissolved;
   (c) Add the contents of the 5 g DAB bottle to a 250 mL volumetric flask; fill to 250 mL with TBS or PBS, and mix by stirring;
   (d) Remove contents to a 500 mL beaker and pipet 4 mL volumes into 4 mL glass Wheaton vials with constant stirring;

(e) The 4 mL vials should be frozen at –70°C until use.

(f) Prepare the working solution in the fume hood by adding one 4 mL vial of DAB to 500 mL of TBS or PBS in a staining dish and then adding 400 µL of 30% H_2O_2. DAB should be prepared directly before use and kept covered in the hood as oxidation begins with the addition of H_2O_2 and will continue if the solution is exposed to the open air. This solution should be made fresh every day and should only be used for 3–4 h or for three racks of slides; it should be discarded when it turns a dark brown color. For a stronger and faster reaction, up to five times the recommended amount of DAB can be used. DAB is a potential carcinogen and should be treated as hazardous waste; 30% H_2O_2 is extremely caustic and can cause burns (*see* the slight variation on conditions in Note 6).

(g) The contaminated glassware and any spills should be cleaned up with a 30% bleach solution, or HRP and H_2O_2. Oxidation should be allowed to occur over 2 or 3 days before handling.

4. As with all immunological procedures, it is important to make sure the specimens stay hydrated throughout. Drying will result in nonspecific immunoglobulin binding. A level chamber rack is also important as in 30 min time, immunoglobulins may, with gravity, flow away from the specimen location.

5. Allow the antibody solutions and the slides to come to room temperature before applying them. Also make sure that the antibodies used are fully dissolved or reconstituted. Sometimes the results are better if the antibody solutions are prepared the day before and left at 4°C overnight. Slight vortexing before application helps to ensure proper solution. To increase reactivity, incubations can be extended in length or temperatures can be raised. This often increases background as well. Sometimes reaction intensity can be increased without background by overnight incubation with primary antibody, at 4°C *(5)*. The inconvenience of using a refrigerator, especially with large volumes of slides, makes room temperature incubations more attractive, and the reduced background benefit sometimes possible with overnight incubations is slight enough to be discounted.

6. Vigorous rinsing is required for reduction of background. Often, when assaying tissue sections that have been proteolytically digested or subjected to microwave retrieval methods, too vigorous a wash may cause the section to dislodge from the slide. Still, it is important to wash as thoroughly as possible. The wash stream should not directly splash the specimen surface as this may dislodge antibodies with low avidity. The

stream should initiate at one end of the slide, and the solution should flow rapidly across the slide surface. Washes are the most important aspect of background reduction and should therefore be extended if too much background is a problem. To reduce background further, 0.25% Triton X-100 or 0.1% Tween 20 (DakoCytomation Corporation, Carpinteria, CA) can be added to the PBS or TBS *(6)*. This will also reduce reactivity in some cases as the charge interactions of antibody-antigen binding will be altered. However, if the antibody has a high avidity, and other unwanted clones are present to a lesser degree, the addition of detergent can reduce background staining. Also, if poly-l-lysine coated or commercially available charged slides are used, it may be necessary to add this detergent to the buffer because of the hydrophobic nature of these slides. The results though, are generally better than with glue, and artifact free. Using prolonged antibody incubation times (60 min for the primary and 45 min for the secondary and PAP incubation steps) along with a compensation in chromogen concentration may offset the effects of the detergent on the signal. The chromogen concentration may be doubled or increased up to five times (0.08%) with a slightly reduced (12 min) incubation time without much increase in background as a result of detergent washes. If there is a substantial background, a preabsorption may be indicated. The antibody may be diluted in buffer containing 2% bovine serum albumin, secondary species serum (swine in the above example), or even 0.5% normal human serum if the contaminating clones are reactive against a serum-based constituent.

7. The 10% secondary species serum incubation allows for protein to bind to charged sites on the specimen. The additional 10 min incubations are extra protection against unwanted antibody sticking nonspecifically. The concentration of the serum solution and the time of incubation may be increased if desired. In some cases, the use of charged slides, pressure cooking with Reveal (Biocare Medical, Concord, CA) (*see* Chapter 13), and special buffer systems such as the TBS plus buffer with Tween 20 added, may alleviate the need for extensive normal serum blocks. Incubations in buffer may be substituted for the 10% serum incubations.

8. It is very important in PAP techniques for the secondary antibody to be applied in excess. This way, one arm of the divalent Fab portion of the immunoglobulin molecule can bind the primary antibody, while the other arm is free to bind the PAP complex. If not in excess, both arms of the molecule may bind the primary antibody creating a prozone-type of effect. Without a free secondary antibody Fab site to capture the PAP complex the assay will not work.

9. It is better if the counterstain is weak, as the principal reaction product may be masked by too much counterstain. Ideally, just enough hematoxylin to identify structure is all that is necessary.
10. These slides are permanent and should not fade with time. If the presence of endogenous pigment is a problem with a particular specimen, or a color other than brown is desired as an indicator, different chromogenic compounds can be used. The compound 3-amino-9-ethylcarbazole (AEC) can be used, for example, to create a red color product at the site of enzyme deposition. This compound can be purchased commercially in kit form and is also thought to be potentially carcinogenic. The AEC chromogen is prepared using the AEC substrate system, beginning at Subheading 3.1, step 17:
    (a) Place 2 mL of acetate buffer in a Wheaton vial.
    (b) Add one drop of AEC to the vial and mix.
    (c) Add one drop of H_2O_2 to the vial and mix.
    (d) Filter if necessary.

    A precipitate may develop which will not affect the results in any way and can be filtered out if desired. The procedure is continued with Subheading 3.1, step 18 in the method. The positive reaction product with this chromogen will be red, with the nuclei a light blue. Rather than being dehydratedin ethanol and xylene, the specimens should be allowed to dry; one drop of Crystal/Mount (Biomeda Corp, Foster City, CA) is added to the specimens, and they are baked in a 60°C oven for 30 min. This preparation is permanent and can be coverslipped with Permount if needed. The Crystal/Mount will form a hard plastic coating on the slide but can be damaged by smudging.

    As an alternative, 1 mL of 1% cobalt or nickel chloride can be added to the DAB solution prior to slide incubation, and the resultant precipitate will be dark blue to black, not brown *(7)*. This can increase the overall sensitivity of the reaction; but it is not popular because of the different color counterstain that is usually required. A 5% solution of Methyl Green used as a counterstain for 5 min provides enough contrast to the blue to be a good background for interpreting assays with a nuclear location. Also, many chromogenic kits are now available from multiple immunohistology companies. The directions are simple, and many color combinations can be achieved that are alcohol insoluble as well. These kits, however, generally provide only enough reagents for a few sections at a time.
11. To use a PAP technique with a mouse monoclonal antibody, the PAP complex must contain mouse immunoglobulin. A good secondary reagent is a rabbit anti mouse IgG, which

necessitates the use of normal rabbit serum for the nonspecific binding blocking solution. To enhance reactivity further, the assay may be repeated following the PAP step, from the secondary antibody step, essentially, reacting the PAP complex with a new secondary antibody incubation, followed by a renewed PAP localization reaction *(8)*.

References

1. Sternberger L (1979) Immunocytochemistry. Wiley, New York
2. Cerio R, MacDonald D (1988) Routine diagnostic immunohistochemical labeling of extracellular antigens in formol saline solution-fixed, paraffin-embedded cutaneous tissue. J Am Acad Dermatol 19:747–753
3. Roche Applied Science (2006) Anti-digoxigenin-POD, Fab fragments, package insert. Roche Diagnostics Corporation, Roche Applied Science, Indianapolis, IN. http://www.roche-applied-science.com/pack-insert/1333062a.pdf
4. Dako Corporation (2004) Dako Envision System Universal Kit Instructions. http://www.dakousa.com/prod_downloadpackageinsert.pdf?objectid=105441004
5. Clements J, Beitz A (1985) The effects of different pretreatment conditions and fixation regimes on serotonin immunoreactivity: a quantitative light microscopic study. J Histochem Cytochem 33:778–784
6. Laitinen L, Laitinen A, Panula P, Partanen M, Tervo K, Tervo T (1983) Immunohistochemical demonstration of substance P in the lower respiratory tract of the rabbit and not of man. Thorax 38:531–536
7. Hsu S, Soban E (1982) Color modification of diaminobenzidine (DAB) precipitation by metallic ions and its application for double immunohistochemistry. J Histochem Cytochem 30:1079–1082
8. Ordronneau P, Lindstrom P, Petrusz P (1981) Four unlabeled antibody bridge techniques: a comparison. J Histochem Cytochem 29: 1397–1404

Chapter 26

The Avidin–Biotin Complex (ABC) Method and Other Avidin–Biotin Binding Methods

Gary L. Bratthauer

Abstract

Immunoenzyme methods can be enhanced by the use of the high affinity molecules, avidin and biotin. The binding of avidin to biotin is almost irreversible. By labeling a detection enzyme such as horseradish peroxidase with biotin, and a secondary antibody (reactive against the antigen detecting primary antibody) with biotin as well, these two compounds can then be linked irreversibly with avidin. For this process, the biotinylated enzyme is complexed with avidin in solution and this avidin–biotin complex (ABC) is then introduced to the biotinylated secondary antibody, where it binds to primary antibody-antigen sites. Also, enzyme-labeled avidin molecules can be used to bind biotinylated secondary antibodies with greater resolution. Finally, biotinylated tyramide used in conjunction with peroxidase precipitates even greater amounts of biotin molecules for detection by enzyme-labeled avidin molecules.

Key words: Avidin, Biotin, Avidin–biotin complex (ABC), Labeled avidin binding (LAB), Biotinylated tyramide, TBS buffer, DAB chromogen

1. Introduction

These methods involve, at their core, the vitamin biotin and the protein avidin, which bind together irreversibly. By establishing a biotin link through avidin, between the horseradish peroxidase enzyme and a secondary antibody reagent, enzyme localization can be achieved at the site of primary antibody interaction with the specimen. These procedures are more universal than most purely immunologic techniques requiring only a biotinylated secondary antibody for each species of primary antibody used. The biotin molecule is small and can be easily conjugated to immunoglobulin by amino substitution at alkaline pH, without the loss of immunoglobulin activity. These secondary antibodies are quite inexpensive,

C. Oliver and M.C. Jamur (eds.), *Immunocytochemical Methods and Protocols*, Methods in Molecular Biology, vol. 588
DOI 10.1007/978-1-59745-324-0_26, © Humana Press, a part of Springer Science+Business Media, LLC 1995, 1999, 2010

readily available commercially, and reactive against immunoglobulin from a wide variety of species. The facts that the binding in this technique is not entirely immunologic, and is almost irreversible due to the high affinity of avidin for biotin, make this technique less prone to errors related to assay conditions than other purely immunologic techniques. While the sensitivity provided by these methods is generally better than that obtained with the peroxidase-anti-peroxidase (PAP) technique (*see* Chapter 25), sometimes due to fixation, or for other reasons, the sample may not be suitable for avidin–biotin methodology (1). Tissues may have endogenous biotin or possess biotin-like binding capabilities, which may result in non-specific binding. The irreversible nature of the binding also allows for the procedure to be undertaken with the most stringent of conditions. The conditions still need to be conducive to antigen-antibody binding, but the strong avidin–biotin interaction makes this procedure slightly more forgiving. The advantages of these techniques lie in the ease of finding suitable secondary reagents. If a primary antibody has been found to be reliable, regardless of the species there probably exists a biotinylated antibody reactive against it, or one could be easily engineered. The need for different PAP reagents appropriate to the primary species is removed (*see* Chapter 25).

The first method to incorporate avidin and biotin was the avidin–biotin complex (ABC) method. This method, described in 1981 by Hsu and associates, makes fundamental use of the covalent and irreversible binding seen between avidin, an egg white protein, and biotin, a vitamin (2). The horseradish peroxidase enzyme can incorporate many biotin molecules without the loss of enzymatic activity. Biotin can also be conjugated to immunoglobulin, which accepts the molecules, as did the enzyme, without the loss of apparent activity (3). The two biotin molecules can be joined via an avidin molecule by creating a complex of avidin and biotinylated enzyme and attaching it to the biotinylated secondary antibody. There are four binding sites for biotin on each avidin molecule and two binding sites for avidin on each biotin molecule. Together, the biotinylated enzyme and avidin molecules form a lattice complex and remain in solution. The ratio is such that there is always an available biotin binding site on the ABC for binding of the biotinylated secondary antibody (Fig. 1). This technology allows for more enzyme to be located at the antigen site through these ABCs, thus increasing the sensitivity. The ABC can also become so large that overall binding is decreased through steric hinderance. This can, in effect, decrease the resolution of the ABC technique.

Variations on the ABC technique can also be used to incorporate different enzymes that result in different chromogenic products. Alkaline phosphatase ABC is one example. The difficulty with this system is the consumption of endogenous alkaline

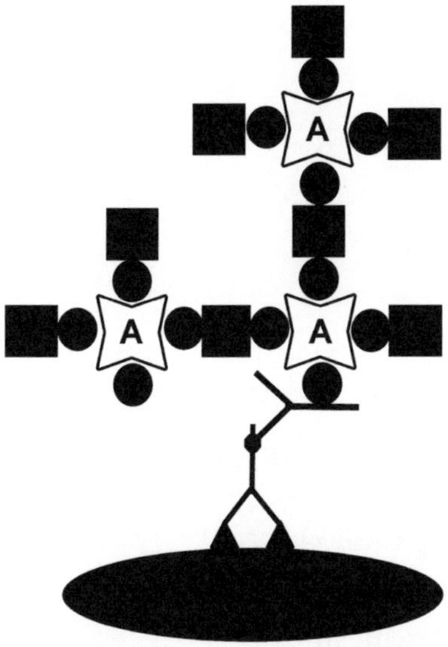

Fig. 1. Diagram illustrating the molecular interactions of the ABC procedure. The primary antibody against the antigen of interest is linked to the avidin-biotinylated peroxidase complex via a biotinylated secondary antibody raised against immunoglobulin of the animal species used to generate the primary antibody (immunoglobulin; ● biotin; A avidin; ■ peroxidase).

phosphatase, which is more prevalent than peroxidase and harder to remove. However, the alkaline phosphatase enzyme does provide more product per unit than does peroxidase and is therefore a slightly more sensitive means of detection. Endogenous alkaline phosphatase can be blocked by incubation in 3 mM levamisole for 15 min, but some enzyme may escape consumption. Alkaline phosphatase has many substrates too, the most popular being BCIP/NBT, which precipitates to a dark blue (*see* Chapter 24).

Finally, an ABC assay system is useful for detecting more than one antibody on an individual specimen. In double labeling, experiments having two completely different assay systems reduce the chances of cross-over reactivity. The first antigen can be detected with the standard ABC procedure, and the second antigen is then detected using the PAP system (*see* Chapter 25). The two technologies provide less chance of cross-over detection, especially if alkaline phosphatase is employed along with the peroxidase enzyme (4).

This method, either standard or "elite" (increased molar ratio), still remains one of the most widely used of the immunocytochemistry methods being performed today and will be the main subject of this chapter. There are other methods, though, that are being used with increased frequency. The labeled avidin binding (LAB) method, sometimes called the streptavidin binding method and a newer catalyzed amplification method that uses avidin, biotin, peroxidase, and a biotinyl tyramide to achieve even more sensitivity, will be discussed at the end of this chapter.

2. Materials

1. Gloves, gowns and masks.
2. Ultra low freezer (–70°C).
3. 45 L carboy.
4. Vortex.
5. Adjustable pipetman pipets with tips.
6. 4 mL glass Wheaton vials (Wheaton Scientific Inc., Millville, NJ)
7. Humid chamber leveling tray with lid, for horizontal antibody application.
8. Absorbent paper towels.
9. Staining racks and dishes for solution incubation.
10. Stirring block with stir bars.
11. Light microscope.
12. Coverslips.
13. Tris-buffered saline (TBS plus, Biocare Medical Corporation, Concord, CA) or phosphate-buffered saline (PBS): pH 7.40–7.8 (TBS) (*see* Note 1).
14. 10 N sodium hydroxide and concentrated hydrochloric acid for adjusting pH.
15. Primary antibody reactive against the desired antigen (*see* Note 2).
16. A secondary antibody labeled with biotin, which is reactive against the species of immunoglobulin used for the primary reagent.
17. 10% normal serum in PBS from the species from which the secondary antibody was generated (For this example: horse serum).
18. Avidin–biotin complex horseradish peroxidase reagent (Vectastain ABC HRP Kit, Vector Laboratories, Inc., Burlingame, CA).
19. Chromogen-substrate solution: 3, 3'diaminobenzidine tetrahydrochloride (DAB) (Sigma-Aldrich., St. Louis, MO), 5 g bottle; 30% hydrogen peroxide (H_2O_2) (*see* Note 3).
20. 30% bleach in water.
21. Counterstain (e.g., Mayer's Hematoxylin).
22. 6 M ammonium hydroxide diluted 1:50 in deionized water.
23. 100% ethanol.
24. Xylene.
25. Permount mounting medium (Fisher Scientific, Pittsburgh, PA).

3. Methods

3.1. The Avidin–Biotin Complex Method

Depending on the starting material, preantibody incubation steps may vary, and are outlined in Chapters 8–14. The following assay begins with the removal of the slides from the overnight 10% normal serum incubation step. Since the ABC technique is universal in application, and a biotinylated secondary antibody exists for virtually any primary antibody, this protocol will assume a monoclonal assay with a primary antibody from a mouse hybridoma. A good secondary antibody to use in this situation is a biotinylated anti-mouse antibody made in horse. Therefore, the overnight serum incubation in this case would have been with 10% normal horse serum in TBS or PBS (*see* Notes 4 and 15).

1. Align a humid staining chamber, leveling the slide bars, and adding water to the chamber (*see* Note 6).
2. Remove the slides from the dish of serum and place them on the bars in the chamber. Cover the specimens with 10% normal horse serum and replace the chamber cover.
3. Prepare the antibody solutions in TBS or PBS. If thawing out fresh frozen reagent, allow plenty of time for aggregates to disperse; likewise for any reconstitution of lyophilized material (*see* Note 2).
4. Blot off the 10% horse serum from each slide by placing the end of the slide on absorbent paper towels.
5. Add the primary monoclonal antibody directed against the antigen desired to the slide making sure to cover the entire specimen. Work quickly to avoid any drying. Cover the chamber and incubate for 30 min (*see* Note 7).
6. Rinse the specimens using TBS or PBS with wash bottle force or a siphon stream. Rinse for several seconds, allowing the buffer to freely flow off the end of the slides sitting on the racks in the chamber. Repeat three times allowing 1 or 2 min between subsequent washings to enable any nonspecifically adherent immunoglobulins to slowly diffuse away (*see* Note 8).
7. Blot off the excess buffer from each slide by placing the end of the slide on the absorbent paper towels.
8. Add more 10% normal horse serum covering the specimens to further guard against nonimmunologic binding. Cover the chamber and incubate for 10 min (*see* Note 4).
9. Rinse with buffer, briefly, then add more 10% normal horse serum and cover the chamber for 10 min incubation.
10. Blot off the 10% horse serum from each slide by placing the end of the slide on the absorbent paper towels (*see* Note 9).

11. Add the biotinylated horse anti-mouse IgG secondary antibody to the slide making sure to cover the entire specimen. Work quickly to avoid any drying. Cover the chamber and incubate for 30 min (*see* Notes 5 and 10).
12. Prepare the ABC reagent according to the manufacturer's instructions. For Vector Laboratories Vectastain Elite kit, add two drops of reagent A to 5 mL of TBS or PBS, and then add two drops of reagent B. Mix and incubate for 30 min at room temperature. Greater volumes may be prepared, if the ratio of reagents is kept constant.
13. Rinse the specimens using TBS or PBS with wash bottle force or a siphon stream. Rinse for several sec, allowing the buffer to flow freely off the end of the slides sitting on the racks in the chamber. Repeat three times, allowing 1 or 2 min between subsequent washings to enable any nonspecifically adherent immunoglobulin to slowly diffuse.
14. Blot off the excess buffer from each slide by placing the end of the slide on the absorbent paper towels.
15. Add the ABC to the slide making sure to cover the entire specimen. Work quickly to avoid any drying. Cover the chamber and incubate for 30 min.
16. Rinse the specimens using TBS or PBS with wash bottle force or a siphon stream. Rinse for several seconds allowing the buffer to flow freely off the end of the slides sitting on the racks in the chamber. Repeat three times, allowing 1 or 2 min between subsequent washings to enable any nonspecifically adherent immunoglobulin to slowly diffuse.
17. Place the slides in a staining slide rack and incubate for 10 min in a dish of TBS or PBS. Do not allow specimens to dry.
18. Prepare the DAB chromogen solution (*see* Note 3).
19. Place the rack of slides into the DAB dish, cover, and incubate for 10–15 min.
20. Remove the slide rack and wash in a dish with three changes of deionized water, for 2 min each.
21. Counterstain with Mayer's hematoxylin 1–5 min, depending on the concentration and color intensity desired (*see* Note 11).
22. Rinse with deionized water, three changes, 2 min each.
23. Develop the nuclei blue with 10 s incubation in ammonium hydroxide in water.
24. Rinse with deionized water, three changes, 2 min each.
25. Dehydrate specimens with 100% ethanol, four changes for 2 min each.
26. Clear specimens with xylene, four changes, for 2 min each.

27. Coverslip with Permount, dry and observe (*see* Note 12). Positive reaction should be visible as a brown precipitate. The nuclei should be light blue.

3.2. Additional Methods

3.2.1. Labeled Avidin Binding Assay

The LAB method provides even more sensitivity than the other popular immunohistochemistry methods (5). The technological change seen with this method is that the enzyme peroxidase is covalently linked directly to the avidin molecule. This enhances sensitivity since the avidin molecule can be labeled extensively with enzyme and the complex remains relatively small. The small size enables many avidin molecules to bind to the biotinylated secondary antibody (6). In addition, the biotin is more accessible since it is positioned on a long carbon arm extension from the secondary antibody, reducing steric hinderance (Fig. 2). With the numerous enzyme-labeled avidin molecules able to attach to any biotin on the secondary antibodies, the sensitivity and the resolution of this technique are superior (7). The avidin molecule in use in this system is generally obtained from *Streptomyces avidinii* bacteria and is called streptavidin, a molecule with a more neutral pH and a reduced tendency toward inappropriate binding (8). There is also another form of avidin developed by Belovo Chemicals called Neutralite Avidin (available from Accurate Chemical and Scientific Corp., Westbury, NY). This avidin molecule has been engineered without sugar residues and modified to have a neutral isoelectric point. When properly labeled with an enzyme marker, this molecule should have a lower tendency to bind nonspecifically to charged sites on the specimen. In addition, like the ABC method,

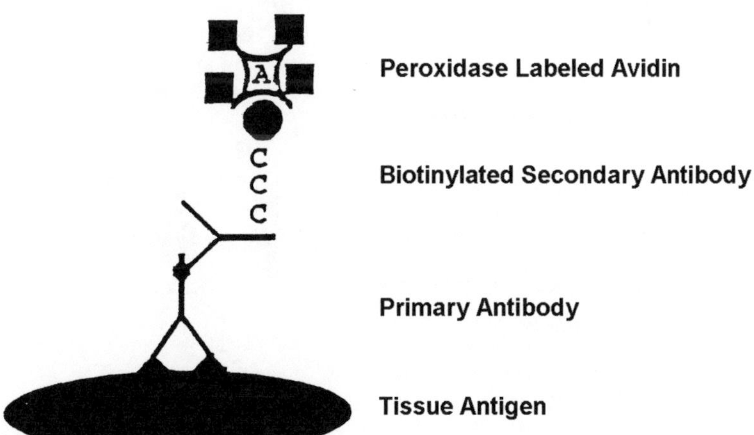

Fig. 2. Diagram illustrating the molecular interactions of the LAB procedure. Horseradish peroxidase is covalently linked to avidin. The primary antibody against the antigen of interest is linked to the enzyme labeled avidin complex (LAB) via a biotinylated secondary antibody raised against immunoglobulin of the animal species used to generate the primary antibody (immunoglobulin; CCC long carbon arm extension; • biotin; A avidin; ▪ peroxidase).

there are alkaline phosphatase labeled streptavidin molecules that can be used to provide different chromogenic products.

For this procedure, a secondary antibody labeled with a long arm spacer biotin reactive against the species of immunoglobulin used for the primary reagent (Kirkegaard & Perry Laboratories, Inc., Gaithersburg, MD) is needed. This reagent is used in Subheading 3.1, step 11 of the above method.

Then, the peroxidase-labeled streptavidin (Kirkegaard & Perry) reagent is used in Subheading 3.1, step 15. Note: The labeled streptavidin is added at the appropriate dilution, which must be experimentally determined (*see* Note 2). It need not be prepared a minimum of 30 min in advance like the ABC reagent.

3.2.2. Amplified Biotin Substrate Assay

The amplified biotin methods involve the use of biotinylated tyramide, which, when subjected to peroxidase enzyme, deposits biotin at the enzyme site. (9) This reagent can be utilized in any detection method incorporating peroxidase. Following the biotin deposition that occurs when this reagent is used in place of DAB or some other chromogen, an additional avidin-enzyme reagent would be employed (Fig. 3). This reagent would bind to all of the deposited biotin, and detection with a subsequent chromogen could increase the sensitivity 1,000-fold. The tremendous increase in sensitivity may require considerable manipulation of an already established technique. Also, the resolution will be far worse than with the ABC type of procedure. However, if used for instances in which the sought-after antigen is in very small quantity, the

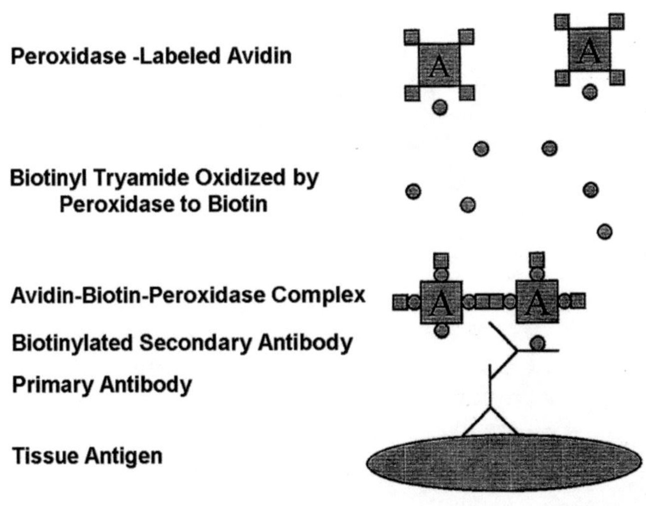

Fig. 3. Diagram illustrating the amplified biotin substrate method. The biotinyl tyramide compound TSA forms biotin when oxidized by peroxidase. The deposition of biotin in the vicinity of the original ABC reagent allows for further amplification by the addition of peroxidase-labeled avidin or more ABC, followed by substrate (immunoglobulin; • biotin; A avidin; ■ peroxidase).

decreased resolution will not be a factor and the increase in sensitivity may allow for the detection of otherwise undetectable substances.

For the procedure, add the biotinyl tyramide (Dupont NEN, Boston, MA; Dako, Carpenteria, CA or Perkin Elmer, Life Science Research, Waltham, MA) solution in place of the DAB solution in Subheading 3.1, step 19 and incubate for 15 min. Rinse as in Subheading 3.1, step 16. Then, return to Subheading 3.1, step 15, and add more ABC solution, or a labeled streptavidin compound. Continue with the procedure from there.

The added steps will increase the overall turn-around time for these procedures, but the potential identification of previously undetectable substances is worth the extra hour or so.

There are other alterations as well to the basic procedures outlined in these chapters that involve combinations of all of these methods, allowing further amplification through the use of antibodies to biotin, avidin or both. For example, a biotinylated antibody can be recognized by an anti-biotin antibody and a linking reagent can be used to bind the anti-biotin antibody to a PAP type of complex. Or, a secondary biotinylated antibody can be employed following the anti-biotin step which could then result in an ABC means of detection. Alternatively, an anti-avidin may be used to further amplify a LAB technique. With each successive step a greater level of amplification can be achieved. However, the possibility of higher background and poorer resolution from severe steric hinderance is also increased.

4. Notes

1. If large volumes of PBS are required, 45 L of a simple buffer with low ionic strength may be prepared as follows:
   (a) Weigh 50 g of sodium phosphate and 150 g of sodium chloride and dissolve in a 4 L flask, filled to within 100 mL of the 4 L mark.
   (b) Bring the pH of the solution to 6.8 with 10 N sodium hydroxide (about 20 mL).
   (c) Fill the remainder of the flask to 4 L and check the pH.
   (d) Dilute the flask to 45 L in carboy.
   (e) Mix well by shaking/rotating the carboy.
   (f) Remove a beaker of solution and check the pH. It should be close to 7.4. If it is not, adjust with appropriate volumes of hydrochloric acid or sodium hydroxide. The final pH of the 0.01 M PBS should be 7.40 ± 0.05.

Alternatively, for smaller volumes and convenience, PBS or TBS buffers may be commercially obtained. These buffers should be prepared according to the manufacturer's recommendations and usually make up 5 L of solution.

2. Antibody solutions are made with TBS or PBS to a predefined dilution. These are experimentally determined on a known positive specimen. Usually, working antibody concentrations are in the range of 10–20 μg/mL. However, depending on the individual reagent, this concentration could vary considerably. For a beginning titration, start at 1:10 and do serial 1:10 dilutions resulting in 10, 100, 1,000, and 10,000-fold dilutions of concentrated or "neat" antibody. Immunoassay a known positive specimen, following the procedure, and examine the sections. Optimum results will occur within a range of the dilutions. Once a range is established another titration can be performed within that range of 1:2 serial dilutions to better optimize the final dilution. The antibodies can be stored concentrated in aliquots in an ultra-low freezer at –70 to –80°C. Antibodies are stable in the freezer indefinitely, but should be thawed once and used, not refrozen. However, the manufacturer recommends that the ABC reagent components be stored in the refrigerator. If desired, antibodies can be thawed and diluted to a concentrated stock solution from which more dilute working solutions can be prepared. These stock solutions can be kept at 4–8°C for a week.
3. The chromogen, DAB, is a potential carcinogen and should be handled accordingly. For small operations, commercially available tablets or prediluted concentrates exist, designed to provide about 100 mL of reagent. These are preferred in those situations where there are few slides because of the reduced contact this type of prepared chromogen offers. However, for large volumes, or in case alterations to the procedure are desired, the following is one method of preparing the DAB chromogen:
   (a) DAB is purchased in 5 g bottles and stored desiccated in a –20°C freezer.
   (b) Working in a fume hood, and wearing the appropriate gloves, gown and mask, add TBS or PBS to the 5 g bottle and mix until dissolved.
   (c) Add the contents of the 5 g DAB bottle to a 250 mL volumetric flask, bring the volume to 250 mL with TBS or PBS and mix by stirring.
   (d) Remove the contents to a 500 mL beaker, and pipet 4 mL volumes to 4 mL glass Wheaton vials, with constant stirring.
   (e) The 4 mL vials should be frozen at –70°C until used.

(f) In the fume hood, add one 4 mL vial of DAB to 500 mL of TBS or PBS in a staining dish, and then add 400 μL of 30% H_2O_2. DAB should be prepared directly before use and kept covered in the hood as oxidation begins with the addition of H_2O_2 and will continue with the exposure to the open air. This solution should be freshly prepared everyday and should only be used for 3–4 h or for three racks of slides, and discarded when it turns to a dark brown color. For a stronger and faster reaction, up to five times the recommended amount of DAB can be used. DAB is a potential carcinogen and should be treated as hazardous waste, and 30% H_2O_2 is extremely caustic and can cause burns. For slight variation in conditions *see* Note 6.

(g) The contaminated glassware and any spills should be cleaned up with a 30% bleach solution, or horseradish peroxidase and H_2O_2. Oxidation should be allowed to occur over 2–3 days before handling.

4. The 10% secondary species serum incubation allows for protein to bind to charged sites on the specimen. The additional 10 min incubations are extra protection against unwanted antibody sticking nonspecifically. The concentration of the serum solution and the time of incubation may be increased if desired. In some cases, the use of charged slides, pressure cooking with Reveal (Biocare Medical, Concord, CA) (*see* Chapter 13), and special buffer systems such as the TBS plus buffer from Biocare Medical with Tween 20 added, may alleviate the need for extensive normal serum blocks. Incubations in buffer may be substituted for the 10% serum incubations.

5. Many biotinylated secondary antibodies from various species reactive against various species immunoglobulin can now be pooled. Some manufacturers provide pooled or universal secondary reagents that can be used regardless of the primary antibody species. The only requirement is that a universal type of blocking serum also be used if the secondary antibody has multiple host species so cross-reactivity will not occur. The various manufacturers also provide these blocking agents, which are protein, milk, or casein-based solutions. While this provides convenience, it does not always produce better results. A universal secondary antibody derived from the same host species is preferred.

6. As with all immunological procedures, it is important to make sure the specimens stay hydrated throughout. Drying will result in nonspecific immunoglobulin binding. A level chamber rack is also important since, in 30 min time, antibodies may flow with gravity away from the specimen location.

7. Allow the antibody solutions and the slides to come to room temperature before applying. Also make sure that the antibodies used are fully dissolved or reconstituted. Sometimes, the results are better if the antibody solutions are prepared the day before and left at 4°C overnight. Slight vortexing before application helps to ensure proper solution. To increase reactivity, incubations can be extended in length, or temperatures can be raised. This often increases background as well. Sometimes reaction intensity can be increased without background by incubation with primary antibody overnight at 4°C (10). The inconvenience of using a refrigerator, especially with large volumes of slides, makes room temperature incubations more attractive; the reduced background benefit, sometimes possible with overnight incubations, is slight enough to be discounted.
8. Vigorous rinsing is required for reduction of background. Often, when assaying tissue sections that have been proteolytically digested or subjected to heat retrieval methods, too vigorous of a wash may cause the section to dislodge from the slide. Still, it is important to wash as thoroughly as possible. The wash stream should not directly splash the specimen surface as this may dislodge antibodies with low avidity. The stream should initiate at one end of the slide and the solution should flow rapidly across the slide surface. Washes are the most important aspect of background reduction and should therefore be extended if too much background is a problem. To further reduce background, 0.25% Triton X-100 or 0.1% Tween 20 (DakoCytomation Corporation, Carpinteria, CA) can be added to the buffer (11). This will also in some cases reduce reactivity as the charge interactions of antibody-antigen binding will be altered. However, if the antibody has a high avidity and other unwanted clones are present to a lesser degree, the addition of detergent can reduce background staining. Also, if poly-L-lysine-coated or commercially available charged slides are used, it may be necessary to add this detergent to the buffer due to the hydrophobic nature of these slides. The results though, are generally better than with glue, and are artifact-free. Using prolonged antibody incubation times (60 min for the primary and 45 min for the secondary and ABC incubation steps) and compensation in chromogen concentration may offset the effects of the detergent on signal. The chromogen concentration may be doubled or increased up to five times (0.08%) with a slightly reduced (12 min) incubation time without much increase in background due to detergent washes. If there is substantial background, a preabsorbtion may be indicated (*see* Chapter 5). The antibody may be diluted in buffer containing 2%

bovine serum albumin, or secondary species serum (horse in the above example), or even 0.5% normal human serum, if the nonspecific contaminating antibodies are reactive against a serum-based constituent.

9. Some tissue samples, especially fresh or frozen ones, can have intrinsic biotin binding capabilities that must first be blocked before using an ABC type of detection. The simple Avidin-Biotin Blocking Kit from Vector Laboratories can be used to add avidin to the specimen to bind biotin, followed by biotin to bind avidin. Incubations of 15 min with brief TBS or PBS rinses should suffice.
10. The ABC complex requires 30 min to form. Make sure the complex is prepared before the secondary antibody addition so it has time to build. The complex is stable in the refrigerator for 72 h.
11. It is better if the counterstain is weak since the principal reaction product may be masked by too much counterstain. Ideally, just enough hematoxylin to identify structure is all that is necessary.
12. These slides are permanent and should not fade with time. If the presence of endogenous pigment is a problem with a particular specimen, or a color other than brown is desired as an indicator, different chromogenic compounds can be used. The compound 3-amino-9-ethylcarbazole (AEC) can be used, for example, to create a red color product at the site of enzyme deposition. This compound can be purchased commercially in kit form, and is also thought to be potentially carcinogenic. Using the AEC substrate system, begin at Subheading 3.1, **step 18** and prepare the AEC chromogen as follows:
    a. Place 2 mL of acetate buffer in a Wheaton vial.
    b. Add one drop of AEC to the vial and mix.
    c. Add one drop of H_2O_2 to the vial and mix.
    d. Filter if necessary. A precipitate may develop, which will not affect the results in any way, but can be filtered out if desired. Apply to the specimen, making sure to cover the specimen and incubate for 15 min and continue with the protocol. Instead of dehydrating in alcohol and xylene, allow specimens to dry, add one drop of Crystal/Mount to each and heat in a 60°C oven for 30 min. This preparation is permanent and can be coverslipped with Permount if needed. The Crystal/Mount will form a hard plastic coating on the slide but can be damaged by smudging. The positive reaction product with this chromogen will be red and the nuclei a light blue.

As an alternative, 1 mL of 1% cobalt or nickel chloride can be added to the DAB solution prior to slide incubation, and the resultant precipitate will be dark blue to black, not brown (12). This can increase the overall sensitivity of the reaction, but is not popular because of the different color counterstain that is usually required. A 5% solution of Methyl Green used as a counterstain for 5 min provides enough contrast to the blue to be a good background for interpreting assays with a nuclear location. Also, many chromogenic kits are now available from multiple immunohistology companies. The directions are simple and many color combinations can now be achieved that are alcohol insoluble as well. These kits, however, generally provide only enough reagents for a few sections at a time.

References

1. Hsu S, Raine L (1981) Protein A, avidin, and biotin in immunohistochemistry. J Histochem Cytochem 29:1349–1353
2. Hsu S, Raine L, Fanger H (1981) The use of avidin-biotin-peroxidase complex (ABC) in immunoperoxidase technique – a comparison between ABC and unlabeled antibody (PAP) procedures. J Histochem Cytochem 29: 577–580
3. Guesdon J, Ternynck T, Avrameas S (1979) The use of avidin-biotin interaction in immunoenzymatic techniques. J Histochem Cytochem 27:1131–1139
4. Gillitzer R, Berger R, Moll H (1990) A reliable method for simultaneous demonstration of two anitgens using a novel combination of immunogold – silver staining and immunoenzymantic labeling. J Histochem Cytochem 38:307–313
5. Elias J, Margiotta M, Gabore D (1989) Sensitivity and detection efficiency of the peroxidase antiperoxidase (PAP), avidin-biotin complex (ABC), and the peroxidase-labeled avidin-biotin (LAB) methods. Am J Clin Pathol 92:62–67
6. Leary J, Brigati D, Ward D (1983) Rapid and sensitive colormetric method for visualining biotin-labeled DNA probes hybridized to DNA or RNA immobilized on nitrocellulose. Proc Natl Acad Sci USA 80:4045–4049
7. Milde P, Merke J, Ritz E, Haussler M, Rauterberg E (1989) Immunohistochemical detection of 1, 25-dihydroxyvitamin D3 receptors and estrogen receptors by monoclonal antibodies: comparison of four immunoperoxidase methods. J Histochem Cytochem 37:1609–1617
8. Ayala E, Matinez E, Enghardt M, Kim S, Murray R (1993) An improved cytomegalovirus immunostaining method. Lab Med 24:39–43
9. Bobrow MN, Litt GJ, Shaughnessy KJ, Mayer PC, Conlon J (1992) The use of catalyzed reporter deposition as a means of signal amplification in a variety of formats. J Immunol Methods 150:145–149
10. Clements J, Beitz A (1985) The effects of different pretreatment conditions and fixation regimes on serotonin immunoreactivity: a quantitative light microscopic study. J Histochem Cytochem 33:778–784
11. Laitinen L, Laitinen A, Panula P, Partanen M, Tervo K, Tervo T (1983) Immunohistochemical demonstration of substance P in the lower respiratory tract of rabbit and not of man. Thorax 38:531–536
12. Hsu S, Soban E (1982) Color modification of diaminobenzidine (DAB) precipitation by metallic ions and its application for double immunohistochemistry. J Histochem Cytochem 30:1079–1082

Chapter 27

Avidin-Biotin Labeling of Cellular Antigens in Cryostat-Sectioned Tissue

Mark Raffeld and Elaine S. Jaffe

Abstract

Advances in immunohistochemical technologies have greatly improved the ability to visualize antigens in formalin-fixed paraffin-embedded tissues. Nonetheless, there are occasions in which there may be no alternative to the use of cryostat-sectioned frozen tissues. While the basic chemistries and techniques used in staining cryostat-sectioned tissues are identical to those employed for staining paraffin-embedded sections, there are some unique issues to consider with frozen sections. Achieving excellent results requires the use of properly prepared and stored frozen tissue blocks embedded in an appropriate mounting compound, properly prepared and mounted cryostat-prepared sections, blocking of endogenous biotin and peroxidases that might interfere with interpretation of specific staining, and a mild postsectioning fixation step. This chapter describes a general frozen-section immunostaining procedure that provides guidelines for handling these special considerations.

Key words: Frozen section immunohistochemistry, Avidin-biotin complex (ABC), Diaminobenzedine (DAB), Monoclonal antibodies, Polyclonal antibodies

1. Introduction

Immunohistochemical staining techniques are widely used for the identification of a variety of diverse antigens in paraffin-embedded tissues (1). Nonetheless, a limitation in the use of paraffin-embedded fixed tissue is that many potentially interesting antigens are denatured and their antigenicity destroyed by the process of tissue fixation. To overcome this problem, many laboratories employ the use of cryostat-cut frozen sections (2–4). The principles of the staining reactions are identical to those used for paraffin sections, and the antigenicity of the majority of cellular proteins and carbohydrate moieties are preserved. The frozen section technique, however, has its own drawbacks. Special equipment is needed for freezing, cutting, and storing the frozen tissue blocks. Second,

C. Oliver and M.C. Jamur (eds.), *Immunocytochemical Methods and Protocols*, Methods in Molecular Biology, Vol. 588, DOI 10.1007/978-1-59745-324-0_27, © Humana Press, a part of Springer Science+Business Media, LLC 1995, 1999, 2010

good morphologic detail requires greater skill in cutting the tissue sections and careful attention to particular steps in the procedure (*see* Subheading 3). Even under optimal conditions, the morphology of the immunostained frozen section will be inferior to the morphology obtained from paraffin-embedded fixed tissue.

As previously mentioned, the principles of staining are identical to those used in paraffin sections. The techniques used may be direct or indirect methods as described in Chapters 16–19. Indirect techniques are generally more sensitive and, therefore, preferable. Indirect techniques can be broken down into three steps. In the first step, an antibody directed against the antigen of interest is applied to the tissue section. In the second step, a labeled secondary antibody directed against the first antibody is applied. The last step consists of a detection step that is composed of linking the secondary antibody to a detection system and an enzymatic reaction that converts a substrate to a colored product (*see* Notes 1 and 2).

The technique described here is for use with monoclonal primary antibodies of mouse origin, but can easily be adapted for use with polyclonal antibodies from other species (i.e., rabbit). This method uses a secondary biotin-labeled antibody and a detection system that employs a biotin-avidin horseradish peroxidase complex linker step, the so-called ABC (avidin-biotin complex) detection system (5) (*see* Chapter 26). In this detection system, avidin acts as a bridge between the biotinylated secondary antibody and a biotin-labeled peroxidase enzyme. The anchored enzyme, in the presence of H_2O_2 can then convert the substrate, diaminobenzidine, to a brown or black reaction product that is easily identifiable in the tissue section.

The ABC detection system has been shown to be more sensitive than most other detection system (5, 6), primarily because of the large size of the preformed ABC complexes, which result in amplification of the signals. Alternative detection systems for immunohistochemical analysis include the peroxidase-antiperoxidase (PAP) (1) and the alkaline phosphatase-antialkaline phosphatase(APAAP) systems (7) (see Chapter 24). More recently, newer commercially available polymer–based detection systems have been developed that combine the secondary antibody and detection enzyme into a single reagent. Polymer-based detection systems overcome problems that may occur with biotin-link based systems, have excellent sensitivity, and can be applied to frozen section immunohistochemistry. Polymer-based detection systems are discussed in other chapters of the manual. (XREF).

2. Materials

1. Freezing solution: 2-methylbutane and dry ice or liquid nitrogen.
2. OCT embedding compound (Sakura Finetek USA, Inc., Torrance, CA).

3. Tris-buffered saline (TBS): 0.05 M Tris-HCl and 0.15 M NaCl, pH 7.6.
4. Acetone.
5. Normal goat serum: 1–3% in TBS.
6. Primary monoclonal antibody (of mouse origin), at appropriate dilution.
7. Secondary antibody: biotin-labeled goat anti-mouse immunoglobulin (Vector Laboratories, Burlingame, CA), at appropriate dilution.
8. Avidin-biotin complex (Vector ABC Elite kit) (Vector Laboratories): ABC solution should be made fresh 10 min before use, so that complexes have time to form according to instructions of manufacturer.
9. Diaminobenzedine (DAB) solution: 100 mg DAB (Sigma, St. Louis, MO) and 0.01% H_2O_2 in 200 mL TBS (optional 1 mL of 8% nickel chloride). DAB is a suspected carcinogen and should be handled with caution. DAB solution should be made fresh, immediately before use (*see* Notes 3 and 4).
10. Dewar flask for snap-freezing tissues.
11. Cryostat for preparing frozen sections; freezing chucks.
12. Clean glass slides previously treated with 3-aminopropyltriethoxysilane (Sigma) or other adhesives, such as gelatin, poly-L-lysine, or glue adhesive.
13. Humid chamber for incubations.
14. Suitable low-temperature freezer or Dewar flask for tissue storage.
15. Absolute alcohol, 95% ethanol, and xylene.
16. Glass coverslips.
17. Permount.

3. Methods

3.1. Preparing the Tissue

1. Place the tissue in normal saline or other media to prevent drying. Do not place tissue on gauze or paper towel since desiccation will occur. Slice the tissue with a sharp scalpel blade or razor. Sections should be 2–3 mm in thickness.
2. Chill the freezing chuck by dipping it briefly into freezing solution, either 2-methylbutane with added dry ice or liquid nitrogen. Use a clamp or other device to hold chuck.
3. Apply a thin layer of OCT embedding compound to the cold chuck. Place the tissue section on the embedding compound,

which by now should have begun to form a solid base. Do not allow the embedding compound to solidify fully. Apply additional OCT compound to cover entire tissue.

4. Immerse the chuck with the tissue slice into the freezing solution. Freezing is indicated by a change in color of the embedding solution from clear to white and will be completed in 5–10 s. After 10 s, remove the chuck and tissue from the freezing solution and place them on dry ice (*see* Note 5).
5. Store the tissue on the chuck if sections are to be cut in the immediate future; if not, wrap the tissue in aluminum foil, and place it in a small sealable plastic bag. Store at –70°C or in the vapor phase of a liquid nitrogen freezer (*see* Note 6).

3.2. Preparing Frozen Section Slides

1. When staining is to be performed, place the chuck containing the frozen tissue slice in the cryostat for preparation of frozen sections.
2. Clean slides, pretreated with 3-aminopropyltriethoxysilane to assist in retaining frozen sections to slide, should be used in the following steps. In addition to silanized slides, other adhesive solutions can be used, including gelatin, amino poly-L-lysine, Histostik (Accurate Chemical & Scientific, Westbury, NY), or glue (10–15% aqueous solution of Elmers Glue-All, Borden, Inc., Columbus, OH). Alternatively, one can purchase charged slides from one of several suppliers of glass microscope slides (Fisher Scientific, Pittsburgh, P A; Baxter Laboratories, McGaw Park, IL).
3. Cryostat sections should be prepared as thin as possible, 4–8 µm in thickness.
4. Air-dry slides for 1–3 h at room temperature (*see* Note 7).
5. Fix sections in acetone for 5 min at room temperature. Place slides in a plastic box, and store at –70°C with desiccant if staining is not to be performed the same day. Alternatively, sections may be kept at 4°C for several days (*see* Notes 8 and 9).

3.3. Staining Procedure (See Note 10)

1. Quickly transfer the slides to TBS and wash, dipping in and out of the solution ten times. Transfer to another Coplin jar containing TBS for 5 min. Transfer to another Coplin jar for a third wash in TBS plus 1–3% normal goat serum for 5 min (*see* Notes 11 and 12).
2. Apply primary antibody at the appropriate dilution, and incubate for 2 h at room temperature in a humid chamber. To keep the chamber humid, a paper towel soaked with H_2O placed at the bottom of the chamber will suffice (*see* Notes 13–18).
3. After incubation with the primary antibody, wash slides two times in TBS for 3 min. Then wash in TBS containing 1–3% goat serum for a third wash for 5 min.

4. Apply secondary biotinylated antibody, and incubate for another 30 min at room temperature.
5. Repeat washing as in **step 3**: two washes in TBS for 3 min each, and a third wash in TBS containing 1–3% goat serum for 5 min.
6. Application of ABC solution: Preform the ABC complex by mixing 10 µL of avidin and 10 µL of biotin-peroxidase (Reagents A and B from Vector ABC Elite kit) in 1 mL of TBS and incubating for 10 min. Apply 100 µL of ABC solution to each tissue section for 30 min at room temperature.
7. Wash slides three times in TBS for 3 min. Do not use the goat serum in the last wash at this step.
8. Incubate slides in DAB solution. The DAB solution should be made up fresh for each staining procedure just before use. Mix 100 µg DAB into 200 mL of TBS, and add H_2O_2 to 0.01%. The DAB development reaction should be monitored under the microscope. The usual development reaction takes 10–20 min. Using a known positive control, monitor development under the microscope to desired level of intensity (*see* Note 19). The brown (or black) reaction product should be specific to the cells bearing the antigen of interest, with little or no background staining, as illustrated in Fig. 1.
9. Wash slides in TBS.
10. Counterstain in hematoxylin. Other counterstains, such as Methyl Green or eosin, may be used (*see* Note 20).
11. Dehydrate the slides in three changes of 95% alcohol and two changes of absolute alcohol, and clear in two changes of xylene.
12. Mount with Permount, and apply a coverslip (*see* Notes 21 and 22).

4. Notes

1. There are many minor variations of the basic method, but the constant features of all indirect immunostaining procedures are:
   (a) A primary antibody incubation.
   (b) A secondary antibody incubation.
   (c) A detection step with color development.
2. If the antigen of interest is abundant and additional sensitivity is not required, then a two-step direct method, rather than a three-step indirect method, can be employed. With the two-step method, the primary antibody is a biotin-labeled

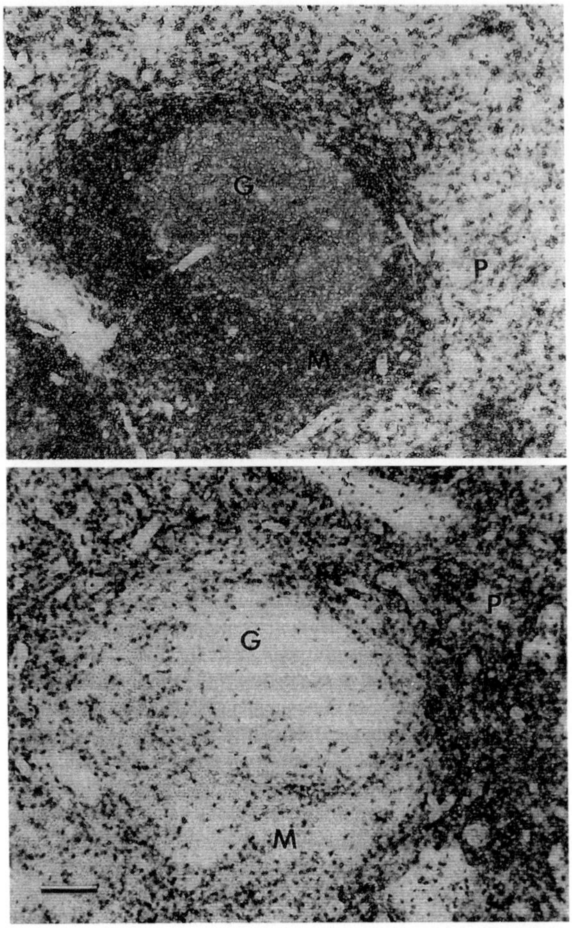

Fig. 1. Photomicrographs of a reactive lymph node follicle with germinal center (*G*), mantle (*M*), and surrounding paracortex (*P*) immunostained using the avidin-biotin complex technique. (*Top*) Follicle stained with an antibody specific to B-cells, B 1 (CD20) (Coulter Immunology, Hialeah, FL), counterstained with Methyl Green. (*Bottom*) Parallel section of the same follicle stained with an antibody specific to T-cells, Leu 4 (CD3) (Becton-Dickinson, Mountain View, CA). Scale bar = 100 μm.

mouse monoclonal antibody, which is followed directly by the ABC incubation step. Due to the abundance of human immunoglobulins in tissue sections, methods for staining immunoglobulin often employ biotin-labeled mouse antihuman immunoglobulin reagents.

3. DAB is a carcinogen and should be handled with care. The powder should be weighed in a chemical hood. Some companies (e.g., Sigma Aldrich) sell preweighed tablets ready to be dissolved in H_2O. Waste from the DAB solution should be collected and disposed of as hazardous waste.
4. Alternate chromogens to DAB can be employed. One such chromogen is aminoethylcarbizol (AEC). AEC is stated to be less carcinogenic than DAB. However, the reaction product is

soluble in organic solvents, such as Permount. Thus, an alternate gelatin-based mounting medium must be employed. These media take longer to dry, and there is often fading with time. Fading of a reaction product is not observed with DAB.

5. If the tissues have not been appropriately snap frozen, ice crystals will be present in the tissue, identifiable as slits or fracture lines through the tissue. Artifactual staining may occur along such fracture lines. Therefore, ice crystal damage should be avoided. The tissues should always be snap frozen. If freezing is performed slowly over dry ice, ice crystals will accumulate in the tissue.
6. Tissue embedded in OCT should also always be maintained in the frozen state. If tissues are allowed to thaw, they cannot be refrozen without resulting in extensive damage to the tissue and often loss of antigenicity.
7. It is often helpful to mark a circle around the tissue section with a diamond glass marking pencil. This allows one to identify the area where the section is located, ensuring that reagents will be applied evenly on the tissue section.
8. Although acetone is a very good general-purpose fixative for preserving antigenicity in frozen sections, other fixatives may be preferable for preserving specific antigens. Alcohol-based fixatives are a widely used alternative to acetone. The fixative of choice for terminal deoxynucleotide transferase (TdT) and certain other nuclear antigens is 4% paraformaldehyde for 30 min (*see* Chapter 8).
9. Frozen sections can be stored dessicated at 4°C for at least 7 days without loss of reactivity of most antigens. For some antigens, slides can be kept for up to 30 days. It is always preferable to stain the slides within a few days of cutting the sections.
10. The entire staining protocol takes about 6 h. Since it is desirable to monitor the final incubation step with DAB, the number of sections stained at any one time should be limited, so that appropriate monitoring can be performed. Most experienced technologists can easily stain up to 50 slides in one run.
11. An optional step is the blocking of endogenous peroxidase activity. This procedure may result in some loss of antigenicity and decreased sensitivity. We recommend omitting this step unless absolutely necessary. Blocking endogenous peroxidase may be required for tissues with high endogenous peroxidase activity, such as spleen or bone marrow. To block endogenous peroxidase, place sections in methanol containing 3% H_2O_2 for 30 min. Blocking should be performed after **step 1** of Subheading 3.3 and should be followed by an additional wash step.

12. Control slides of known reactivity should be run with each set of slides immunostained. Appropriate controls should include an irrelevant antibody of the same immunoglobulin class at an equivalent concentration.
13. Most primary commercial monoclonal antibodies are used at titers ranging from 1:40 to 1:100. Antibodies should be diluted in TBS. Concentrated monoclonal antibodies should be stored with 0.1 % sodium azide to prevent contamination. Most antibodies may be frozen down in concentrated form. Rare antibody preparations will lose activity on freezing.
14. Freezing and thawing of the monoclonal antibodies should be avoided. Most monoclonal antibodies are stable for months at 4°C if stored at an adequate protein concentration. Dilute antibodies in small aliquots, and use the diluted aliquot for a month or so, rather than diluting a large amount of the antibody at once. Use sterile technique when handling expensive antibodies.
15. Each primary antibody should be titered before its use in the laboratory against a known tissue expressing the antigen of interest.
16. If the reagents are not evenly applied, artifacts of staining will occur. The most common artifact is an "edge" effect or a rim of false positivity around the edge of the tissue section. This usually results from some drying of the antibodies at the edge of the tissue section. If any portion of the tissue has not been coated with reagents at any step in the procedure, this area will appear unstained. Usually a sharp line demarcates such artifactually negative areas. Once the primary antibody has been applied to the test slide, the section should never be allowed to dry.
17. Alternate staining protocols provide for incubation of the tissue sections with the primary antibody at 4°C overnight. This sometimes results in enhanced staining without an increase in background.
18. The method presented may be easily modified to accommodate primary polyclonal heteroantisera prepared in goats, rabbits, or other species. The advantages of monoclonal antibodies are the high specificity of these reagents and their standardization from laboratory to laboratory. Monoclonal antibodies will react only with specific and crossreacting epitopes. Serum-derived antibodies (including some sold as "affinity-purified" antibodies) may be reactive with many irrelevant antigens.
19. Nickel chloride (1 mL, 8% solution) may be added to the DAB solution. Without nickel chloride, the reaction product is brown. Nickel chloride produces a black reaction product that

may be preferable for black and white photography of stained slides.

20. Methyl Green is the preferable counterstain if black and white photography is to be performed because the positive black reaction product will be clearly evident against the pale green background. If photography is not anticipated, hematoxylin may be desirable, since it provides better nuclear detail. Eosin may be preferable if one is staining nuclear antigen, such as TdT, Ki-67, or p53.
21. The pattern of anticipated results will vary with the tissue antigen identified. It is important to know the cellular distribution of the antigen of interest. Some staining patterns will be membranous. Others will be cytoplasmic or concentrate in the Golgi region. Yet others will be nuclear in their distribution. Knowledge of the cellular localization of the antigen of interest will help one to judge whether an observed staining pattern is appropriate for that antigen or whether the observed staining pattern may be the result of some artifact. Some antigens are restricted to cells, whereas others are also found in interstitial spaces, appearing to produce a high background. For example, antibodies against immunoglobulins will not only stain B cells; they will also stain interstitial tissues because of free immunoglobulins present in serum and interstitial spaces.

References

1. Stemberger LA (1978) Immunocytochemistry. Prentice-Hall, Englewood Cliffs, NJ
2. Hsu SM, Cossman J, Jaffe ES (1983) Lymphocyte subsets in normal human lymphoid tissues. Am J Clin Pathol 80:21–30
3. Sheibani K, Tubbs RR (1984) Enzyme immunohistochemistry: technical aspects. Semin Diagn Pathol 1:235–251
4. Wamke RA, Rouse RV (1985) Limitations encountered in the application of tissue section immunodiagnosis to the study of lymphomas and related disorders. Hum Pathol 16:326–331
5. Hsu SM, Raine L, Fanger H (1981) The use of avidin-biotin-peroxidase complex (ABC) in immunoperoxidase technique: a comparison between ABC and unlabeled antibody PAP procedures. J Histochem Cytochem 29:577–580
6. Hsu SM, Cossman JC, Jaffe ES (1983) A comparison of ABC, unlabeled antibody and conjugated antibody methods with monoclonal and polyclonal antibodies-an examination of germinal center of tonsils. Am J Clin Pathol 80:429–435
7. Cordell JL, Falini B, Erber WN, Ghosh AK, Abdulaziz Z, MacDonald S, Pulford KAF, Stein H, Mason DY (1984) Immunoenzymatic labeling of monoclonal antibodies using immune complexes of alkaline phosphatase and monoclonal anti-alkaline-phosphatase (AP AAP complexes). J Histochem Cytochem 32:219–229

Chapter 28

Multiple Antigen Immunostaining Procedures

Tibor Krenacs, Laszlo Krenacs, and Mark Raffeld

Abstract

Detection of multiple antigens in the same tissue section can be done by combining a range of immunohisto/cytochemical techniques based either on light microscopic chromogenic precipitates or fluorochrome labeling. Light microscopic techniques preferred for this purpose use combinations of immunogold silver staining (black precipitate), immunoperoxidase, immunoalkaline phosphatase and immunogalactosidase methods using chromogens of different colors. Fluorochrome labels favored for these combinations include AMCA (blue), FITC (green), rhodamine (orange-red) and Cy5 (far red), their matching synthetic members from the Alexa series, or quantum dots. Antibodies directly labeled or those from noncross-reacting animal species (e.g., mouse, rabbit, goat, guinea pig etc.) can be applied simultaneously. When the antigens of interest are in separate cells or cell compartments (e.g., in cell membrane, cytoplasm or nucleus), and only cross-reacting antibodies are available, there have also been ways of avoiding unwanted cross-talk. These include the exploitation of the shielding effect of chromogens; inactivation of immuno-sequences of the first staining by using either acidic elution, formaldehyde fixation or microwave heating; combining unlabeled and hapten-labeled antibodies; or using labeled monovalent F(ab) secondary antibodies. In this chapter we briefly discuss the principle of multiple antigen immunolabeling and provide useful protocols for its performance.

Key words: Multiple antigen immunostaining, Immunoenzymatic methods, Immunofluorescence, Noncross-reacting antibodies, Simultaneous antigen detection

1. Introduction

The immunohistological demonstration of multiple antigens in a single tissue section has many applications and is commonly used to elucidate the topographic relationships of antigenically defined cell populations, and to correlate phenotypic information with functional or prognostic markers, or with microbial infection (1). In addition, single or double label immunohistochemistry may be combined with in situ hybridization to identify genes or

C. Oliver and M.C. Jamur (eds.), *Immunocytochemical Methods and Protocols*, Methods in Molecular Biology, Vol. 588, DOI 10.1007/978-1-59745-324-0_28, © Humana Press, a part of Springer Science+Business Media, LLC 1995, 1999, 2010

mRNAs, and translated protein side-by-side (2–4). The combination of these techniques depends primarily on the compatibility of the antigen retrieval techniques required for the individual antigens, and the stability of the RNA and DNA sequences in question (4).

Two basic strategies have evolved for the detection of multiple antigens in a tissue section. One strategy is to combine immunoenzymatic methods that use different chromogenic-substrate reactions (5–7) (*see* Chapter 24) and/or the silver-enhanced immunogold technique (IGSS) (8–10) (*see* Chapter 30). The different colored reaction products can easily be studied against the recognizable background structure with a conventional light microscope, particularly when traditional histological stains such as hematoxylin for nuclei or PAS for basement membranes are additionally applied. With careful balancing of the subsequent chromogenic reactions, up to four antigens situated in separate cell populations or within different compartments of the same cell (nucleus, cytoplasm, or cell membrane) can be distinguished in a single tissue section (7, 10).

The second strategy uses combinations of different antibodies detected with fluorochromes of distinct emission maxima (at least 40 nm difference) recognized as discernible colors (11, 12). The visualization of fluorochromes requires the use of fluorescence or confocal laser scanning microscopes with special filters. The combinations of noncross-reacting immunoreagents labeled with distinct fluorochromes allow for the clear demonstration of overlapping fluorescence signals of merged colors characteristic of antigen coexpression in the same tissue/cell compartment (13, 14). With proper fluorochrome and filter combinations up to four antigens can be selectively immunostained side by side in the same tissue sections (11).

Multiple antigen staining protocols can be further subdivided depending on whether antibodies of one immunoreaction can interact with those used in the subsequent immunoreaction(s). When such "cross-talk" between the multiple staining reactions can be excluded (e.g., when mouse and rabbit antibodies are combined in a dual labeling experiment), the immunoreagents of identical layers (e.g., primary antibodies or link/detection antibodies) may be mixed and used simultaneously. If crosstalk cannot be avoided in the experimental design (i.e., when two monoclonal mouse primary antibodies of the same subclass are used), the reaction steps for each antigen have to be completed consecutively, including some blocking steps. In this chapter we present guidelines and describe protocols suitable for performing immunohistochemical double and triple antigen detection. Although we have not detailed specific protocols for double/multiple staining using immunofluorescence, the principles of staining are identical, and suggestions for immunofluorescent antigen detection are provided.

1.1. Double/multiple Antigen Immunostaining

1.1.1. Principles of Reagent Combination

The principles followed for multiple antigen staining are identical to those for single antigen staining. The primary difference is that one must prevent unwanted cross-reactions (cross-talk) between the different staining sequences. Thus, the combination of primary and secondary antibodies is a major determinant of the appropriate double/multiple antigen detection protocol. Cross-talk is not expected when the primary antibodies originate from different species such as mouse, rabbit, goat, sheep, guinea pig or monkey (7, 11), the secondary antibodies are species-specific and purified from cross-reacting elements, and the chromogen-substrate reactions are distinct. The same is true for combinations consisting of antibodies of different immunoglobulin isotypes (i.e., IgG and IgM), or subclasses (i.e., IgG_1 and IgG_2) that are detected with isotype/subclass-restricted secondary antibodies (15). Cross-talk will also not occur if the primary antibodies are of identical species or isotype and are directly coupled to different enzymes or fluorochromes (4, 16). Another method to reduce cross-talk is to apply preformed complexes of the primary antibodies and their cognate enzyme or fluorochrome coupled secondary reagents (17, 18). This approach, however, can be laborious as one must first determine the optimal saturation for the complexes or eliminate uncomplexed reagents prior to performing the immunoreaction.

In all of the above combinations, reagents of identical layers (primary and secondary) may be applied simultaneously in the same incubation steps. Only the chromogenic-enzyme reactions, if relevant, need to be carried out consecutively, (e.g., alkaline phosphatase activity revealed first followed by peroxidase development).

1.1.2. Combining Immunofluorescence Techniques

Immunofluorescence methods can be combined only if cross-talk between the immunological sequences can be excluded, regardless of whether the antigens are situated in the same or different cells/compartments. Fluorochrome molecules are small, usually below the molecular range of 1 kDa, and thus, unlike chromogenic precipitates (discussed below), they cannot mask antigenic epitopes to prevent cross-reacting secondary detection reagents from binding to primary antibodies of prior reaction layers (12). On the other hand, immunofluorescence methods are ideal for co-localization studies at the light microscopic level, where mixed colors of intermediate emission wavelength indicate two antigens in the same structure (12, 13). Fluorochrome labeling is also the method of choice for double fluorescence in situ hybridization (FISH) and has gained widespread use for detecting chromosomal abnormalities in diagnostic pathology (19). The Alexa series of recently designed fluorochromes represent a pH- and relatively photo-stable alternative to the traditional fluorescing dyes with significantly brighter light emission at the same wavelength

(12). The fluorochromes most commonly used for combined antigen detection and their absorption and emission maxima and fluorescent color are summarized in Table 1. More recently fluorescent semiconductor nanoparticles called quantum dots (Q-dot® nanocrystals, Invitrogen, Molecular Probes, Carlsbad, CA) have been used for dual antigen detection in tissue sections (20). These cadmium-based nanoparticles can be coupled to a variety of secondary detection reagents, including anti-immunoglobulins, streptavidin, and protein A. Q-dots® are available in multiple emission spectra (a function of their size and composition), have very intense and narrow emission characteristics, and are highly stable over time, eliminating several of the major problems of dye-based fluorescent detection technologies.

Significant improvements in microscopic resolution and color contrast can be achieved when the fluorescence signals are studied with confocal laser scanning microscopy and the optical layers generated are digitally merged, magnified and the color channels are assigned to artificial colors using commercially available software programs (Fig. 1). In this way, the cellular distribution of objects as small as 0.2–0.5 μm such as desmosomes and gap junctions can be analyzed in known tissue volumes of identical sections,

Table 1
The most common fluorochromes used for multiple antigen immunostaining

Fluorochrome	Alexa® series	Abs. max. (nm)	Emiss. max. (nm)	Color	References
AMCA (7-aminomethyl-4-methylcoumarin-3-acetic acid)	Fluor 350	350/346	450/445	Blue	(12, 13, 34, 38)
DAPI[a] (4′6-diamidino-2-phenylindole, dihydrochloride)		348	461	Blue	(12)
FITC (fluorescein-5-isothiocyanate)	Fluor 488	494	518	Yellow-green	(12, 13, 18, 34, 38, 39)
TRITC (tetramethyrhod-amine-5-isothiocyanate)	Fluor 546	545/556	580/573	Orange-red	(12)
Cy3 (cyanin 3)		550	570	Orange-red	(13, 38, 39)
Texas Red®	Fluor 594	590	615	Red	(12, 13, 18, 34)
7-AAD[a] (7-aminoactino-mycine D)		546	647	Red	
Cy5 (cyanin 5)	Fluor 647	650	670	Far red	(18)

[a]DNA/nuclear stains

well beyond the resolution of the light microscope (14). The same principle of analyzing the two signals in separate recording channels is utilized in double epi-illumination microscopy (epi-polarization for gold-silver and epi-fluorescence for Fast Red) (21), or when CCD camera-captured individual images either of immunofluorescence of immunoenzyme nature are enhanced, filtered and then merged using imaging software (22, 23).

1.1.3. Combining Immunostains Based on Catalytic Chromogenic Precipitation

Noncross-reacting antibodies, however, are not always available in the laboratory. Methods based on catalytic chromogenic precipitation, including immunoenzyme techniques and immunogold silver staining (IGSS), can be used for combinations of either noncross-reacting or cross-reacting immune sequences, provided the antigens to be detected are in separate cells/compartments (6). In cases, however, when cross-talk is expected, it is essential that the immunostains are performed sequentially and certain precautions are taken.

Preventing Cross-Talk Based on the Shielding Effect of Chromogenic Precipitates

In enzyme reactions, catalytic precipitates will be formed as long as the enzyme is active, and has not been concealed by the accumulating precipitate. In the IGSS method although autocatalysis is continuous, the appearance of silver grains in the developer solution limits further intensification. In both cases catalytic precipitates form permanent shells shielding the immunological sequences used, which can be exploited to avoid potential but unwanted cross-talk in multiple antigen detection protocols. The silver shell of IGSS and the compact 3, 3′-diaminobenzidine tetra-hydrochloride (DAB) precipitate can completely block the immunological sequences of the associated antigen/antibody complex (10). Therefore, when the antigens of interest are expected in different cell populations or in different cellular compartments, primary antibodies of the same animal species may be used in consecutive immunoreactions. IGSS (black) or immunoperoxidase (IPO)/DAB (brown) should be used to reveal the first immunoreaction, followed by the application of either IPO/3-amino-9-ethylcarbazole (AEC; red), immunoalkaline phosphatase (IAP)/Fast Blue (blue), nitro-blue-tetrazolium (NBT; purple-black), Fast Red (magenta/red), or New Fuchsine (magenta/red) to demonstrate additional antigen(s) (8–10, 24) (*see* Chapter 24).

DAB is probably the most versatile chromogen in immunohistochemistry. Its brown color can be modified when used in the presence of nickel-chloride (purple-black), cobalt-chloride (dark-blue) or copper sulfate (dark brown) (25). Also, DAB and its metallic complexes can be further contrasted to form a black precipitate with silver intensification (26). Immunoreactions resulting in electron-dense precipitates, such as immunogold, IGSS, and IPO/DAB-complexes, have also been used widely for double/multiple antigen detection at the ultrastructural level (1, 27). For light microscopy, one of our preferred double labeling techniques

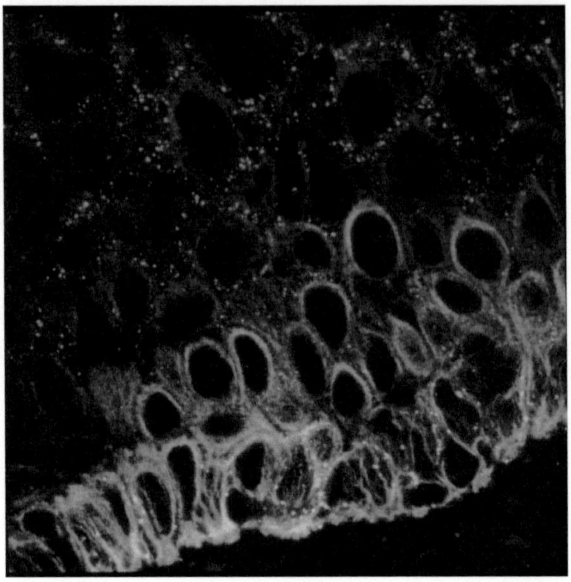

Fig. 1. Double immunofluorescence detection of cytoplasmic cytokeratin 19 intermediate filaments (CK19) (FITC, green/filamentous) and the cell-membrane associated connexin 43 (Cx43) gap junction protein (Cy3, red/dot-like) in the stratified squamous epithelium of human cervix. Combination of mouse monoclonal (CK19) and rabbit polyclonal (Cx43) antibodies and distinct fluorochrome-labeled secondary antibodis. Confocal laser scanning microscopy, a projection of five optical layers.

combines two IPO/DAB detections, whereby the first enzyme label is developed with DAB-Ni to form a purple-black precipitate that provides excellent contrast with the light-brown DAB "only" precipitate used for the second immunodetection (Fig. 2). IPO techniques used with different chromogenic reactions (e.g., DAB-Ni, DAB and V-VIP) may allow clear distinction of as many as three antigens in the same section (28). Chromogenic precipitates, most commonly used for combined antigen immunodetection, are summarized in Table 2.

Preventing Cross-Talk by Inactivation, Hapten-Labeling, Using Monovalent Ig Fab, or Tyramide Amplification

Alternative protocols that combine potentially cross-reacting antibodies focus on either inactivating the immunological layers following the first immunostaining, combining unlabeled and labeled primary antibodies, using monovalent Fab secondary antibodies, or utilizing the sensitivity advantage of tyramide amplification. For inactivating immunological layers of the first sequence, sections may be treated with low pH (pH 1–2) solutions such as 0.01 M hydrochloric acid, a mixture of $KMnO_4$-H_2SO_4, or oxalic acid (29–31). Other protocols use formaldehyde fixation (32), or microwave heating in an antigen retrieval buffer, between the stains (33, 34). Acidic solutions elute interfering antibodies from the first immunoreaction, however, their effect is not consistent (31). The intermediate application of formaldehyde may either be insufficient, or reduce the antigenicity of the targeted epitopes in the subsequent immunoreactions (34). Although microwave heating between immunostains does not eliminate tissue-bound antibodies, 1–2 × 5 min. of boiling in a 0.01 M citrate buffer (pH 6.0) denatures immunoglobulins to prevent their further reaction in either immunoenzyme or immunofluorescent methods (33, 34). For these reasons, microwave heating between immunostains is the method we favor for minimizing the chance of unwanted color mixing due to potential cross-reaction. Standardized, ready to use, double staining kits with an intermediate blocking step for detecting primary antibodies of the same species are also commercially available, such as the EnVision Double stain kit (Dako, K1395).

Monovalent polyclonal Fab fragments of enzyme coupled secondary immunoglobulins have also been used to reduce or eliminate cross-reactions when using more than one primary antibody from the same species. The polyclonal nature of the secondary allows it to saturate all possible epitopes on the first primary antibody, while the monovalent property of the Fab fragment eliminates the possibility that an unsaturated arm on a divalent secondary may bind subsequent primary antibodies of the same species during their application (35).

The use of directly labeled primary antibodies is also an effective method to eliminate potential cross-reactions (*see* Chapter 6). Following the detection of the first antibody (e.g., a mouse monoclonal) using a traditional protocol, a FITC- or biotin-labeled second (mouse) monoclonal antibody is applied and detected through its hapten label (i.e., anti-FITC or -biotin) using a different enzyme reaction (24, 36). Here, an intermediate step for saturating anti-mouse Ig binding sites of the first sequence secondary using normal mouse serum is necessary. The

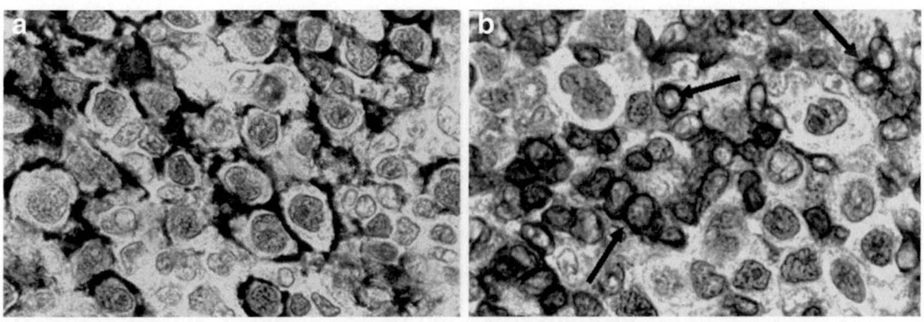

Fig. 2. Double staining of membrane and nuclear antigens using consecutive immunoreactions. (**a**) Depicts a large B-cell lymphoma (LBCL) doubly stained for the B-cell-associated membrane antigen CD20 and the B-cell-associated nuclear antigen B-cell-specific activator protein (BSAP). Note the colocalization of BSAP and CD20 in the tumor cells. (**b**) Depicts the same LBCL doubly stained for BSAP and the membrane-associated T-cell-associated antigen CD3 (*arrows*). Note the divergence of nuclear BSAP staining of the tumor cells and membrane CD3 staining of reactive T-cells. Double-staining method used: IOP/DAB (*brown*) (first antibody) and IP)? DAB + NiCl (*black*) (second antibody). Abbreviations are as in text.

Table 2
The most common catalytic chromogenic precipitates used for multiple antigen immunostaining

Method	Label	Chromogen	Substrate	Color	References
IGSS	Colloidal gold	(Hydroquinone-silver acetate)		Black	(8–10, 24)
IPO	Peroxidase	3,3′-diaminobenzidine (DAB)	Hydrogen peroxide	Light brown	(5–8, 10, 15, 28–31, 35)
		DAB-nickel chloride		Purple blue	(25, 27)
		DAB-cobal chloride		Dark blue	(7, 25)
		DAB-copper sulfate		Dark brown	(25)
		DAB-nickel chloride-silver nitrate		Grey-black	(26)
		Vector-VIP		Deep violet	(28)
		4-chloro-1-naphthol (4-CN)		Blue	(29, 30)
		3-amino-9-ethylcarbazole (AEC)		Red	(8–10, 15, 36, 37)
IAP	Alkaline phosphatase	Fast red TR	Naphthol-AS-MX-Phosphate	Red	(6, 8, 10, 15)
		Fuchsin		Magenta	(7, 9, 22, 24)
		Fast blue BB		Blue	(6–10, 24, 35–37)
		Nitro-blue-tetrazolium (NBT)	5-Bromo-4-chloro-indoxyl-phophate (BCIP)	Purple blue	(15, 36)
IGal	β-D-galactosidase	Ferro-ferri-cyanide	5-Bromo-4-chloro-indoxyl-β-D-galactose	Turquoise	(7, 22, 36)

commercialization of easy to use mouse Ig biotinylation kits utilizing biotin-coupled monovalent goat anti-mouse-Fab Ig fragments has greatly facilitated this approach (37).

Another method takes advantage of significant differences in detection sensitivities of two immunostaining procedures. For example, the streptavidin-biotin method with biotinylated-tyramide amplification can detect antigens at such a low concentration of the primary antibody, that they can't be detected with the traditional indirect methods used in the subsequent immunoreactions (38, 39). The principles of double/multiple immunostaining techniques are summarized in Table 3.

The protocols we provide below take advantage of the chromogen shielding effect and the microwave denaturation of immu-

Table 3
Principles of double/multiple immunostaining techniques using simultaneous or sequential immunostaining procedures

Source and type of primary antibody	Blocking of unwanted cross-links	References
Simultaneous procedures (mixing of identical layers)		
Noncross-reacting antibodies (e.g., mouse, rabbit, goat etc.)	None	(5, 7, 8, 15)
Same species but different subclass/isotype (IgG1, IgG2, IgM etc.)	Detection with isotype-restricted labeled antibodies	(15)
Antibodies of the same species origin	Direct labeling with enzymes or fluorochromes	(4, 16)
	Using preformed complexes with	
	Enzyme-labeled anti-immunoglobulins or	(17)
	Alexa-labeled protein A (rabbit Igs)	(18)
Sequential procedures (consecutive immunostainings)		
Cross-reacting antibodies (e.g., same species of origin)		
Utilizing chromagen shielding effect		(1, 6, 8–10, 24–26, 28)
	IGSS, DAB, DAB-Ni/Co/Cu, DAB-Ni/Ag	
Inactivating immune sequences by		
	Acidic elution	(29, 30)
	Denaturation with formaldehyde	(32)
	Denaturation by microwave	(33, 34)
Combining unlabeled and hapten-labeled abs		
	FITC-labeled, detected with anti-FITC	(24, 36)
	Biotin-labeled, detected with Streptavidin-PO	(36)
	ARK biotinylation with anti-mouse Ig F(ab)	(37)
Using monovalent enzyme labeled F(ab) fragments		(35)
Utilizing sensitivity advantage of tyramide amplification		(38, 39)

nological sequences to minimize unwanted color mixing, when potentially cross-reacting sequences are used for double or triple immunolabeling.

2. Materials

With the assistance of wet-heat mediated antigen retrieval, most antigens of interest to a general histopathology laboratory can be detected in archival tissues that have been fixed in either 10% buffered formalin (4% formaldehyde) or B5, and embedded in paraffin wax (*see* Chapter 14). If one or more antigens of interest can not be detected in paraffin embedded tissues, or if the necessary retrieval procedure is incompatible with the detection of another antigen, frozen tissue sections may be used instead (*see* Chapter 10). Antibodies, immunoreagents, chemicals, and equipment needed are identical to those used for single antigen detection (*see* Chapters 15–19 and 24–27).

1. Tissue sections of 5 μm thickness. Paraffin sections mounted on commercially available silane-coated glass slides, such as standard SuperFrost Plus (Fischer Scientific, Pittsburgh, PA) or on slides prepared using a home-made APES coating; or frozen sections mounted on silanized, gelatin-coated or poly-L-lysine-coated slides (*see* Notes 1–4).
2. Lugol's iodine: 1% iodine and 2% potassium iodine in distilled water.
3. 2.5% and 5% sodium thiosulfate in distilled water.
4. Methanol with 0.5% hydrogen peroxide.
5. Acetone.
6. Antigen retrieval solution (TRS): Target retrieval solution, pH 6.1 (Dako, Carpinteria, CA; catalog number: S1699).
7. Antigen retrieval buffer (citrate): 0.01 M citric acid-sodium citrate, pH 6.0.
8. TBS: 0.05 M Tris–HCl and 0.15 M sodium chloride, pH 7.6.
9. Blocking solution (BS): TBS with 1% bovine serum albumin (BSA), 0.1% sodium azide with 5% normal goat serum.
10. TBS with 0.1% Tween-20; TBS with 0.05% Tween-20.
11. Mouse monoclonal or rabbit polyclonal primary antibodies.
12. Secondary antibodies: goat anti-mouse or anti-rabbit antibodies (1) conjugated with colloidal gold (1.4 nm gold: Nanogold, Stony Brook, NY or 5 nm gold: GE Health Care Life Sciences, Piscataway, NJ; both diluted 1:30 in TBS with 0.05% Tween-20); (2) conjugated with horseradish peroxidase (PO) or alkaline phosphatase (AP) (1:50 dilution in TBS; Dako, Carpinteria, CA); (3) conjugated with separate fluorochromes, e.g., AMCA, FITC, TRITC, Texas Red, Cy-5 (1:50 dilution in TBS; Vector Labs, Burlingame, CA; Jackson

ImmunoResearch, West Grove, PA) or with the corresponding Alexa® dyes (1:200 dilution in TBS; Invitrogen, Molecular Probes) (*see* Tables 1 and 2, Notes 5 and 6).

13. Double-distilled water.
14. Silver acetate developer: ***part *a*: 250 mg hydroquinone in 50 mL 0.1 M citrate buffer, pH 3.5 (*see* Note 7); and part *b*: 100 mg silver acetate (Sigma Aldrich) in 50 mL double distilled H_2O (*see* Note 8).
15. DAB chromogen-substrate solution: 20 mg DAB (Sigma Aldrich); 100 mL 0.05 M Tris–HCl buffer, pH7.6; and 100 μL 30% H_2O_2. Alternatively, standardized DAB+ chromogen-substrate kit (e.g., Dako, code: K3467) (*see* Subheading 3.3.2).
16. Nickel chloride salt (Sigma Aldrich).
17. AEC chromogen-substrate solution: AEC (Sigma Aldrich); N,N-dimethylformamide; 0.1 M acetate buffer pH4.6; and hydrogen peroxide. Alternatively, standardized AEC+ chromogen-substrate kit (e.g., Dako, code: K3461) (*see* Subheading 3.3.4).
18. Fast Blue chromogen-substrate solution: Fast Blue BB Salt (Sigma); Naphthol AS-MX-phosphate (Sigma); N,N-dimethylformamide; 0.1 M Tris–HCl buffer, pH9.0; and 1 M Levamisole (*see* Note 9) (*see* Subheading 3.3.5).
19. BCIP/NBT standardized chromogen-substrate kit (e.g., Dako, code: K0598).
20. Fast Red-naphthol phosphate standardized chromogen-substrate kit (e.g., Dako, code: K0597).
21. Fuchsin-naphthol phosphate standardized chromogen-substrate kit (e.g., Dako, code: K0624).
22. Glycerol-based mounting medium containing antifading agent, e.g., Vectashield (Vector Labs.); or glycerol-gelatin based mounting medium, e.g., Faramount (Dako) (*see* Note 10).

3. Methods

3.1. Sequential Antigen Detection

In sequential detection protocols (*see* Note 11), the immunohistochemical detection of each antigen is performed separately and sequentially. As discussed above in Subheading 1.1.3.1, the precipitated reaction products of IGSS, IPO or IAP can mask the immunological sequences of their associated antigen-antibody complex, thereby preventing secondary antibodies used in the subsequent detections from binding to primary antibodies of identical species. Microwaving between the stains in citrate buffer (pH 6.0) can optionally be used to inactivate previously applied reagents. Primary antibodies of the same animal species and/or cross-reacting antibodies can be combined, provided that the antigens are localized in different cell types or in different areas of the same cell. Immunofluorescence methods should not be used in combinations with cross-reacting antibodies.

For paraffin sections begin with step 1 and skip steps 5 and 6; for frozen sections begin with step 5 (*see* Notes 1–4 and 12) (*see* Chapters 10 and 13).

1. Dewax paraffin sections in three changes of xylene and ethanol for 2 min each.
2. Apply wet-heat mediated antigen retrieval in TRS, pressure cooking or microwaving when appropriate (*see* Chapter 14).
3. Place sections in Lugol's iodine for 5 min, then in 2.5% sodium thiosulfate for 30 s if IGSS method is to be used.
4. Block endogenous peroxidase in methanol containing 0.5% hydrogen peroxide for 15 min.
5. Allow freshly cut frozen sections to dry for ~15 min at room temperature.
6. Fix in acetone for 5–10 min and let sections dry again for at least 2 h at room temperature before use. Drying can be shortened to 3–5 min by using a hair dryer with constant agitation from a 5–10 cm distance.
7. Wash dewaxed or frozen sections in TBS for 3 min and incubate in blocking solution (BS) for 5–10 min. Use BS for diluting primary antibodies and TBS for diluting all other immunoreagents.
8. Apply primary antibody (mouse monoclonal or rabbit polyclonal) for 2 h on paraffin sections and for 30 min on frozen sections at room temperature (*see* Note 13).
9. Wash slides for three times for 2 min each in TBS containing 0.1% Tween-20. Acetone-fixed frozen sections must be washed with neat TBS.
10. Apply goat anti-mouse or anti-rabbit secondary antibody labeled either with colloidal gold or horseradish peroxidase for 30 min (*see* Notes 5 and 14).
11. Wash for two times for 2 min each in TBS containing 0.1% Tween 20. Acetone-fixed frozen sections must be washed with neat TBS.
12. Before silver amplification of gold particles rinse the sections three times for 30 s and then wash three times for 2 min each in double-distilled water.

13. Use silver development for IGSS (*see* Notes 15 and 16) or DAB chromogenic-substrate reaction for IPO as detailed in Subheadings 3.3.1 and 3.3.2.
14. Optional for paraffin sections if cross-reacting antibody follows: Rinse slides in TBS and apply an intermediate microwave heating at 300 W power in 150 mL of citrate buffer (pH 6) for 10 min. Cool in flowing tap water.
15. Incubate sections in BS for 5–10 min then apply the primary antibody of the second immunological sequence for 2 h on paraffin sections or for 30 min on frozen sections.
16. Wash three times for 2 min each with TBS and apply the appropriate secondary antibody; that is goat anti-rabbit or anti-mouse Ig coupled either to peroxidase or alkaline phosphatase, for 30 min (*see* Note 17).
17. Wash slides three times for 2 min each in TBS.
18. Develop the chromogenic reaction of the second sequence using either AEC chromogenic substrate reaction for IPO or naphthol phosphate/Fast Blue, NBT/BCIP, Fast Red or New Fuchsin for IAP development as detailed in Subheading 3.3 (*see* Note 18 for triple labeling).
19. Mount sections, without dehydrating when any IPO/AEC or any IAP detection method was involved, using Faramount (Dako).

3.2. Simultaneous Antigen Detection

In this method, the primary antibodies are combined into a single cocktail and applied simultaneously in a single-reaction step. The same can be done for labeled secondary antibodies. Antibodies of different animal species, or different immunoglobulin isotypes (noncross-reacting) detected with isotype-restricted labeled immunoglobulins, or antibodies of the same species directly coupled to different enzymes/fluorochromes are required. Immunofluorescent methods are particularly suited for this method.

Steps 1–7 are identical to those described in Subheading 3.1.

1. Mix primary antibodies (e.g., a rabbit polyclonal with a mouse monoclonal) in BS. Prepare double concentrations of half the needed volume from each primary antibody, mix equal volumes, and apply the primary antibody mixture onto the sections. Incubate paraffin sections for at least 2 h and frozen sections for 30 min.
2. Wash slides for three times for 2 min each in TBS containing 0.05% Tween-20. Acetone-fixed frozen sections must be washed in neat TBS.
3. Apply appropriate, labeled secondary antibodies together, (e.g., goat anti-mouse and anti-rabbit immunoglobulins),

labeled either with colloidal gold, horseradish peroxidase or alkaline phosphatase, respectively. Alternatively, use secondary antibodies labeled with separate fluorochromes (see Table 1). Incubate paraffin sections for 1–2 h and frozen sections for 30 min or less.

4. Wash for three times for 2 min each in TBS.
5. Use the relevant visualization steps described in Subheading 3.3 to develop chromogenic precipitates for IGSS, IAP, or IPO techniques, sequentially.
6. Cell nuclei may be counterstained either with DAPI (blue) or 7-AAD (red) after immunofluorescence stainings (*see* Note 19), or with hematoxylin or methyl green after immunoenzyme techniques.
7. Rinse slides and mount them with glycerol-gelatin based Faramount (Dako) without dehydration.

3.3. Visualization of Reaction Products for Light Microscopy

The wide range of chromogenic-substrate systems available allows one to obtain excellent color contrast for double/multiple antigen detection (*see* Tables 1 and 2). (*see* Note 20).

3.3.1. IGSS

1. Prepare silver acetate developer (40) solution *a* by dissolving 250 mg hydroquinone in 50 mL 0.1 M citrate buffer, pH 3.5; and solution *b* by dissolving 100 mg silver acetate in 50 mL double-distilled water (*see* Notes 7 and 8).
2. Mix *a* and *b* above just before use.
3. Immerse sections in developer and place the jar in a dark place. After 5–8 min monitor the intensity of the gray-black product under the microscope.
4. When desired intensity is achieved, wash slides in distilled water for 2 min, and then in 5% sodium thiosulfate for 2 min.

3.3.2. IPO/DAB

1. Dissolve 20 mg DAB in 100 mL 0.05 M Tris–HCl buffer, pH 7.6, and mix 100 µL 30% hydrogen peroxide in it just before use.
2. Place slides into DAB solution in Coplin jar and develop for 5–15 min under microscopic control to obtain a yellow-brown product.

Alternatively, use DAB+ chromogen-substrate kit available from Dako (or other comparable kit) by mixing 20 µL of DAB chromogen per 1 mL of substrate buffer. Pipette 100 µL mixture on the horizontally placed sections and develop for 5–15 min.

3.3.3. IPO/DAB-Ni

1. Dissolve 20 mg DAB and 0.5% nickel chloride in 100 mL 0.05 M Tris–HCl buffer, pH 7.6, and mix 100 µL hydrogen peroxide in it just before use.

2. Develop slides for 5–15 min under microscopic control to obtain a purple-black product (*see* Note 21).

3.3.4. IPO /AEC

1. Mix 2.5 mL of AEC dissolved in dimethylformamide into 90 mL of 0.1 M acetate buffer, pH4.6. Mix 100 μL 30% hydrogen peroxide with the AEC solution before use.
2. Place slides into AEC solution in a Coplin jar and develop for 5–15 min under microscopic control to obtain a red-brown product. Alternatively, drop AEC+ "ready-to-use" chromogen/substrate solution available from Dako (or other comparable kit) onto the sections and develop for 5–15 min.

3.3.5. IAP/Fast Blue

1. Dissolve 2 mg naphthol AS-MX phosphate (Sigma) in 200 μL N,N-dimethylformamide, mix solution with 9.8 mL 0.1 M Tris–HCl buffer (pH9.0) and add one drop of 1 M levamisole (*see* Note 9).
2. Before use, add 10 mg of Fast Blue BB salt, shake to dissolve, filter, and drop the mixture onto the sections. A blue product will form in 5–15 min.

3.3.6. IAP/NBT-BCIP (See Note 22*)*

1. Apply "ready-to-use" reagent mix available from Dako (or other comparable kit) onto the section, and develop between 10 min and several hours to produce a purple blue reaction product on the specific antigenic sites (*see* Note 23).

3.3.7. IAP/Fast Red (See Note 22*)*

1. Using a commercial kit available from Dako (or other comparable kit) dissolve one tablet containing the Fast Red chromogen and levamisole in 3 mL of 0.1 M Tris–HCl, pH8.2 substrate buffer provided in the kit.
2. Drop the mixture onto the sections and develop for 5–30 min to get a *magenta-red* reaction product.

3.3.8. IAP/Fuchsin (See Note 22*)*

1. Using a commercial kit available from Dako (or other comparable kit) add one drop Tris-buffer concentrate (vial a) and one drop of substrate concentrate (vial b) to 2 mL of distilled water.
2. Mix one drop Fuchsin (vial c) with one drop sodium nitrite (vial d). After 2 min, mix the chromogen solution with the substrate-buffer. Cover tissue sections with the solution. A magenta-red product will form in 5–15 min.

4. Notes

1. 3-aminopropyl-triethoxysilane (APES) coating: Clean glass slides by immersing in ethanol for 5 min. After drying, immerse

the slides for 5 min in 2% APES dissolved in acetone. Rinse the slides briefly in distilled water, and keep them at 56°C overnight before use. Once the sections are mounted heat activate the slides at 60°C for 2 h to prevent detachment of tissue sections during antigen retrieval. (The latter also applies to sections mounted on commercial SuperFrost Plus slides.)

2. When IGSS is used for color development, sections should be mounted on high purity gelatin or poly-L lysine coated slides instead of silane-coated slides. Silane may take part in silver reduction causing background in the reaction. This background can be reduced by careful washing and by the addition of detergent to the wash buffer and diluent. Silane is the preferable "gluing" agent for sections when harsh antigen retrieval is used.
3. Frozen-sections fixed in acetone are vulnerable to washing and soaking. Therefore, the immunostaining protocol should be kept as short as possible to avoid structural damage. Overnight drying of frozen sections at RT following acetone fixation is recommended to help protect section integrity during the longer double/triple staining procedure. Most antigens will survive the overnight drying step.
4. Epoxy resin-embedded semithin sections of 1–2 μm may also be used following extraction of the resin with a sodium meth(eth)oxide treatment for 5–8 min. Sodium meth(eth) oxide is prepared by saturating methanol or ethanol with sodium hydroxide pellets.
5. Sodium azide inhibits peroxidase enzyme, therefore it should be left out from the diluents used with PO-immunoglobulin conjugates. Use TBS containing 0.05% Tween-20 for diluting gold reagents, and neat TBS for diluting fluorochrome-labeled antibodies.
6. Streptavidin-fluorochrome conjugates provide higher sensitivity than two-step indirect techniques. The use of Alexa® dyes instead of the traditional fluorochromes enhances brightness and detection sensitivity of immunofluorescence methods several-fold (12).
7. Prepare citrate buffer pH 3.5 as follows: Dissolve 2.56 g citric acid and 2.36 g tri-sodium citrate in 50 mL double-distilled water. Stir with magnetic stirrer for 15 min. The buffer may be stored at 4°C for approximately 2 months.
8. Use a magnetic stirrer for 15 min to dissolve the silver acetate.
9. The Fast Blue substrate solution can be stored at –20°C for 2 months.
10. Faramount hardens 20–30 min after mounting, which facilitates handling and immersion studies of the immunostained

slide. Vectashield does not provide adequate adhesion of the coverslip to the slide requiring the use of an adhesive to secure the coverslip to the slide (e.g., nail polish).

11. In general, the accompanying two-step indirect methods provide sufficient sensitivity to successfully complete double/triple immunolabeling procedures in 1 day.
12. F(ab) fragments of both conjugated and unconjugated antibodies are preferred in frozen section immunohistochemistry of lymphoid tissues in order to avoid nonspecific binding of antibodies through their FC fragments to Fc receptors (present on B lymphocytes) (17).
13. Antibody concentration and detectability of antigens need to be tested in single immunostainings and should be considered when deciding the order and sensitivity of detection systems to be used. Usually, the detection of "difficult" antigens with highly sensitive methods (e.g., ABC, EnVision or tyramide amplification) precedes those, which are more easily accessible or present in abundance and detectable with average sensitivity techniques using, e.g., labeled anti-immunoglobulins. Thus, the final results may not necessarily reflect the real proportions of the detected antigens.
14. As a negative control, the cross-reactivities of the secondary antibodies may be tested by exchanging them in single immunostainings.
15. The silver development step of the IGSS is very sensitive to the ambient temperature in the laboratory. There can be significant differences in the reaction speed in summer and winter depending on air conditioning or heating.
16. A further advantage of the IGSS method is that its reaction product can clearly be differentiated from immunoenzyme products with epi-polarization microscopy (*see* Chapter 30).
17. When increased sensitivity without extended time is needed, Dako's EnVision (indirect) reagents are recommended. These products consist of long dextran polymers coupled to tens of enzyme and immunoglobulin molecules. Monospecific EnVision+ conjugates are most useful, but dual specificity reagents (i.e., anti-mouse and -rabbit) labeled with both PO and AP may also be combined following the elution or blocking of the cross-reacting or irrelevant sequence after the first staining.
18. Double labeling with IGSS and IPO may be followed by the detection of a third antigen consecutively with an indirect IAP method as detailed above. Recommended combinations for sequential triple antigen detection are:
    (a) IGSS (black) + IPO (AEC, red-brown) + IAP (Fast Blue, blue)

(b) IGSS (black) + IPO (DAB, brown) + IAP (Fast Red or Fuchsine, magenta-red)

(c) IPO (DAB, brown) +IPO (AEC, red) + IAP (Fast Blue, blue; or NBT-BCIP, dark-blue)

19. Fluorescent nuclear counterstains such as DAPI (blue), or 7-AAD (red) can substantially improve recognition of morphological details. Dilute any of these dyes 1:1000 in TBS and incubate between 30 s and 2 min.

20. Preconditioning of the sections for 3–5 min in the neat substrate-chromogen buffers is important in order to avoid formation of unexpected precipitation of the chromogens due to sudden changes in pH or salt molarity.

21. Commercial DAB chromogen-substrate kits, such as DAB+ from Dako may also be used with metallic salt solutions, such as nickel-, cobalt- and copper-, but this need to be tested in advance. However, only a small volume of concentrate metal salt solution (e.g., 10 %) should be added to the developer to avoid its over-dilution.

22. Development of IAP products is very hard to standardize; therefore, the use of commercial kits are highly recommended.

23. The NBT-BCIP is probably the most stable chromogen-substrate system, and does not form precipitates in the developing solution for several hours. It is well suited for overnight development in nonradioactive in situ hybridization also.

References

1. Krenacs T, Krenacs L (1994) Immunogold-silver staining (IGSS) for immunoelectron microscopy and in multiple detection affinity cytochemistry. In: Gu J, Hacker GW (eds) Modern methods in analytical morphology. Plenum, New York, pp 225–251
2. Brahic M, Ozden S (1992) Simultaneous detection of cellular RNA and proteins. In situ hybridization. Oxford University Press, Oxford, UK, pp 85–102
3. Speel JM, Herbergs J, Ramaekers CS, Hopman AHN (1994) Combined immunocytochemistry and fluorescence in situ hybridization for simultaneous tricolor detection of cell cycle, genomic, and phenotypic parameters of tumor cells. J Histochem Cytochem 42: 961–966
4. Martinez-Ramirez A, Cigudosa JC, Maestre L, Rodriguez-Perales S, Haralambieva E, Benitez J, Roncador G (2004) Simultaneous detection of the immunophenotypic markers and genetic aberrations on routinely processed paraffin sections of lymphoma samples by means of the FICTION technique. Leukemia 18:348–353
5. Mason DY, Sammons R (1978) Alkaline phosphatase and peroxidase for double immunoenzymatic labeling of cellular constituents. J Clin Pathol 31:454–460
6. Falini B, Abdulaziz Z, Gerdes J, Canino S, Ciani C, Cordell JL, Knight PM, Stein H, Grignani F, Martelli MF, Mason DY (1986) Description of a sequential staining procedure for double immunoenzymatic staining of pairs of antigens using monoclonal antibodies. J Immunol Methods 93:265–273
7. Van Noorden S, Stuart MC, Cheung A, Adams EF, Polak JM (1986) Localization of pituitary hormones by multiple immunoenzyme staining procedures using monoclonal and polyclonal antibodies. J Histochem Cytochem 34:287–292

8. Krenacs T, Dobo E, Laszik Z (1990) Characteristics of endocrine pancreas in chronic pancreatitis as revealed by simultaneous immunocytochemical demonstration of hormone production. J Histotechnol 13:213–218
9. Krenacs T, Krenacs L, Bozoky B, Ivanyi B (1990) Double and triple immunocytochemical labeling at a light microscopic level in histopathology. Histochem J 22:530–536
10. Krenacs T, Laszik Z, Dobo E (1989) Application of immunogold-silver staining and immunoenzymatic methods in multiple labeling of human pancreatic Langerhans islet cells. Acta Histochem 85:79–85
11. Ferri G-L, Gaudio RM, Castello IF, Berger P, Giro G (1997) Quadruple Immunofluorescence: a direct visualization method. J Histochem Cytochem 45:155–158
12. Panchuk-Voloshina N, Haugland RP, Bishop-Stewart J, Bhalgat MK, Millard PJ, Mao F, Leung W-Y, Haugland RP (1999) Alexa dyes, a series of new fluorescent dyes that yield exceptionally bright, photostable conjugates. J Histochem Cytochem 47:1179–1188
13. Farstad IN, Halstensen TS, Kvale D, Fausa O, Brandtzaeg P (1997) Topographic distribution of homing receptors on B and T cells in human gut-associated lymphoid tissue. Am J Pathol 150:187–199
14. Krenacs T, Rosendaal M (1995) Immunohistological detection of gap junctions in human lymphoid tissue: connexin 43 in follicular dendritic and lymphoendothelial cells. J Histochem Cytochem 43:1125–2237
15. Chaubert P, Bertholet M-M, Correvon M, Laurini S, Bosman FT (1997) Simultaneous double immunoenzymatic labeling: a new procedure for the histopathologic routine. Mod Pathol 10:585–591
16. Boorsma DM (1984) Direct immunoenzyme double staining applicable for monoclonal antibodies. Histochemistry 80:103–106
17. Krenacs T, Uda H, Tanaka S (1991) One-step double immunolabeling of mouse interdigitating reticular cells: Simultaneous applications of preformed complexes of monoclonal rat antibody M1–8 with horseradish peroxidase-linked anti-rat immunoglobulin and of monoclonal mouse anti Ia antibody with alkaline phosphatase coupled anti-mouse immunoglobulins. J Histochem Cytochem 39:1719–1723
18. Morris TJ, Stanley EF (2003) A simple method for immunocytochemical staining with multiple rabbit polyclonal antibodies. J Neurosci Methods 127:149–155
19. Muehlmann M (2002) Molecular cytogenetics in metaphase and interphase cells for cancer and genetic research, diagnosis and prognosis. Application in tissue sections and cell suspensions. Genet Mol Res 1:117–127
20. Wu X, Liu H, Liu J, Haley KN, Treadway JA, Larson JP, Ge N, Peale F, Bruchez MP (2003) Immunofluorescent labeling of cancer marker Her2 and other cellular targets with semiconductor quantum dots. Nat Biotechnol 21:41–46
21. Van der Loos CM, Becker AE (1994) Double epi-illumination microscopy with separate visualization of two antigens: a combination of epi-polarization for immunogold-silver staining and epi-fluorescence for alkaline phosphatase staining. J Histochem Cytochem 42:289–295
22. Lehr H-A, Van der Loos CM, Teeling P, Gown AM (1999) Complete chromogen separation and analysis in double immunohistochemical stains using photoshop-based image analysis. J Histochem Cytochem 47:119–125
23. Mason DY, Micklem K, Jones M (2000) Double immunofluorescence labelling of routinely processed paraffin sections. J Pathol 191:452–461
24. Gillitzer R, Berger R, Moll H (1990) A reliable method for simultaneous demonstration of two antigens using a novel combination of immunogold-silver staining and immunoenzymatic labeling. J Histochem Cytochem 38:307–313
25. Hsu SM, Soban E (1982) Color modification of diaminobenzidine (DAB) precipitation metallic ions and its application for double immunohistochemistry. J Histochem Cytochem 30: 1079–1082
26. Merchenthaler I, Stankovics J, Gallyas F (1989) A highly sensitive one-step method for silver intensification of nickel-diaminobenzidine end product of peroxidase reaction. J Histochem Cytochem 37:1563–1565
27. Van den Pol AN (1986) Tyrosine hydroxylase immunoreactive neurons throughout the hypothalamus receive glutamate decarboxylase immunoreactive synapses: a double pre-embedding immunocytochemical study with particulate silver and HRP. J Neurosci 6:877–891
28. Lanciego JL, Goede PH, Witter MP, Wouterlood FG (1997) Use of peroxidase substrate vector VIP for multiple staining light microscopy. J Neurosci Methods 74:1–7
29. Nakane PK (1968) Simultaneous localization of multiple tissue antigens using the peroxidase-labeled antibody method: a study on pituitary glands of the rat. J Histochem Cytochem 16:557–560
30. Tramu G, Pillez A, Leonardelli J (1978) An efficient method of antibody elution for the successive or simultaneous localization of two

antigens by immunocytochemistry. J Histochem Cytochem 26:322–324

31. Gown AM, Garcia R, Ferguson M, Yamanaka E, Tippens D (1986) Avidin-biotin-immunoglucose oxidase: use in single and double labelling procedures. J Histochem Cytochem 34:403–409
32. Wang BL, Larsson LI (1985) Simultaneous demonstration of multiple antigens by indirect immunofluorescence or immunogold staining. Novel light and electron microscopic double and triple staining method employing primary antibodies from the same species. Histochemistry 83:47–56
33. Lan HY, Mu W, Nikolic-Paterson DJ, Atkins RC (1995) A novel, simple, reliable, and sensitive method for multiple immunoenzyme staining: use of microwave oven heating to block antibody cross-reactivity and retrieve antigens. J Histochem Cytochem 43:97–102
34. Tornehave D, Hougard DM, Larsson L-I (2000) Microwaving for double indirect immunofluorescence with primary antibodies from the same species and for staining of mouse tissues with mouse monoclonal antibodies. Histochem Cell Biol 113:19–23
35. Negoescu A, Labat-Moleur F, Lorimier P, Lamarcq L, Guillermet C, Chabaz E, Brambilla E (1994) F(ab) secondary antibodies: a general method for double immunolabeling with primary antisera from the same species. Efficiency control by chemiluminescence. J Histochem Cytochem 42:433–437
36. Van der Loos CM, Das PK, Van der Oord JJ, Houthoff HJ (1989) Multiple immunoenzyme staining techniques. Use of fluoresceinated, biotinylated and unlabelled monoclonal antibodies. J Immunol Methods 117:45–52
37. Van der Loos CM, Gobel H (2000) The animal research kit (ARK) can be used in a multistep double staining method for human tissue specimens. J Histochem Cytochem 48:1431–1437
38. Hunyady B, Krempels K, Harta GY, Mezey E (1996) Immunohistochemical signal amplification by catalyzed reporter deposition and its application in double immunostaining. J Histochem Cytochem 44:1353–1362
39. Shindler KS, Roth KA (1996) Double immunofluorescent staining using two unconjugated primary antisera raised in the same species. J Histochem Cytochem 44:1331–1335
40. Hacker GW, Grimelius L, Danscher G, Bernatzky G, Muss W, Adam H, Thurner J (1988) Silver acetate autometallography: an alternative enhancement technique for immunogold-silver staining (IGSS) and silver amplification of gold, silver, mercury and zinc in tissues. J Histotechnol 11:213–221

Chapter 29

Immunoenzymatic Quantitative Analysis of Antigens Expressed on the Cell Surface (Cell-ELISA)

Elaine Vicente Lourenço and Maria-Cristina Roque-Barreira

Abstract

Cell-enzyme-linked immunosorbent assay (cell-ELISA) is an useful technique for the quantitative analysis of cell surface antigen expression that was developed on the basis of enzyme immunohistochemistry (EIH) and ELISA. Since its development, which was made possible by the establishment of monoclonal antibody technology, a wide range of cell types and surface molecules were analyzed by cell-ELISA. Here we show four variants of this method and provide a brief comparison of cell-ELISA with flow cytometry (FACS) and radioimmunobinding assay (RIA), which are other methods for the quantitative detection of cell-surface molecules. We describe step-by-step procedures for both direct and indirect cell-ELISA using either adherent or nonadherent live cells.

Key words: Cell-ELISA, Surface antigen, Intracytoplasmic antigen, Diagnosis, Adherent, Endogenous enzyme, FACS, RIA

1. Introduction

Cell-enzyme-linked immunosorbent assay (cell-ELISA) is an immunoenzymatic technique for the quantitative analysis of molecules expressed on the cell surface. The technique was developed (1) on the basis of two earlier immunoenzymatic methods: (1) enzyme immunohistochemistry (EIH), developed in the mid-sixties for the identification and localization of antigens in histological preparations, and (2) ELISA, which allows for the quantification of soluble antigens or antibodies by immobilizing one of the immunoreactants on a solid phase (2). The most important motivation for cell-ELISA development was the establishment of monoclonal antibody (mAb) technology (3), which created the necessity for rapidly screening, after a single fusion procedure, several hundreds of antibody secreting clones specific

C. Oliver and M.C. Jamur (eds.), *Immunocytochemical Methods and Protocols*, Methods in Molecular Biology, Vol. 588, DOI 10.1007/978-1-59745-324-0_29,

for cell-surface antigens. Since the eighties, a wide range of cell types and surface molecules were analyzed by cell-ELISA and several variants of this method were developed, showing that the applications of this technique go beyond hybridoma screening (3). Today, the cell-ELISA technique is widely used in many diverse situations, such as the detection of intracytoplasmic and endoplasmic reticulum-located antigens (4), differential diagnosis between tuberculous and pyogenic meningitis (5), and quantifying GPI- and transmembrane-anchored proteins (6).

Considering the purpose of this book, it is important to briefly compare cell-ELISA with other methods for the quantitative detection of cell-surface molecules, such as flow cytometry (FACS, *see* Chapters 31–36) and radioimmunobinding assay (RIA) (1, 7). In spite of their sensitivity, these methods present some disadvantages associated with cost, handling of radioactive materials, difficulty in performing a large number of analyses, and, in the case of FACS, the impossibility of determining antigen expression in adherent cells. Cell-ELISA, besides avoiding these negative aspects, is a simple, rapid, inexpensive, and highly sensitive alternative to quantify cell-surface molecules (8–11). However, unlike FACS analysis, cell-ELISA is not appropriate for analyzing mixed cell populations. In cell-ELISA, labeling of immunoreactant molecule is provided by an enzyme, such as horseradish peroxidase (HRP), alkaline phosphatase or β-galactosidase. In this manner, the assays take advantage not only from the discriminatory capacity of the antibodies, but also from the high catalytic power and specificity of enzymes (1). Chromogenic substrates may be detectable with great ease by inexpensive photometric equipment. The antibody/enzyme conjugates, unlike fluorochrome and radioisotope-coupled reagents, have a long shelf-life. In addition, antibody/enzyme conjugates do not represent health or environmental hazards, as radioactive reagents do. Nevertheless, in the case of cells with endogenous enzyme activity (i.e., granulocytes or macrophages), it may be necessary to inhibit the endogenous enzyme or select a secondary antibody that is coupled to an enzyme that is not endogenously expressed.

In this chapter, we describe four variants of the cell-ELISA procedure using viable cells. The choice of the appropriate assay will basically depend on the adhesion characteristics of the cells to be assayed.

2. Materials

2.1. Cell Culture

1. Culture medium (e.g., RPMI) supplemented with 5% fetal calf serum, 10 mM HEPES, 2 mM L-glutamine, all from Sigma-Aldrich, St. Louis, MO, USA; and 1% non-essential

amino acids, 1 mM sodium pyruvate, gentamicin (50 μg/mL), all from Invitrogen, GIBCO, Carlsbad, CA, and 50 μM β-mercaptoethanol. The medium choice will depend on the cell type used.

2. Fetal bovine serum (FBS–Sigma) heat-inactivated at 56°C for 30 min.
3. Flat-, cone- or round-bottomed 96 multiwell plates (Corning Life Sciences, Lowell, MA).
4. Culture flasks, cell scraper, conical centrifuge tube (Corning).

2.2. Cell-ELISA

1. Cell sample.
2. Positive-control antibodies (i.e., those that react with the experimental cells).
3. Negative-control antibodies (i.e., those that do not react with the experimental cells, IgG from the same species as the primary antibody, or no antibody).
4. HRP-conjugated specific antibody (*see* Note 5).
5. Phosphate-buffered saline (PBS), pH 7.4: 8 g sodium chloride (NaCl), 200 mg potassium chloride (KCl), 200 mg monobasic potassium phosphate (KH_2PO_4), 1.15 g anhydrous dibasic sodium phosphate (Na_2HPO_4), bring volume to 1 L with deionized glass-distilled water (dH_2O).
6. ELISA buffer: PBS containing 1% bovine serum albumin (BSA); 1 g BSA (Sigma) and 100 mL PBS. Make fresh daily or aliquot and store at –20°C.
7. Washing buffer: 0.5% BSA and 100 mL PBS.
8. Substrate buffer, pH 4.5: *Solution A* (0.1 M citric acid [0.48 g/25 mL dH_2O]), *Solution B* (0.2 M Na_2HPO_4 [0.852 g/30 mL dH_2O]). Mixture: 24.3 mL of solution A, 25.7 mL of solution B, bring volume to 100 mL with dH_2O. Store at 4°C in the dark. Stable for up to 1 month.
9. TMB chromogen Stock: 41.6 mM 3,3′,5,5′ tetrametilbenzidine (TMB) (10 mg/mL dimethyl sulfoxide (DMSO-Sigma)]. Light sensitive. Stable at 4°C for 1 month.
10. Substrate solution: 4.95 mL of substrate buffer, 0.05 mL of TMB chromogen stock, 0.01 mL of 3% H_2O_2 (0.01 mL of 30% H_2O_2/mL dH_2O). Make fresh as required. Alternatively, use TMB single solution cat. # 00-2023 from Zymed Laboratories.
11. Stop solution: 2 M sulfuric acid (H_2SO_4); 2 mL sulfuric acid, bring volume to 18 mL with dH_2O.
12. 0.2% Trypan blue (Merck): 0.2 g of Trypan blue powder and 100 mL PBS.

3. Methods

3.1. Indirect Cell-ELISA for Adherent Cells

1. If cells are growing in a culture flask, detach them from the surface using a cell scraper. Centrifuge the cell suspension 5 min at 500×*g*, 4°C, in a 15 mL conical centrifuge tube.
2. Re-suspend cells in 3–5 mL of culture medium containing 5% FBS, wait 3 min to allow clumps to settle, and transfer to another tube the upper portion of the cell suspension, leaving the clumps behind.
3. Count viable cells mixing an aliquot of the cell suspension with trypan blue. Adjust the suspension to give a density of 1×10^6 cells/mL.
4. Add 100 μL of the cell suspension (1×10^5 cells *see* Note 1) into wells of flat-bottomed 96 multiwell plates and incubate in 5% CO_2, at 37°C, at least 24 h for cells to attach.
5. Remove residual culture medium by inversion and gently tapping the inverted plate on a paper towel.
6. Dispense the primary antibody (50 μL) diluted in ice-cold ELISA buffer at the optimal concentration (*see* Note 1), holding the pipette tips against the walls of the wells.
7. Incubate 1 h at 4°C. (*see* Note 2).
8. Remove the unbound primary antibody by vacuum aspiration, being careful to avoid drying. Wash the plate by gently adding 200 μL of ice-cold washing buffer by holding the pipette tips against the walls of the wells to prevent detachment and loss of cells.
9. Repeat the washing step four more times (*see* Note 3). After the last washing step, remove the washing buffer by inversion and gently tapping the inverted plate on a paper towel.
10. Add the HRP-conjugated to antibody specific for the primary antibody (50 μL) diluted in ice-cold ELISA buffer at the optimal concentration and incubate the plate for 1 h at 4°C (*see* Notes 4–7).
11. Wash the plate wells five more times as above.
12. Add 50 μL freshly prepared substrate solution to the wells. Keep the plate at room temperature and allow enzyme activity to proceed until the signal has reached the desired levels.
13. Stop the enzyme reaction by adding 25 μL stop solution and measure the enzyme activity using a microtiter plate reader at A_{450} nm.

3.2. Indirect Cell-ELISA for Cells in Suspension

1. Centrifuge cell samples 5 min at 500×*g*, 4°C, in a 15 mL conical centrifuge tube. Re-suspend cells in 3–5 mL of culture medium and wait 3 min to allow clumps to settle.

2. Transfer the upper portion of the cell suspension to another tube, leaving the clumps behind and count viable cells by mixing an aliquot of the cell suspension with trypan blue.
3. Adjust the suspension to give a density of 1×10^6 cells/mL. Pipet 100 µL of the cell suspension (1×10^5 cells) (*see* Note 1) into wells of round- or cone-bottomed 96 multiwell plates that had been pretreated with 200 µL/well of ELISA buffer for 1 h at room temperature.
4. Centrifuge the plate in a centrifuge with adapters holding microtiter plates at $1,000 \times g$ for 1 min at 4°C.
5. Remove the supernatant by vacuum aspiration, being careful to avoid drying, and loosen the cell pellet by briefly shaking the multiwell plate.
6. Re-suspend cells in 50 µL of the primary antibody diluted in ice-cold ELISA buffer at the optimal concentration (*see* Note 1). Incubate 1 h at 4°C, re-suspending cells by gently shaking at 15 min intervals.
7. Centrifuge the plate 1 min at $1,000 \times g$ at 4°C. Remove the unbound antibodies by vacuum aspiration, being careful to avoid drying. Loosen the cell pellet by briefly shaking the multiwell plate.
8. Wash the plate by adding 200 µL of ice-cold washing buffer to the wells, centrifuge the plate at $1,000 \times g$ for 1 min at 4°C.
9. Remove the washing buffer by vacuum aspiration, being careful to avoid drying, and gently tapping the inverted plate on a paper towel. Loosen the cell pellet by briefly shaking the multiwell plate and repeat the wash step four times.
10. Re-suspend the loosened cell pellet in 50 µL HRP-conjugated to antibody specific for the primary antibody diluted in ice-cold ELISA buffer at the optimal concentration (*see* Notes 4–7).
11. Incubate 1 h at 4°C, re-suspending cells by gently shaking at 15 min intervals.
12. Wash the cells five times as above.
13. Add 50 µL freshly prepared substrate solution to the loosened cell pellet. Keep the plate at room temperature, re-suspending cells by gently shaking at 5 min intervals. Allow enzyme activity to proceed until the signal has reached the desired levels.
14. Stop the enzyme reaction by adding 25 µL of stop solution and measure the enzyme activity using a microtiter plate reader at A_{450} nm

3.3. Direct Cell-ELISA for Adherent Cells

1. If cells are growing in culture flask, detach them from the surface using a cell scraper. Centrifuge the cell suspension 5 min at 500 × *g*, 4°C, in a 15 mL conical centrifuge tube.
2. Re-suspend cells in 3–5 mL of culture medium containing 10% FBS, wait 3 min to allow clumps to settle, and transfer the upper portion of the cell suspension to another tube, leaving the clumps behind.
3. Count viable cells mixing an aliquot of the cell suspension with trypan blue. Adjust the suspension to give a density of 1×10^6 cells/mL.
4. Add 100 μL of the cell suspension (1×10^5 cells *see* Note 1) to wells of flat-bottomed 96 multiwell plates and incubate in 5% CO_2, at 37°C, at least 24 h for cells to attach.
5. Remove residual culture medium by inversion and gently tapping the inverted plate on a paper towel.
6. Add the antibody, specific for the epitope of interest, directly conjugated to HRP (50 μL) diluted in ice-cold ELISA buffer at the optimal concentration (*see* Notes 4–7), holding the pipette tips against the walls of the wells. Incubate 1 h at 4°C.
7. Remove the unbound conjugate by vacuum aspiration, being careful to avoid drying. Wash the cells by gently adding 200 μL of ice-cold washing buffer by holding the pipette tips against the walls of the wells to prevent detachment and loss of cells.
8. Repeat the washing step four more times (*see* Note 3). After the last washing step, remove the washing buffer by inversion and gently tapping the inverted plate on a paper towel.
9. Add 50 μL freshly prepared substrate solution to the wells. Keep the plate at room temperature and allow enzyme activity to proceed until the signal has reached the desired levels.
10. Stop the enzyme reaction by adding 25 μL stop solution and measure the enzyme activity using a microtiter plate reader at A_{450} nm.

3.4. Direct Cell-ELISA for Cells in Suspension

1. Centrifuge cell samples 5 min at 500 × *g*, 4° C, in a 15 mL conical centrifuge tube. Re-suspend cells in 3–5 mL of culture medium and wait 3 min to allow clumps to settle.
2. Transfer the upper portion of the cell suspension to another tube, leaving the clumps behind and count viable cells mixing an aliquot of the cell suspension with trypan blue.
3. Adjust the suspension to give a density of 1×10^6 cells/mL. Pipet 100 μL of the cell suspension (1×10^5 cells *see* Note 1) into the wells of round- or cone-bottomed 96 multiwell plates that had been pretreated with 200 μL/well of ELISA buffer for 1 h at room temperature.
4. Centrifuge the plate in a centrifuge with adapters holding microtiter plates at 1,000 × *g* for 1 min at 4°C.

5. Remove the supernatant by vacuum aspiration, being careful to avoid drying, and loosen the cell pellet by briefly shaking the multiwell plate.
6. Re-suspend cells in antibody, specific for the epitope of interest, directly conjugated to HRP (50 μL) diluted in ice-cold ELISA buffer at the optimal concentration (*see* Notes 4–7).
7. Incubate 1 h at 4°C, re-suspending cells by gently shaking at 15-min intervals.
8. Centrifuge the plate 1 min at 1,000 × *g* at 4°C. Remove the unbound antibodies by vacuum aspiration, being careful to avoid drying, loosen the cell pellet by briefly shaking the multiwell plate.
9. Wash the plate by adding 200 μL of ice-cold washing buffer into the wells, centrifuge the plate at 1,000 × *g* for 1 min at 4°C.
10. Remove the washing buffer by vacuum aspiration, being careful to avoid drying, and gently tapping the inverted plate on a paper towel. Loosen the cell pellet by briefly shaking the multiwell plate and repeat the wash step four times.
11. After washing, re-suspend the loosened cell pellet with freshly prepared substrate solution. Keep the plate at room temperature, re-suspending cells by gently shaking at 5-min intervals. Allow enzyme activity to proceed until the signal has reached the desired levels.
12. Stop the enzyme reaction by adding 25 μL stop solution and measure the enzyme activity using a microtiter plate reader at A_{450} nm.

4. Notes

1. The optimal number of cells, as well as the primary antibody concentration should be determined in preliminary experiments by serial-dilution assays. A range of 0.1–1 × 10^5 cells/well and primary antibody at 1–10 μg/mL for purified antibody. When the antibody is hybridoma supernatant, a 1:2 dilution may be used. Both negative and positive controls should be included to account for any nonspecific binding.
2. This temperature is indicated for both antibody incubations and washing steps to minimize the endocytosis of cell surface molecules.
3. An alternative washing protocol may be used to minimize the loss of adherent cells (12). The plate is immersed in a tray containing 1 L of washing buffer, gently agitating the submerged plate for 1 min. The plate should be transferred to another tray containing fresh washing buffer three more times.

4. The optimal antibody-conjugate concentration should be determined in preliminary experiments by serial-dilution assays. Titrate conjugate initially at 1–10 μg/mL.
5. Since HRP, as well as alkaline phosphatase can be expressed by eukaryotic cells (*see* Zymed recommended ELISA methods, http://www.invitrogen.com/content.cfm?pageid=10702), test cells must be assayed in preliminary experiments by incubation with TMB substrate alone. If the test shows unacceptable background, detection antibody conjugated to HRP should be replaced with the bacterial enzyme β-galactosidase (BG). BG is preferable to HRP and alkaline phosphatase because in eukaryotic organisms as lower endogenous enzyme activity is detected in some cell populations (12, 13). Kits are now commercially available for both peroxidase and alkaline phosphates based ELISA. A final alternative may be to adapt the ELISA to use an antibody conjugated to a fluorophore and use a fluorescent plate reader (BMG Labtech Inc, Durham, NC; Global Medical Instrumentation Inc., Ramsey, MN; Turner Biosystems, Sunnyvale, CA).
6. Alternatively, fixation of the cells can be used to minimize the enzyme background problems, because this step may inactivate endogenous HRP or alkaline phosphatase activity (14). Furthermore, fixation ensures adhesion of cells to the plate well and minimizes cell loss during washing steps (15, 16). However, the use of this procedure it is not advised because it can modify the outcome of the experiment, leading to false positive and false negative results (17, 18). Nevertheless, if the surface antigen is fixation-resistant, cells may be fixed at the beginning of the experiments with 0.05% glutaraldehyde in PBS at 4°C for 30 min. Glutaraldehyde should not be used as a fixative if you are using a fluorescent assay. Remove the fixation solution and wash the cells three times with 0.1 M glycine in PBS. Block nonspecific-binding sites with ELISA buffer before performing the assay.
7. Another background problem may be due to nonspecific binding of the conjugate to Fc receptors in the test cells. To prevent this, enzyme conjugated to $F(ab')_2$ fragments are preferable. Since these fragments have had the Fc portion of the antibody enzymatically removed they no longer bind to Fc receptors. Another alternative is to use Fc block (BD Biosciences, Franklin Lakes, NJ). This is a mixture of antibodies against CD16 (FcγRIII) and CD32 (FcγRII) that blocks binding of the Fc portion of IgGs to these receptors. Chicken IgY may also be used in place of IgG. The Fc portion of chicken IgY does not bind to mammalian IgG receptors. IgY is commercially available as both unconjugated or conjugated primary and secondary antibodies. Alternatively, normal serum or normal IgG from the same species as the conjugate may prevent nonspecific reaction with Fc receptors.

References

1. Tijssen P (ed) (1985) Practice and theory of enzyme immunoassays. Elsevier, Amsterdam
2. Köhler G, Milstein C (1975) Continuous cultures of fused cells secreting antibody of predefined specificity. Nature 256:495–497
3. Sedgwick JD, Czerkinsky C (1992) Detection of cell-surface molecules, secreted products of single cells and cellular proliferation by enzyme immunoassay. J Immunol Methods 150:159–175
4. Ogino T, Wang X, Ferrone S (2003) Modified flow cytometry and cell-ELISA methodology to detect HLA class I antigen processing machinery components in cytoplasm and endoplasmic reticulum. J Immunol Methods 278:33–44
5. Kashyap RS, Kainthla RP, Satpute RM, Agarwal NP, Chandak NH, Purohit HJ, Taori GM, Daginawala HF (2004) Differential diagnosis of tuberculous meningitis from partially-treated pyogenic meningitis by cell ELISA. BMC Neurol 4:16–21
6. Bumgarner GW, Zampell JC, Nagarajan S, Poloso NJ, Dorn AS, D'Souza MJ, Selvaraj P (2005) Modified cell ELISA to determine the solubilization of cell surface proteins: applications in GPI-anchored protein purification. J Biochem Biophys Methods 64:99–109
7. Loken MR, Herzenberg LA (1975) Analysis of cell populations with a fluorescence-activated cell sorter. Ann NY Acad Sci 254:163–171
8. Avrameas S, Guilbert B (1971) A method for quantitative determination of cellular immunoglobulins by enzyme-labeled antibodies. Eur J Immunol 1:394–396
9. Buchanan D, Kamarck M, Ruddle NH (1981) Development of a protein A enzyme immunoassay for use in screening hybridomas. J Immunol Methods 42:179–185
10. Aida Y, Onuma M, Kasai N, Izawa H (1987) Use of viable-cell ELISA for detection of monoclonal antibodies recognizing tumor-associated antigens on bovine lymphosarcoma cells. Am J Vet Res 48:1319–1324
11. Posner MR, Antoniou D, Griffin J, Schlossman SF, Lazarus H (1982) An enzyme-linked immunosorbent assay (ELISA) for the detection of monoclonal antibodies to cell surface antigens on viable cells. J Immunol Methods 48:23–31
12. Liu Z, Gurlo T, von Grafenstein H (2000) Cell-ELISA using beta-galactosidase conjugated antibodies. J Immunol Methods 234:153–167
13. Cobbold SP, Waldmann H (1981) A rapid solid-phase enzyme-linked binding assay for screening monoclonal antibodies to cell surface antigens. J Immunol Methods 44:125–133
14. Douillard JY, Hoffman T, Herberman RB (1980) Enzyme-linked immunosorbent assay for screening monoclonal antibody production: use of intact cells as antigen. J Immunol Methods 39:309–316
15. Nibbering PH, Van de Gevel JS, Van Furth R (1990) A cell-ELISA for the quantification of adherent murine macrophages and the surface expression of antigens. J Immunol Methods 131:25–32
16. Hatayama H, Imai K, Kanzaki H, Higuchi T, Fujimoto M, Mori T (1996) Detection of antiendometrial antibodies in patients with endometriosis by cell ELISA. Am J Reprod Immunol 35:118–122
17. Feit C, Bartal AH, Tauber G, Dymbort G, Hirshaut Y (1983) An enzyme-linked immunosorbent assay (ELISA) for the detection of monoclonal antibodies recognizing surface antigens expressed on viable cells. J Immunol Methods 58:301–308
18. Drover S, Marshall WH (1986) Glutaraldehyde fixation of target cells to plastic for ELISA assays of monoclonal anti-HLA antibodies produces artefacts. J Immunol Methods 90:275–281

Chapter 30

Use of Immunogold with Silver Enhancement

Constance Oliver

Abstract

Although gold particles are readily detectable by transmission electron microscopy, they can be difficult to visualize by bright-field light microscopy. However when the gold is silver-enhanced it is easy to see. During silver-enhancement, the colloidal gold serves as a nucleation site for the deposition of metallic silver. The enhancing solutions are physical developers that contain both silver ions and a reducing agent, buffered to an acid pH. The silver-enhancement method has also been used successfully to enlarge small-diameter gold particles for visualization by scanning electron microscopy. Silver-enhancement has been applied to a wide variety of tissues and antigens for both light and scanning electron microscopy.

Key words: Silver enhancement, Colloidal gold, Scanning electron microscopy, Light microscopy, Epipolarization, Immunomicroscopy

1. Introduction

Although gold particles are readily detectable by transmission electron microscopy, they can be difficult to visualize by bright-field light microscopy. If the particle size is large enough and the labeling dense enough, the gold particles will stain tissue red (1, 2). However, unless the gold is silver-enhanced to help visualize it, the sensitivity of the staining is fairly low. During silver-enhancement, the colloidal gold serves as a nucleation site for the deposition of metallic silver. The silver layer increases the size of the gold and imparts a black color to the stained tissue when viewed by bright-field microscopy (Fig. 1a). The silver-enhanced gold particles can also be visualized using epipolarization, where they appear bright against a dark background (Fig. 1b). The silver-enhancement method has its basis in nineteenth-century photographic techniques. The enhancing solutions are physical developers that contain both silver ions and a reducing agent,

C. Oliver and M.C. Jamur (eds.), *Immunocytochemical Methods and Protocols*, Methods in Molecular Biology, Vol. 588, DOI 10.1007/978-1-59745-324-0_30, © Humana Press, a part of Springer Science+Business Media, LLC 1995, 1999, 2010

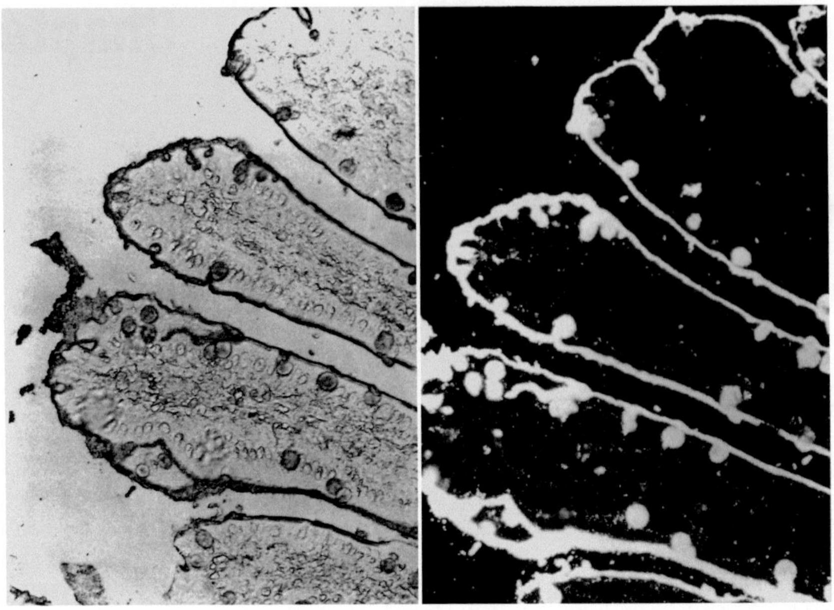

Fig. 1. Small intestine: formaldehyde-fixed paraffin-embedded. Section was stained with Concanavalin A conjugated to 5-nm colloidal gold. The gold was then silver-enhanced. Staining of mucous on the cell surface and in goblet cells is seen. **(a)** Bright field microscopy. The silver-enhanced gold appears as a dark stain. **(b)** Epipolarization microscopy. The silver-enhanced gold appears bright against a dark background.

buffered to an acid pH. The developers most commonly used contain silver lactate as the source of silver ions (3). The silver lactate has a low dissociation coefficient that allows for more control of the reduction. Hydroquinone (1,4-dihydroxybenzene) is the only reducing agent that has been used in silver-enhancement techniques. A protective colloid, such as gum arabic, bovine serum albumin, dextran, polyethylene glycol (PEG), or polyvinylpyrrolidone (PVP), is frequently added in order to inhibit the autocatalytic reaction between the silver salt and the reducing agent. The protective colloid also helps in providing even distribution of the components during the development. The developing solution is very unstable and must be protected from light. The samples should also be protected from light during silver-enhancement. Commercial silver-enhancing kits are also available. These kits have the advantage that their components are stable and may be stored in the refrigerator for months. They are also insensitive to light, so that the enhancement procedure can be monitored by light microscopy. The use of silver-enhancement for detecting gold in tissue sections was introduced in 1935 by W. J. Roberts, who published a photochemical method for detecting injected gold salts in animal tissues (4). By the 1980s, immunogold staining was firmly established for electron microscopy. Danscher's (3, 5) evaluation of photochemical methods to visualize gold for light and electron microscopy, and the application of these methods by Holgate et al. (6, 7) demonstrated the feasibility of applying physical development methods to localize immunogold-stained sites. The silver-enhancement method has also been used successfully to enlarge small-diameter gold particles for visualization by scanning electron microscopy (SEM) (8, 9). Although the use of small gold particles will increase the efficiency of the reaction, particles smaller than 20 nm are too small to be easily seen using standard scanning electron microscopic methods. The use of silver-enhancement to enlarge the smaller gold particles overcomes this problem. When combined with backscattered imaging, the ability to resolve immunogold by SEM is further increased. Silver-enhancement has been applied to a wide variety of tissues and antigens for both light and SEM (10–12).

2. Materials

1. Sections cut onto aminosilane-coated slides and rehydrated to water (*see* Note 1).
2. Tris-buffered saline (TBS): 2.4 g Tris and 8.76 g NaCl. Adjust the pH to 7.4 with HCl then bring volume to 1 L with deionized glass-distilled water.
3. 1% Bovine serum albumin (BSA): 1 g BSA and 100 mL TBS, pH7.4. Add BSA to TBS while stirring.
4. Primary antibody diluted in 1% BSA in TBS.
5. Silver-enhancing solution (11): 60 mL protective colloid (25% gum arabic or 50% PEG [20,000 mol. wt.] or PVP), 10 mL 2 M citric acid or sodium citrate, and 850 mg hydroquinone dissolved in 15 mL deionized glass-distilled water; mix thoroughly; adjust pH to 3.8; immediately before use, add 110 mg silver lactate dissolved in 15 mL deionized glass-distilled water (*see* Note 2).
6. Commercially available silver enhancement kit (see Note 3).
7. Colloidal gold conjugate (*see* Note 4).

3. Methods

3.1. Silver-Enhancement for Light Microscopy

Immunogold staining can be used successfully at the light microscopic level if the gold is silver-enhanced. Enhancing solutions may be made up in the laboratory, but because of their instability and light sensitivity, the commercially available silver-enhancing kits are preferable.

1. Block tissue for 15 min in TBS containing 1–5% BSA.
2. Rinse five times in TBS containing 1% BSA.
3. Incubate slides in a moist chamber in primary antibody diluted in TBS plus 1% BSA for 1–2 h at room temperature. Plastic-embedded sections may need to be incubated for 2 h at 37°C.
4. Rinse five times in TBS containing 1% BSA.
5. If required, incubate 30 min at room temperature in bridging antibody diluted in TBS plus 1% BSA, and rinse five times in TBS plus 1% BSA.
6. Incubate slides for 30 min at room temperature in colloidal gold conjugate diluted in TBS plus 1% BSA.
7. Rinse the sections five times in TBS, and then rinse five times in deionized glass-distilled water (*see* Note 5).
8. Prepare silver-enhancing solution immediately prior to use, and cover the sections with the solution (*see* Note 6) and incubate at room temperature.
9. Rinse the sections five times in deionized glass-distilled water (*see* Note 7).
10. Counterstain and mount. All commonly used counterstains and mounting media can be used.

3.2. Silver Enhancement for Scanning Electron Microscopy

The procedure given above may be used successfully to surface-label cells or tissue for examination by SEM.

1. Immunolabel samples either before or after fixation. Any size gold can be used for SEM. The size of the gold particles is limited by the resolution of the instrument.
2. After fixation and labeling, silver-enhance the gold using a commercially available kit. Generally, the time needed for enhancement for SEM is around 5 min.
3. Dehydrate the samples, and critically point-dry.
4. The silver-enhanced gold can be detected in the scanning electron microscope using backscattered electron imaging.

4. Notes

1. Do not use coatings, such as poly-L-lysine or chrome-alum, since the charge will interfere with the silver intensification reaction. For paraffin sections, remove paraffin with xylene

and rehydrate to water. Penetration of reagents into plastic-embedded sections may be improved by treating the sections for 15 min with xylene and rehydrating to water. Following rehydration, the sections should not be allowed to dry.

2. All components, except the protective colloid, should be prepared immediately before use. Protect hydroquinone, silver lactate, and complete developer from light.
3. Commercially available kits, such as IntenSE™ Silver Enhancement reagents from GE Healthcare Life Technologies, are more stable and not as light-sensitive as enhancing solutions prepared in the laboratory.
4. The colloidal gold should be conjugated to an antibody raised against the species of the primary antibody or to Protein A, such that it will bind to the primary antibody (*see* Chapter 39). For light microscopy, 1- and 5-nm colloidal gold conjugates are used most frequently. The 1-nm gold may be somewhat more difficult to silver-enhance. For SEM, the size of the gold depends on the resolution of the instrument: 10–20 nm gold is the size most frequently used for SEM.
5. The ions from the buffer must be removed, or they will serve as nucleation sites for the silver and increase the background. If rinsing the samples in distilled water damages the tissue or if the acid pH of the enhancing solution removes antibodies with low affinities, the samples may be briefly fixed and quenched before rinsing in water and proceeding to the next steps.
6. For commercial enhancing solutions, incubate the sections 5–15 min. With these solutions, the optimal incubation time may be determined by monitoring the deposition of the silver by light microscopy. For developing solutions prepared in the laboratory, development should be done in a dark room with a safety light. The samples are immersed in the developer for 10–45 min. For longer development times, the solution may have to be changed.
7. After development, the slides must be thoroughly washed in deionized glass-distilled water to stop development.

References

1. DeMey J, Moeremans M, Geuens G, Nuydens R, DeBrander M (1981) High resolution light and electron microscopic localization of tubulin with the IGS (immuno-gold staining) method. Cell Biol Int Rep 5: 889–899
2. Geoghegan WD, Scillian JJ, Ackerman GA (1978) The detection of human B lymphocytes by both light and electron microscopy utilizing colloidal gold labeled anti-immunoglobulin. Immunol Commun 7:1–12
3. Danscher G (1981) Histochemical demonstration of heavy metals. A revised version of the sulphide silver method suitable for both light and electron microscopy. Histochemistry 71:1–16

4. Roberts WJ (1935) A new procedure for the detection of gold in animal tissues: physical development. Proc R Acad Sci Amsterdam 38:540–544
5. Danscher G (1981) Localization of gold in biological tissue. A photochemical method for light and electron microscopy. Histochemistry 71:81–88
6. Holgate CS, Jackson PI, Cowen PN, Bird CC (1983) Immunogold-silver staining: new method of immunostaining with enhanced sensitivity. J Histochem Cytochem 31:938–944
7. Holgate CS, Jackson P, Lauder I, Cowen P, Bird CC (1983) Surface membrane staining of immunoglobulins in paraffin sections of non-Hodgkin's lymphomas using immunogold-silver staining technique. J Clin Pathol 36:742–746
8. Goode D, Maugel TK (1987) Backscattered electron imaging of immunogold labeled and silver-enhanced microtubules in cultured mammalian cells. J Electron Microsc Tech 5:263–273
9. de Harven E (1989) Backscattered electron imaging of the colloidal gold marker on cell surfaces. In: Hayat MA (ed) Colloidal gold, vol. 1. Academic, New York, NY, pp 229–249
10. Larsson L-I (1988) Immunocytochemical detection systems. In: Larsson L-I (ed) Immunocytochemistry: theory and practice. CRC, Boca Raton, FL, pp 77–146
11. Scopsi L (1989) Silver-enhanced colloidal gold method. In: Hayat MA (ed) Colloidal gold, vol. 1. Academic, New York, NY, pp 251–295
12. Hacker GW (1989) Silver-enhanced colloidal gold for light microscopy. In: Hayat MA (ed) Colloidal gold, vol. 1. Academic, New York, NY, pp 297–321

Part IV

Fluorescence-Activated Cell Sorter (FACS) Analyses

Chapter 31

Overview of Flow Cytometry and Fluorescent Probes for Flow Cytometry

Robert E. Cunningham

Abstract

This chapter provides an introduction to the use of fluorescent probes in flow cytometry. Sample preparation for the use of surface labeling with antibodies as well as for the use of nucleic acid probes is discussed. The utility of cell sorting is also discussed.

Key words: Flow cytometry, Fluorescent probe, Nucleic acid probe, Sample preparation, Cell sorting

1. Introduction

It was shown by Creech and Jones (1), in 1940, that proteins, including antibodies, could be labeled with a fluorescent dye (phenylisocyanate) without biological or immunological effect on the intended target. In theory, fluorescent reporters (tracers, probes, antibodies, stains, etc.) can be used to measure any cell constituent, provided that the tag reacts specifically and stoichiometrically with the cellular constituent in question (2). Today, the repertoire of fluorescent probes is expanding almost daily. One area that has benefited from the ever increasing number of fluorescent probes is flow cytometry. One of the most interesting new dyes is green fluorescent protein (GFP). This is a green protein fluorophore that is used to study genetically modified cells (transgenic), and it essentially forms a fusion product with any protein and then retains its fluorescent properties (3). This allows for protein localization in living cells without the concomitant problems of injection and protein handling. This becomes an elegant way to track a constructed genetic expression vector and subsequent intracellular modification. Also, mutants

C. Oliver and M.C. Jamur (eds.), *Immunocytochemical Methods and Protocols*, Methods in Molecular Biology, Vol. 588,
DOI 10.1007/978-1-59745-324-0_31, © Humana Press, a part of Springer Science+Business Media, LLC 1995, 1999, 2010

of GFP allow for varied spectral properties and differing emission and excitation frequencies. I expect that more dyes of this type will be developed in the future.

Flow cytometry is a high-precision technique for rapid analysis and sorting of cells and particles. This fluorescent detection technique provides statistical accuracy, reproducibility, and sensitivity and allows the simultaneous measurement of several constituents on a cell-by-cell basis. Extrinsic and intrinsic fluorescent probes allow selective examination of both functional and structural components of cells. Detection of intracellular proteins is less well-developed and has some potential problems. Because antibodies can bind nonspecifically to dead cell components, there may be considerable biological noise. This noise reduces the sensitivity for detecting the desired protein within the cell. Information is derived from optical responses of the fluorescent probe. This can be done directly with fluorescent probes that bind to cellular constituents or indirectly by first attaching the fluorescent probe to a protein, e.g., antibody, and then locating the protein with a second protein labeled with a fluorescent marker. By using a combination of specific antibodies that are each labeled with a different fluorochrome, panels can be designed to follow residual disease with greater precision than any other method. When flow cytometric results are combined with histologic results, the confidence in pathologic interpretation is far greater than what either can provide alone. It is likely that the future application of these approaches will significantly improve diagnosis and patient care.

One major drawback of flow cytometry is the lack of visual control and structural information, without a specific probe, in the cell suspension. This drawback might come to an end. One aspect of flow cytometry that is changing is data acquisition. Data acquisition for flow cytometry was described to me as a bucket brigade. Imagine that we are watering our lawns using a bucket. The bucket is filled and passed on where the contents of the bucket are dumped onto the lawn. Now imagine watering the lawn with a hose! There is no stopping the water flow to fill the bucket up or to empty it, just constant watering. This is the new data acquisition. Our computing power has become so fast and so robust that we will soon be able to continuously collect data and process that data at a much faster rate. This means no cells will be lost in counting, as we will not be filling and dumping the bucket. No sorting events will be lost. This is particularly important in "rare event" sorting projects.

Careful sample preparation, quality control of all staining and instrumentation procedures, and the use of immunohistologic or cytologic controls are essential for high-quality flow cytometric analysis. The technique has been used successfully for simultaneous measurement of DNA and tumor-associated antigens, oncogene products, proliferation markers, and cell surface markers in cultured cell lines and in cell suspensions prepared from solid tumors.

The development of nucleic acid probes, other reporters, and techniques within molecular biology has been of revolutionary significance in the biological and medical sciences (4). These probes offer the promise of disease diagnosis through direct genomic analysis and the detection of genomic products at an unprecedented level of sensitivity. cDNA probes have been used for the diagnosis of infectious diseases, genetic diseases, and neoplasia. The combination of FCM and fluorescent molecular biology techniques has unprecedented power in the biological sciences and combines the ability of the flow cytometer to identify, quantify, and separate rare cell populations with the unique specificity of cDNA probes for genetic sequences in cells or microbial organisms (5). One technique that was exclusively used for slide based assays has recently become available to FCM. Fluorescence in situ hybridization (FISH) techniques demonstrate great promise for detecting specific sequences of nucleic acid by FCM, particular in instances where multiple copies of the nucleic acid sequence are present. Detection of a single gene copy remains difficult due to poor signal-to-noise ratios and limits the application of FCM assays for direct examination of individual nucleic acid sequences such as point mutations of oncogenes (6). It is quite possible that this technical obstacle will be overcome in the near future.

One of the most eloquent techniques in the realm of molecular biology is a micro technique known as the polymerase chain reaction (PCR) and when combined with FCM has further expanded the technique of cell sorting (7). Nuclei can be sorted on the basis of cell cycle, digested to single stranded DNA and the desired segment of DNA amplified. PCR has the end result of making DNA from a complementary DNA template. Further, sorting does not necessarily require live cells for post sorting analysis and/or PCR, thereby decreasing the complexity of the sorting process. The requirement for live cells can be replaced by a retrospective analysis of paraffin embedded tissue. Another molecular technique that utilizes FCM and sorting is cytogenetics, which is the study of karyotype anomalies by loss or gain of chromosomal material and structural changes. Molecular biology provides the means to recognize chromosome losses and especially to study oncogenic or antioncogenic mutations (8). Sorting also allows for the separation of individual chromosomes. Studying these alterations allows better prediction of high risk subjects in cancer families (9). Lastly, the integration of FISH and FCM analysis provides more information on the chromosomal abnormalities of these neoplasms (10). A large number of methods for staining and measuring properties of individual cells are available (11). New protein and DNA dyes have made it possible to analyze large number of cells individually for multiple properties. These techniques have had a large impact on cellular immunology and the study of cell proliferation. New fluorescent molecules that report on intracellular conditions are used increasingly to study cell physiology. Chromosome analysis and sorting by FCM are becoming a valuable tool, and refinements in the techniques for manipulating small quantities of DNA will increase the application of chromosome sorting in molecular biology. The analysis of rare cell populations is still hampered by shortcomings in the present generation of commercial instruments. Finally, FCM can be used for the study of multi drug resistance (MDR), which is the study of the capacity of modulating agents to result in overexpression of the P-glycoprotein and the functional aspect of MDR in expulsion of the cytotoxic agents (12).

2. Sources

To find additional fluorescent probes or to enhance the rendering of existing probes, journal articles, books, and manufacturers data sheets are valuable entities. I have listed selected review journal articles (13–24) and books that have broad based applications in fluorescence as applied to biology and specifically flow cytometry as well as useful web sites (25–54). The utility of these fluorescent probes has become routine enough that some database utilities use fluorescent probes as headings. In fact, some of the most used probes have become headings within the MEDLINE system of the National Library of Medicine's online database. These probes are noted with an asterisk (*) following the probe name. Another source of information and protocols is the Internet. The Internet supplies not only sources, but also valuable protocols and hints. A particularly useful site is the Purdue University Cytometry group, (http://www.cyto.purdue.edu), which has links to many other flow cytometry sites.

I have listed below some of the more popular probes used in flow cytometry (Table 1). This is by no means a complete listing of probes, but it is a good starting point (also see http://pingu.salk.edu/flow/fluo.html). Particular attention has been paid to the excitation capability of the argon (blue) laser, which is the most widely used light source on flow cytometers. The (EX) is the peak excitation wavelength in nanometers. The (EM) is the peak emission wavelength in nanometers.

Table 1
Commonly used probes for flow cytometry

Fluorescent probe	EX	EM
Adriamycin	472	570
7-Aminoactinomycin D	550	650
Acridine Orange*	480	520, 640
Acriflavine*	480	550–600
Allophycocyanin	650	660
Alexa® Fluors	346–680	445–702
Bodipys®	490–647	515–676
Cyanine dyes	489–675	506–805
DAPI	354	470
Dansyl chloride	340	578
DiL-Cns	515–646	485–668 505
Eosins*	527	550
Erythrosin*	530	540
Ethidium Bromide	518	610
FDA	475	530
Fluoresceins (FITC)*	494	517
Fura-2*	335	515
Green Fluorescent Protein	395/489	509
Hoechst 33258*	365	480
Hoechst 33342	355	465
Image-Orange	545	585
Indo-1	330	400
Mithramycin	421	575
Nile red (acetone)	530	605
PE-Texas Red®	488	615
PE-Cy5	488	670
Phycocyanin-C +	620	640
Phycoerythrin-B +	546	575

(continued)

Table 1 (continued)

Fluorescent probe	EX	EM
Phycoerythrin-R +	566	575
Propidium Iodide	520	610
Pyronin Y(G)	555	571
Quinacrine*	440	510
RITC	540	550
Red Dye 613	488	613
Red Dye 670	488	670
Rhodamines*	496–530	520–605
SITS	350	420
SYTOs®	488–652	527–676
TOPRO-1®	515	531
TO-PRO-2®	642	661
TO-PRO-3®	747	770
TOTO-1®	514	533
TOTO-3®	642	660
TRITC®	540	550
Texas Red®	595	615
Thiazole orange	453	480
YO-PRO-1®	491	509
YO-PRO-3®	613	629
YOYO-1®	491	509
YOYO-3®	612	631
XRITC	580	605

References

1. Creech HJ, Jones RN (1940) The conjugation of horse serum albumin with 1, 2-benzanthryl isothiocyanate. J Am Chem Soc 62:1970–1975
2. van Dam PA, Watson JV, Lowe DG, Shepherd JH (1992) Flowcytometric measurement of cell components other than DNA: virtues, limitations, and applications in gynecologic oncology. Obstet Gynecol 79:616–621
3. Chalfie M, Tu Y, Euskirchen G, Ward WW, Prasher DC (1994) Green fluorescent protein as a marker for gene expression. Science 263:802–805
4. Keren DF (1989) Clinical molecular cytometry: merging flow cytometry with molecular biology in laboratory medicine. In: Keren DF, Hanson CA, Hurtubise PE (eds) Flow cytometry in clinical diagnosis. ASCP Press, Chicago, IL, pp 614–634

5. Tim EA, Stewart CC (1992) Fluorescence in situ hybridization in suspension, (FISHES) using digoxigenin-labeled probes and flow cytometry. Biotechniques 12:362–367
6. Bauman J, Bentvelzen P, van Bekkum D (1987) Fluorescent in situ hybridization of MRNA in bone marrow and leukemic cells measured by flow cytometry. Cytometry Suppl 1:4
7. Gyllensten UB (1989) PCR and DNA sequencing. Biotechniques 7:700–708
8. Milan D, Yerle M, Schmitz A, Chaput B, Vaiman M, Frelat G, Gellin J (1993) A PCR-based method to amplify DNA with random primers: determining the chromosomal content of porcine flow-karyotype peaks by chromosome painting. Cytogenet Cell Genet 62:139–141
9. Gray JW, Cram LS (1990) Flow karyotyping and chromosome sorting. In: Melamed MR, Lindmo T, Mendelsohn M (eds) Flow cytometry and sorting. Wiley-Liss, New York, pp 503–530
10. Carrano AV, Gray JW, Langlois RG, Burkhart SK, Van Dilla DM (1979) Measurement and purification of human chromosomes by flow cytometry and sorting. Proc Natl Acad Sci USA 76:1382–1384
11. Cram LS, Bartholdi MF, Ray FA, Meyne J, Moyzis RK, Schwarzacher-Robinson T, Kraemer PM (1988) Overview of flow cytogenetics for clinical applications. Cytometry Suppl 3:94–100
12. Herzog CE, Bates SE (1994) Molecular diagnosis of multidrug resistance. Cancer Treat Res 73:129–147
13. Darzynkiewicz Z, Bruno S, Del Bino G, Gorczyca W, Hotz MA, Lassota P, Traganos F (1992) Features of apoptotic cells measured by flow cytometry. Cytometry 13:795–808 Review Article: 63 Refs
14. Zola H, Flego L, Sheldon A (1992) Detection of cytokine receptors by high-sensitivity immunofluorescence/flow cytometry. Immunobiology 185:350–365 Review Article: 58 Refs
15. Hashimoto K (1992) [Flow karyotyping and chromosome sorting]. Nippon Rinsho 50:2484–2488
16. Mitsui H (1992) [AgNORs (Ag nucleolar organizer regions)]. Nippon Rinsho 50:2349–2354 Review Article: 18 Refs
17. Wakita A, Kaneda T (1992) [Detection of proliferative cells by DNA polymerase a as a proliferation associated marker]. Nippon Rinsho 50:2338–2342 Review Article: 15 Refs
18. Loken MR, Brosnan JM, Bach BA, Ault KA (1990) Establishing optimal lymphocyte gates for immunophenotyping by flow cytometry. Cytometry 11:453–459 Review Article: 31 Refs
19. van Dam PA, Watson JV, Lowe DG, Shepherd JH (1992) Flow cytometric measurement of cell components other than DNA: virtues, limitations, and applications in gynecologic oncology. Obstet Gynecol 79:616–621 Review Article: 74 Refs
20. Morrell JM (1991) Applications of flow cytometry to artificial insemination: a review. Vet Rec 129:375–378 Review Article: 37 Refs
21. Gray JW, Kuo WL, Pinkel D (1991) Molecular cytometry applied to detection and c haracterization of disease-linked chromosome aberrations. Baillieres Clin Haematol 4:683–693 Review Article: 37 Refs
22. Vindel LL, Christensen IJ (1990) A review of techniques and results obtained in one laboratory by an integrated system of methods designed for routine clinical flow cytometric DNA analysis. Cytometry 11:753–770 Review Article: 44 Refs
23. Garratty G (1990) Flow cytometry: its applications to immunohaematology. Baillieres Clin Haematol 3:267–287 Review Article: 74 Refs
24. Packman CH, Lichtman MA (1990) Activation of neutrophils: measurement of actin conformational changes by flow cytometry. Blood Cells 16:193–205 Review Article: 39 Refs
25. The handbook – a guide to fluorescent probes and labeling technologies (http://probes.invitrogen.com/handbook/), ↑ Invitrogen, Molecular Probes contains detailed information describing the use of more than 3000 products and is available from Invitrogen, Molecular Probes, Carlsbad, CA
26. International Society for Analytical Cytology, http://www.isac-net.org/ (n.b. many internet links)
27. Purdue University, Cytometry Laboratories, http://www.cyto.purdue.edu/ (n.b. many internet links)
28. Catalog of Free Flow Cytometry Software, http://bio.umas.edu/mcbfacs/flowcat-old.html, University of Massachusetts, Amherst, MA
29. Flow Cytometry on the Web, http://flowcyt.salk.edu/sitelink.html
30. Wikipedia, Flow Cytometry, http://en.wikipedia.org/wiki/Flow_cytometry (many definitions and internet sources)
31. Brink PR, Dewey MM (1981) Diffusion and mobility of substances inside cells. Elsevier-North Holland, New York
32. Foskett JK, Grinstein S (1950) Noninvasive techniques in cell biology. Wiley-Liss, New York
33. Givan AL (2001) Flow cytometry: first principles. Wiley-Liss, Wilmington, DE

34. Givan AL (2004) Flow cytometry: an introduction. In: Hawley TS, Hawley RG (eds) Methods in Molecular Biology. Humana, Totowa, NJ, pp 1–32
35. Hawley TS, Hawley RG (eds) (2004) Flow cytometry protocols. Methods in molecular biology. Humana, Totowa, NJ
36. Kohen E (1981) Examination of single cells by microspectrophotometry and microspectrofluorometry. Elsevier-North Holland, New York
37. Lang M (1978) Interaction of fluorescent probes with rat liver microsomes and drug metabolizing enzymes. University of Kuopio, Kuopio, Finland, Dept. of Physiology
38. Lay CL (1952) An evaluation of fluorescent staining for detection of cancer cells in vaginal smears. Lafayette, Minneapolis, MN
39. Lee A (1982) Membrane studies using fluorescence spectroscopy. Elsevier, County Clare, Ireland
40. Loew LM (1988) Spectroscopic membrane probes. CRC, Boca Raton, FL
41. Ockleford CD (1990) An atlas of antigens – fluorescence microscope localization patterns in cells and tissues. Stockton, New York
42. Osborn M (1981) Localization of proteins by immunofluorescence techniques. Elsevier-North Holland, New York
43. Sanborn WR (1968) Immunofluorescence, an annotated bibliography. Aerobiology and Evaluation Laboratory, Technical Information Division, Fort Detrick, Frederick MD.
44. Seiler FR, Johannsen R, Sedlacek HH (1976) Immunochemical analysis of various biological structures. Behringwerke, Marburg, Germany
45. Sernetz M, Thaer A (1973) Fluorescence techniques in cell biology. Proceedings of the conference on quantitative fluorescence techniques as applied to cell biology, Battelle Research Center, Seattle. Springer, New York
46. Shapiro HM (2003) Practical flow cytometry. Wiley-Liss, Wilmington, DE
47. Taylor DL, Wang Yu-li (1969) Fluorescence microscopy of living cells in culture, methods in cell biology. Vol. 30. Academic, New York
48. Taylor DL (1986) Applications of fluorescence in the biomedical sciences, Proceedings of a meeting held in Pittsburgh, Pennsylvania, April 12–15, 1985. Alan R. Liss, New York
49. Watson JV (2004) Introduction to flow cytometry. Cambridge University Press, New York
50. Watson JV (2005) Flow cytometry data analysis: basic concepts and statistics. Cambridge University Press, New York
51. Wampler JE (1989) New methods in microscopy and low light imaging. Proceedings of a Conference held August 8-11 San Diego. Society of Photo-Optical Instrumentation Engineers, CA
52. Willingham MC, Pastan IH (1985) An atlas of immunofluorescence in cultured cells. Academic, Orlando, FL
53. Wolf DE, Edidin M (1981) Diffusion and mobility of molecules in surface membranes. Elsevier-North Holland, New York
54. Voss EW (1984) Fluorescein hapten. CRC, Boca Raton, FL

Chapter 32

Tissue Disaggregation

Robert E. Cunningham

Abstract

A conventional flow cytometry procedure for creating single cell suspensions is provided. Methods of tissue disaggregation to create single-cell suspensions from formalin fixed tissue are also given. Chemical, mechanical, and enzymatic multistep methods for separating single cells from tissue are discussed. These procedures are very tissue dependent.

Key words: Flow cytometry, Tissue disaggregation, Single-cell suspension, Mechanical dissociation, Enzymatic dissociation, Chemical dissociation

1. Introduction

The extracellular matrix of mammalian tissue is composed of a complex mix of constitutive proteins. This matrix must be broken down to effectively recover single cells for culture and/or staining (1). Tissue dissociation and its associated problems were described and defined over 70 years ago by Rous and Jones (2). More recent reviews (3, 4) have revealed newer methods of creating single-cell suspensions. Numerous procedures exist for dissociating solid tumors. They are usually multistep procedures involving one or a combination of mechanical, enzymatic, or chemical manipulations. Ideally, the dissociation protocol is individualized for the tissue of interest and evaluated relative to both optimal and representative cell yield. In our laboratory, we employ a modified mechanical/enzymatic method to isolate cells. Mechanical dissociation of tissue may involve repeated mincing with scissors or sharp blades, scrapping the tissue surface, homogenization, filtration through a nylon or steel mesh, vortexing, repeated aspiration through pipettes or small gauge needles, abnormal osmolality

C. Oliver and M.C. Jamur (eds.), *Immunocytochemical Methods and Protocols*, Methods in Molecular Biology, Vol. 588, DOI 10.1007/978-1-59745-324-0_32,

stress, or any combination of these techniques. These methods result in variable cell yields and cell viability. There are various enzymes that can be used, alone or in combination, to digest desmosomes, stromal elements, and extracellular and intercellular adhesions. Enzymes commonly used include trypsin, pepsin, papain, collagenase, elastase, hyaluronidase, pronase, chymotrypsin, catalase, and dispase. The most routinely used enzymes are collagenase and dispase. DNase is used with these proteolytic enzymes to hydrolyze the DNA-protein complexes, which often entrap cells and can lead to reaggregation of suspended cells. The different specificities of these enzymes for intercellular components allow one to design a dissociation protocol for a specific tumor and for specific purposes. Many enzymes are crude extracts that contain varying amounts of contaminating proteolytic enzymes. The enzymatic method (5, 6) is probably the method of choice as a starting point for most tissue types for its ability not only to release a large number of cells but also to preserve cellular integrity and viability (7). Lastly, chemical dissociation is commonly used in conjunction with mechanical or enzymatic procedures. Chemical methods are designed to omit or sequester the Ca^{2+} and Mg^{2+} ions needed for maintenance of the intercellular matrix and cell surface integrity. Ethylene-diaminoacetate (EDTA) or citrate ion is commonly used to remove these cations, but does not adequately dissociate all types of tissue. Dissagregation protocols must be individualized for each tissue type. A general protocol, outlining the individual steps, is given below (*see* Note 1).

2. Materials

1. Tissue, fresh.
2. Enzyme Cocktail: collagenase, 0.5 mg/mL, trypsin or dispase, 0.25% w/v, DNAse, 0.002% w/v.
3. Dulbecco's Phosphate Buffered Saline, pH 7.0–7.2 without Ca^{2+} and Mg^{2+}, but with 1.0 g/L glucose: 2.7 mM KCl, 1.2 mM KH_2PO_4, 138 mM NaCl, 8.1 mM Na_2HPO_4 and 5.6 mM d-glucose.
4. Flask, Erlenmeyer, 25 mL.
5. Hot plate/stirrer.
6. Forceps.
7. Razor blades.
8. Ice bath.
9. Centrifuge, low speed.
10. Collection tubes, e.g., 100× 13 polypropylene.
11. Cell counter.

12. Trypan blue 0.4% (w/v).
13. Hemocytometer

3. Methods

1. Chop tissue into 2–3 mm diameter pieces (*see* Note 2).
2. Transfer tissue pieces into a 250 mL Erlenmeyer flask.
3. Add 100 mL (*see* Note 3) of enzyme cocktail (collagenase, trypsin, DNAse) and stir at 200 rpm – 30 min at 37°C (*see* Note 4).
4. Allow fragments to settle; collect supernatant.
5. Centrifuge supernatant at 500 × *g* for 5 min.
6. Resuspend pellet in complete media with serum (*see* Note 3).
7. Store cells on ice.
8. Add fresh digestion cocktail (*see* Note 3).
9. Repeat steps 3–7 until disaggregation is complete (*see* Note 5).
10. Collect, pool, and count cells (*see* Note 6).
11. Determine viability using trypan blue: Place 0.5 mL of cell suspension (dilute cells to an approximate concentration of 1×10^5 to 2×10^5 cells per mL) in a screw cap test tube. Add 0.1 mL of 0.4% trypan blue stain. Mix thoroughly. Allow to stand for 5 min to 10 min at room temperature. Using a hemocytometer, under a microscope, determine the per cent of nonviable (stained) and viable cells (*see* Note 7).

4. Notes

1. Specialized protocols can be found by searching the literature or on the internet at various companies web sites such as Worthington Biochemical Corporation, Worthington Tissue Dissociation Guide, http://www.tissuedissociation.com/; Phoenix Flow Systems, Protocol for the use of ACCUMAX™ in Primary Tissue Dissociation, http://www.phnxflow.com/pdfs/Accumax.primary.pdf; Roche Applied Bioscience, Tissue Dissociation, http://www.roche-applied-science.com/collagenase/home.html; Sigma-Aldrich, Enzymes for Cell Detachment and Tissue Dissociation, http://www.sigmaaldrich.com/Area_of_Interest/Biochemicals/Enzyme_Explorer/Key_Resources/Cell_Detachment.html; StemCell Technologies, Technical Bulletin, A Guide to Solid Tissue Dissociation, http://www.stemcell.com/technical/29107_Tissue%20Dissociation.pdf.

2. This protocol can be used as a first-run attempt at tissue disaggregation. Further experience with tissue will probably yield insights as to the best enzyme types, enzyme concentration, and digestion time and temperature.
3. The volume of enzyme solution needed will depend on the enzymes being used and on the amount of tissue to be digested.
4. This technique uses enzymes to disrupt the tissue. Alliteratively, mechanical methods, such as passing the tissue through metal mesh (50–100 μm opening) or through a commercially available BD Falcon™ Cell Strainers (http://www.bdbiosciences.com/) or disrupting the tissue by passing small pieces through sequentially smaller needles (e.g., 16, 20, 23 gauge), can be employed. Chemical methods involve procedures such as changing the pH, use of chelators, such as EDTA or EGTA, or the increase or decrease in the salt concentration of the digestion buffer. The most suitable disaggregation procedure usually involves the combination of enzymatic and mechanical techniques, although permutations of all three techniques are possible.
5. The number of times these steps need to be repeated will depend on the amount and type of tissue. Prolonged tissue digestion will result in lowered viability.
6. If the yield of cells has decreased viability: reduce the exposure time to enzyme; reduce the amount of mechanical disruption; readjust the pH of the digestion cocktail often; increase digestion cocktail concentration, thereby decreasing the exposure time to the enzymes; add albumin or serum to the digestion cocktail; be gentle in all aspects of the disaggregation process; remove separated cells from the digestion cocktail more frequently.
7. If the yield of viable cells is low: be sure that the enzymes are stored cold and dry and that the aliquots of enzyme are stored frozen; use more collagenase; depending upon tissue type, additional enzymes may be needed, e.g., elastase, protease.

References

1. Berwick L, Corman DR (1962) Some chemical factors in cellular adhesion and stickiness. Cancer Res 22:982–986
2. Rous P, Jones FS (1916) A method for obtaining suspensions of living cells from the fixed tissues and for the plating of individual cells. J Exp Med 23:549–555
3. Waymouth C (1974) To disaggregate or not to disaggregate. Injury and cell disaggregation, transient or permanent? In Vitro 10:97–111
4. Freshney RI (2005) Culture of animal cells. A manual of basic technique. Wiley-Liss, New York
5. Lewin MJM, Cheret AM (1989) Cell isolation techniques: use of enzymes and chelators. Methods Enzymol 171:444–461
6. Cerra R, Zarbo RJ, Crissman JD (1990) Dissociation of cells from solid tumors. Methods Cell Biol 33:1–12
7. Costa A, Silvestrini R, Del Bino G, Motta R (1987) Implications of disaggregation procedures on biological representation of human solid tumors. Cell Tissue Kinet 20:171–180

Chapter 33

Indirect Immunofluorescent Labeling of Viable Cells

Robert E. Cunningham

Abstract

A recognized flow cytometry procedure for standard indirect antibody staining for cellular analysis and cell sorting is discussed. A protocol for cell surface or intracellular antibody staining of viable cells is provided.

Key words: Flow cytometry, Viable cell, Fluorescence detection, Monoclonal antibody, Epitope

1. Introduction

The combination of the specificity of the antigen-antibody interaction with the exquisite sensitivity of fluorescence detection and quantitation yields one of the most widely applicable analytical tools in cell biology (1). Within the last decade, flow cytometry (FCM) has become an integral part of basic immunological research. Elaboration of this technology has been intensively stimulated by a rapidly growing sophistication in monoclonal antibody technology and vice versa (2).

The added specificity of monoclonal antibodies in immuncytochemical technology provides a consistent and reliable method for exploiting the range of pure antibodies and subclasses of antibodies. These antibodies provide a means of defining cell surface, intracellular, and membrane epitopes for single cells as well as tissue sections. When these antibodies are "tagged" with a fluorescent reporter antibody, it makes multiple markers possible. In particular, methods using protein A or the avidin-biotin complexed with alternative fluorescent tags as second steps have added significant latitude to the immunofluorescence technique (3). An increasing number of clinical laboratories are using flow

C. Oliver and M.C. Jamur (eds.), *Immunocytochemical Methods and Protocols*, Methods in Molecular Biology, Vol. 588,
DOI 10.1007/978-1-59745-324-0_33, © Humana Press, a part of Springer Science+Business Media, LLC 1995, 1999, 2010

cytometry to analyze cells stained with fluorescent antibodies, dyes or receptors (4, 5). Today, choices have to be made for the most appropriate fluorochromes, reagents, equipment, and preparative procedure. In the following example, a primary antibody (mouse anti-human monoclonal) will be followed by a tagged secondary antibody (fluoresceinated anti-mouse) to render a green fluorescent product. This procedure can also be used for cell enrichment techniques utilizing cell sorting (*see* Notes 1 and 2).

2. Materials

1. Sample (cell suspension of at least 10^6 cells).
2. Primary antibody (usually a monoclonal antibody) (*see* Note 3).
3. Secondary antibody (usually antimouse conjugated with a fluorochrome).
4. Bovine serum albumin (BSA).
5. Dulbecco's Phosphate Buffered Saline (PBSG), pH 7.0–7.2 without Ca^{2+} and Mg^{2+}, but with 1.0 g/L glucose: 2.7 mM KCl, 1.2 mM KH_2PO_4, 138 mM NaCl, 8.1 mM Na_2HPO_4 and 5.6 mM d-glucose.
6. Test tubes, e.g., 100× 13 polypropylene.
7. Pipettor(s) 20-100 μL, 100-1,000 μL.
8. Disposable pipet tips.
9. Ice bath.
10. Centrifuge, low speed.
11. Vortex mixer.
12. Propidium Iodide, stock 50 mg/mL PBS (*see* Note 4).

3. Methods

1. Harvest and count cells (*see* Note 5).
2. Wash cells two times: Centrifuge at $300\times g$ for 5 min (*see* Note 6); Decant supernatant; Vortex pellet; Resuspend pellet in 2 mL PBS (4 C).
3. Add 100 μL PBS (4 C) per 10^6 cells.
4. Add appropriate amount of primary (monoclonal) antibody.
5. Incubate 30 min on ice.
6. Wash cells twice.
7. Add 100 μL PBS (4 C).

8. Add appropriate amount of secondary (fluorescently conjugated) antibody.
9. Incubate 30 min on ice.
10. Wash cells twice.
11. Resuspend the pellet to a concentration of 1–2 million cell/mL of PBSG or other medium. Add propidium iodine (PI) to a final concentration of 500 ng/mL (*see* Note 7).

4. Notes

1. Alternative techniques are available, especially in the area of hematology, where isolation of cell types may be deemed necessary to give good immunocytochemical results.
2. Human genes coding cell surface molecules can be introduced into host cells using a variety of somatic cell genetic techniques (6). FCM can then be used to monitor the effectiveness of the genetic techniques.
3. The working concentration of antibody must be determined empirically by serial dilution of the stock solution in PBSG with 10% BSA. Usual concentrations range from 1–20 μg/mL. Depending on the individual reagent, this could vary considerably. *See* Chapter 25 for additional instructions on performing titrations.
4. Propidium iodide is a possible *carcinogen* and should be handled appropriately. The stock solution should be stored and refrigerated in the dark.
5. If the cells are tissue culture cells intended for cell sorting, I use tissue culture media in which the cells have been growing as the wash solution. We refer to this media as "spent media." The tissue culture supernatant is withdrawn from the tissue culture flask and filtered through a 0.22 μm filter to ensure sterility. The addition of this media helps cells recover after sorting and increases the growth of cells when they are placed back into tissue culture.
6. One major pitfall is the centrifugation of the suspension. If centrifugation is not long enough or not enough centrifugal force has been created, the cells can be "poured off." Conversely, if the centrifugation is too long or too much force was created, then the cells may clump.
7. It is useful to resuspend the stained cell pellet in 1 mL PBS w/500 ng/mL propidium iodide (PI) to detect dead cells by the inclusion of PI and its red resultant fluorescence on the flow cytometer. The use of red fluorescence (PI) versus light scatter is used to exclude dead cells before collecting the green (FITC) signals of the viable cell population.

References

1. Bosman FT (1983) Some recent developments in immunocytochemistry. Histochem J 15: 189–200
2. Kung PC, Talle MA, DeMarie ME, Butler MS, Lifter J, Goldstein G (1980) Strategies for generating monoclonal antibodies defining human T lymphocyte differentiation antigens. Transplant Proc 3:141–146
3. Othmer M, Zepp F (1992) Flow cytometric immunophenotyping: principles and pitfalls. Eur J Pediatr 151:398–406
4. Haaijman JJ (1988) Immunofluorescence: quantitative considerations. Acta Histochem Suppl 35:77–83
5. Zola H, Flego L, Sheldon A (1992) Detection of cytokine receptors by high-sensitivity immunofluorescence/flowcytometry. Immunobiology 185:350–365
6. Kamarck ME, Barbosa JA, Kuhn L, Peters PG, Shulman L, Ruddle FH (1983) Somatic cell genetics and flow cytometry. Cytometry 4:99–108

Chapter 34

Indirect Immunofluorescent Labeling of Fixed Cells

Robert E. Cunningham

Abstract

Flow cytometry protocols for defining cell surface or intracellular antibody staining are discussed. Various staining protocols are provided. Routine cell surface and intracellular techniques as well as more advanced signal enhancement techniques are detailed.

Key words: Flow cytometry, Intracellular protocol, Permeabilization, Fixation, Stain, Antigen

1. Introduction

One of the major advantages of flow cytometry is the simultaneous evaluation of multiple markers, especially surface markers (1). The detection of intracellular proteins is less well-developed, in large part because antibodies can bind nonspecifically to dying cells and dead cell components, which leads to considerable biological noise in the fluorescent detectors. There is also noise caused by the intra and/or intermolecular ionic interactions during the process of fixation, which reduces the sensitivity of detecting the desired protein(s) within the cell. This is a double-edged sword for labeling cells. It is very important to start the staining procedure with a viable cell suspension. If the starting material is viable, at least one of the two problems associated with cell fixation and staining is remedied. The fixation protocols are varied not only for their uses of cross-linking agents, permeabilization agents, and/or precipitating agents but also for time and temperature of the protocols. I have included some protocols for unfixed staining, fixation followed by surface staining and fixation followed by intracellular staining. These techniques have worked well for us, and I believe they are, at least, a workable starting protocol.

C. Oliver and M.C. Jamur (eds.), *Immunocytochemical Methods and Protocols*, Methods in Molecular Biology, Vol. 588.
DOI 10.1007/978-1-59745-324-0_34,

The permeabilization/fixation conditions used to prepare cells for antibody application are assumed to preserve the distributions of the protein(s) being examined (2). Soluble proteins can be redistributed into inappropriate locations and can be differentially extracted from native locations during the permeabilization and fixation of the cells before antibody application (3, 4). Further, no cell aggregation or alteration of the intracellular antigenicity should occur in the permeabilization/fixation treatment. The fixation/stain methodology, with and without permeabilization, can be accomplished in various ways depending upon the exact site of the organelle or cell constituent to be stained.

The stain/fixation method is usually used for surface markers that can withstand fixation, and is followed by the application of a DNA-binding fluorochrome. The fixation/stain method is used not only for surface markers that can withstand fixation but also for intracellular constituents such as cytoplasmic proteins, membrane and cytoplasmic antigens, nuclear membrane and nuclear protein staining. This is accomplished by using a cross-linking fixative (e.g., paraformaldehyde (PFA), or formalin) followed by a permeabilization agent such as Triton X-100, Tween 20, saponin, or lysolecithin. Some of the precipitating agents (e.g., ethanol, methanol, acetone) can also be used for permeabilization after the initial fixation with PFA or formalin, or they can be used alone for both fixation and permeabilization.

Finally, there are numerous techniques for signal enhancement such as avidin – biotin – complexes and tyramide signal amplification methods. All of these tertiary procedures obviously add to the time parameter of any test, but can add significant staining intensity that is critical in samples with low numbers of antibody binding sites. Determination of methodology for cell staining must be evaluated on the basis of tissue/cells samples to be examined.

2. Materials

1. Sample (Cell suspension).
2. Fixatives: Cross-linkers – paraformaldehyde; Precipitators - ethanol, methanol.
3. Permeabilizers: Triton-X100, Tween 20, saponin, l-lysophosphatidylcholine, n -octyl-beta-d-glucopyranoside.
4. Primary Antibody (e.g., monoclonal antibody to surface antigen or intracellular antigen).
5. Secondary Antibody (e.g., anti-mouse antibody fluorescent conjugated).
6. Bovine serum albumin (BSA).

7. Dulbecco's Phosphate Buffered Saline (PBSG), pH 7.0–7.2 without Ca^{2+} and Mg^{2+}: 2.7 mM KCl, 1.2 mM KH_2PO_4, 138 mM NaCl, and 8.1 mM Na_2HPO_4.
8. Test tubes (e.g., 100× 13 polypropylene).
9. Pipettor(s) 100-1,000 μL, with disposable tips.
10. Ice bath.
11. Centrifuge, low speed.
12. Vortex mixer.
13. Propidium Iodide, stock 50 mg/mL PBSG stored dark at 5 C.

3. Methods

3.1. Staining Cell-Surface Antigens Prior to Fixation for Flow Cytometric Analysis

It is entirely possible that surface staining cannot be accomplished before fixation. Some antibody/receptor complexes cannot withstand chemical fixation and/or permeabilization. This is an empirical evaluation of surface, cytoplasmic, or nuclear antigen/receptor sites, and each must be evaluated before staining or fixation can be accomplished. In this example I, first stain with a monoclonal antibody against a cell surface receptor, fix the cells with ethanol then stain the DNA, and analyze the cells for two colors of fluorescence, red (DNA) and green (surface marker). This approach works for antibody-antigens that are unaffected by fixation.

1. Harvest and count cells.
2. Wash cells twice: Centrifuge at $300 \times g$ for 5 min; decant supernatant; vortex pellet; resuspend pellet in 2 mL PBSG (4 C).
3. Add 100 μL PBSG per 10^6 cells.
4. Add appropriate amount of primary (monoclonal) antibody.
5. Incubate 30 min on ice.
6. Wash cells twice.
7. Add 100 μL PBSG.
8. Add appropriate amount of secondary (fluorescent) antibody.
9. Incubate 30 min on ice.
10. Wash cells twice; *do not resuspend* pellet in PBSG.
11. Fix cells following surface staining: Centrifuge cells at $300 \times g$ and decant supernatant; while vortexing the cell pellet, add 1 mL 100% EtOH (-20 C) dropwise; store at 4 C up to 2 weeks.
12. Stain with Propidium iodide (*see* Note 1): Centrifuge cells and decant supernatant; for 10^6 cells, add 15 μg propidium

iodide, 1,000-2,000 units of RNase A in 1 mL of PBSG; Incubate at 4 C overnight for best results; analyze sample in "soup," do not wash (*see* Notes 2 and 3).

3.2. Fixation and Permeabilization for Antigen Staining for Flow Cytometric Analysis

The following protocol can be used for both intracellular and surface markers.

1. Fix for 60 min in 0.25%, w/v paraformaldehyde in PBSG at 4 C (*see* Note 4).
2. Wash in PBSG.
3. Permeablize for 15 min in 0.2%, v/v Tween 20 in PBSG at 37 C (*see* Note 5).
4. Wash in PBSG.
5. Immunostain (*see* Subheading 3.1, steps 4–9).
6. Rinse twice in PBSG.
7. Cells may be stained with Propidium iodide (Subheading 3.1, step 11).

3.3. Fixation and Permeabilization for Intracellular Antigen Staining for Flow Cytometric Analysis (see Note 6 and Chapter 9)

3.3.1. Method 1: Methanol/Triton X-100

1. Fix for 2 min in 1%, w/v paraformaldehyde in PBS at 20 C (*see* Note 4).
2. Wash in PBS.
3. Permeabilize for 10 min with methanol at -20 C.
4. Wash in PBS containing 0.1% Triton X-100 v/v.
5. Immunostain (*see* Subheading 3.1, steps 4–9).
6. Rinse twice in PBSG.
7. Cells may be stained with Propidium iodine (Subheading 3.1, step 11).

3.3.2. Method 2: Triton X-100

1. Wash in PBS with 0.1% Triton X-100 v/v (*see* Note 7).
2. Wash in PBS.
3. Fix for 2 min 1%, w/v paraformaldehyde in PBS at 20 C.
4. Wash in PBS.
5. Immunostain (*see* Subheading 3.1steps 4–9).
6. Rinse twice in PBSG.
7. Cells may be stained with Propidium iodide (Subheading 3.1, step 11)

3.3.3. Other Fixation Methods (see Chapter 8)

Several different methods of cytological fixation can be used (*see* Note 8):

1. Acetone (15 min).
2. 95% ethanol (15 min).
3. Methanol (3 min, -20 C).
4. Bouin's fixative (5 h), followed by 1.0% trypsin (15 min, 37 C).

5. 10% buffered neutral formalin (24 h), followed by 1.0 % trypsin (15 min 37 C).
6. 4% paraformaldehyde, followed by permeabilization with 1% saponin in PBS containing 20% human serum (0 C).

4. Notes

1. If Propidium iodide is used as the nuclear stain, the red excitation is at 488 nm and the emission at >665 nm.
2. If there is too much background staining, use Tween 20 in washes.
3. 0.65 M–1.0 M NaCl in the staining solution can enhance staining.
4. After fixation, the cells can be rinsed in 0.1% $NaBH_4$ or 0.1 M glycine to quench free aldehyde groups and reduce background fluorescence.
5. Permeabilization of cells with 0.1% detergent after paraformaldehyde fixation can leave an uneven cytoplasmic distribution of the labeled proteins, and some of the larger proteins are redistributed to the nuclei.
6. The choice of method will depend on the susceptibility of a given antigen to detergent extraction (*see* Note 7).
7. Extraction with 1% detergent prior to fixation removes most but not always all of the exogenous proteins from the cell remnants.
8. The choice of fixative depends on the susceptibility of the antigen of interest to a fixative.

References

1. Vyth-Dreese FA, Kipp JBA, DeJohn TAM (1980) Simultaneous measurement of surface immunoglobulins and cell cycle phase of human lymphocytes. In: Laerum OD, Lindo T, Thorn E (eds) Flow Cytometry IV. Universitetsforlaget, Oslo, Norway, pp 207–212
2. Labalette-Houache M, Torpier G, Capron A, Dessaint JP (1991) Improved permeabilization procedure for flow cytometric detection of internal antigens. Analysis of interleukin-2 production. J Immunol Methods 138: 143–153
3. Pollice AA, McCoy JP Jr, Shackney SE, Smith CA, Agarwal J, Burholt DR, Janocko LE, Hornicek FJ, Singh SG, Hartsock RJ (1992) Sequential paraformaldehyde and methanol fixation for simultaneous flow cytometric analysis of DNA, cell surface proteins, and intracellular proteins. Cytometry 13:432–444
4. Schmid I, Uittenbogaart CH, Giorgi JV (1991) A gentle fixation and permeabilization method for combined cell surface and intracellular staining with improved precision in DNA quantification. Cytometry 12:279–285

Chapter 35

Fluorescent Labeling of DNA

Robert E. Cunningham

Abstract

A well-defined method for staining cellular DNA especially for cell cycle determination is provided. Emphasis is placed on utilizing DNA content and cell sizing measurement to further define cell populations.

Key words: Flow cytometry, DNA, Fluorescent distribution, Cell cycle

1. Introduction

Flow cytometry (FCM) is a high-precision technique for rapid analysis and sorting of cells and particles. In theory, it can be used to measure any cell component, provided that a fluorescent tracer that reacts specifically and stoichiometrically with that constituent is available. The technique provides statistical accuracy, reproducibility, and sensitivity.

The quantitative cytochemical determination of DNA has been carried out using cytofluorochemical stains, and it offers a direct measurement of the DNA content of individual cells in a population (1, 2). The fluorescent distribution produced by a cell suspension provides a representation of the cell cycle distribution of this population. Based upon histograms generated from FCM data of the DNA content of individual cells, three groups can be identified in an asynchronous and mitotically active cell population. Most cells are in a resting (G0/G1) phase, also known as Gap0 and Gap1. As cells enter the synthesis (S) phase, the amount of cellular DNA increases resulting in increased fluorescence. After S phase, cells enter the Gap2/Mitosis (G2/M) phase where very little additional DNA is synthesized and cell division occurs. Now the cells contain twice the amount of DNA with approximately twice the staining intensity of the G0/G1 phase (*see* Note 1).

C. Oliver and M.C. Jamur (eds.), *Immunocytochemical Methods and Protocols*, Methods in Molecular Biology, Vol. 588,
DOI 10.1007/978-1-59745-324-0_35, © Humana Press, a part of Springer Science+Business Media, LLC 1995, 1999, 2010

In this example, I use propidium iodide (PI) as the fluorescent tracer for DNA content (3–6). PI binds to both double-stranded DNA and double-stranded RNA. Therefore, RNAse will be used to reduce the amount of double-stranded RNA, resulting in only DNA staining. Finally, although flow cytometric DNA staining has been regarded as an objective prognostic parameter in several types of human cancer, it is important to remember that this is a "snapshot" of the cell cycle. From a DNA content histogram, it cannot be determined if a cell is actively moving through the cell cycle, it has slowed, or even stopped its traverse through the cell cycle.

2. Materials

1. Sample (cell suspension).
2. Ethanol, stock 100%, store at -20 C.
3. DNA fluorochrome: propidium iodide, stock 50 mg/mL PBS, store in the dark at 4 C (*see* Note 2).
4. Dulbecco's Phosphate Buffered Saline (PBS), pH 7.0–7.2 without Ca^{2+} and Mg^{2+}: 2.7 mM KCl, 1.2 mM KH_2PO_4, 138 mM NaCl, and 8.1 mM Na_2HPO_4 without CA++ and MG++, pH 7.2.
5. RNase, DNase free.
6. Centrifuge, low speed.
7. Test tubes (e.g., 13× 100 polypropylene).
8. Ice bath.
9. Pipettors e.g., 1-20 μL, 20-100 μL, 100-1,000 μL with tips.
10. Vortex mixer.

3. Method

1. Fixation with ethanol can begin immediately after a suitable cell suspension pellet is available, e.g., 2×10^6 cells per tube (*see* Note 3).
2. 0.3 mL of PBS is added to the pellet followed by the drop-wise addition of 0.9 mL of cold 100% ethanol while the cell suspension is being vortexed.

3. Continue to add EtOH, and vortex the suspension until the EtOH concentration reaches 70% (v/v).
4. At this time, the sample can be stored at 4 C.
5. Centrifuge the suspension.
6. Decant the EtOH/PBS mix.
7. Add staining solution (1.0 mL/10^6 cells) consisting of 50 µg/mL propidium iodide and 1,000 units/mL Ribonuclease A per mL of PBS (*see* Notes 4 and 5).
8. Incubate 20 min at room temperature before analysis (*see* Note 6).
9. Analyze sample (*see* Note 7).

4. Notes

1. DNA content can be paired with cell size to better define the progression of cells through the cell cycle and to distinguish between G0 and G1 cells and occasionally between G2 and M cells.
2. Wear gloves when handling PI as it is a possible carcinogen.
3. There are other fixatives that can be used for DNA staining. In addition to ethanol, methanol and paraformaldehyde are used most commonly.
4. The concentration of the PI can vary according to the material being evaluated. For dual staining of DNA and a surface marker, I routinely use a concentration of 15 µg/mL. For DNA staining, I use up to 50 µg/mL.
5. There are other fluorochromes that can be used for DNA analysis. The following three are the most straight forward and reproducible in ease of application: Mithramycin, 4′, 6-Diamidino-2-phenylindole hydrochloride (DAPI), and Hoechst 33258.
6. The 20 min stain time at room temperate for PI is the minimum required for reproducible DNA staining. I prefer to allow the cell suspension to incubate in the refrigerator overnight before analysis on the flow cytometer. The control values are usually better and the control size measurements more univariate.
7. Doublets, higher aggregates, and cell debris can be excluded from analysis by using correlated area/peak measurements of DNA content histograms (7).

References

1. Joensuu H, Kallioniemi OP (1989) Different opinions on classification of DNA histograms produced from paraffin-embedded tissue. Cytometry 10:711–717
2. van Dam PA, Watson JV, Lowe DG, Shepherd JH (1992) Flow cytometric measurement of cell components other than DNA: virtues, limitations, and applications in gynecologic oncology. Obstet Gynecol 79:616–621
3. Vindelov LL, Christensen IJ, Nissen NI (1983) A detergent-trypsin method for the preparation of nuclei for flow cytometric DNA analysis. Cytometry 3:323–327
4. Krishan A (1975) Rapid flow cytofluorometric analysis of mammalian cell cycle by propidium iodide staining. J Cell Biol 66: 188–193
5. Deitch AD, Law H, Vere De, White R (1982) A stable propidium iodide staining procedure for flow cytometry. J Histochem Cytochem 30:967–972
6. Taylor IW (1980) A rapid single step staining technique for DNA analysis by flow microfluorimetry. J Histochem Cytochem 28: 1021–1024
7. Sharpless TF, Traganos F, Darzynkiewicz Z, Melamed MR (1975) Flow cytofluorimetry: discrimination between single cells and cell aggregates by direct size measurements. Acta Cytol 19:577–581

Chapter 36

Deparaffinization and Processing of Pathologic Material

Robert E. Cunningham

Abstract

Methods for preparation of whole nuclei from paraffin embedded tissue are given. The combination of cell sorting of isolated nuclei combined with the polymerase chain reaction can be used to investigate other cellular parameters such as nuclear proteins and proliferation factors.

Key words: Flow cytometry, DNA, Fluorescent distribution, Cell cycle

1. Introduction

Paraffin-embedded tissue (PET) can be examined by flow cytometric methods (FCM) for total DNA content and aneuploidy with respect to the classification of the original pathologic diagnosis. The relative significance of studies on archival material permits retrospective analysis on a great number of cases, studying different specimens of a tumor for intratumor heterogeneity while comparing results from previous pathologic evaluations (1). DNA content as measured in PET is closely related to that obtained from fresh specimens. Still, a major drawback in the procedure is that only nuclei are recovered for analysis of DNA content. DNA content has become an important diagnostic, as well as prognostic, method for clinical pathology and investigative oncology.

A modification of the Hedley technique (2, 3) has been used to prepare nuclear suspensions from the paraffin-embedded tissue samples. Microtome sections were dewaxed, hydrated, and incubated in pepsin with intermittent vortexing and mechanical disruption to release the nuclei. After completion of the tissue digestion, the nuclei were either suspended in 70% EtOH for storage or stained with propidium iodide (PI) for FCM analysis

C. Oliver and M.C. Jamur (eds.), *Immunocytochemical Methods and Protocols*, Methods in Molecular Biology, Vol. 588, DOI 10.1007/978-1-59745-324-0_36, © Humana Press, a part of Springer Science+Business Media, LLC 1995, 1999, 2010

Another use of the nuclei isolated from PET is to study low number of nuclei by polymerase chain reaction (PCR). Nuclei can be sorted on the basis of cell cycle, digested to single stranded DNA, and the desired segment of DNA amplified. PCR has the ability to make DNA from a complementary DNA template. Lastly, the isolated nuclei can not only be stained for DNA content but also be stained for nuclear proteins, proliferation factors, and other nuclear proteins.

There are three techniques differing primarily in the initial handling of the paraffin embedded tissue sections. In the first, paraffin-embedded tissue sections are placed on glass microslides (*see* Subheading 3.1), the second involves placing the paraffin-embedded tissue sections into bags for digestion (*see* Subheading 3.2), and the last uses a test tube to hold the paraffin-embedded tissue sections during processing (*see* Subheading 3.3). The "tea bag" and test tube methods give a higher yield of nuclei. Basically, the "tea bag" technique provides a way of controlling the yield of a nuclear extraction from paraffin embedded tissue. The "tea bag" has pores that are slightly smaller than the size of the nuclei. Therefore, the nuclei stay inside the tea bag and are not washed away during digestion and subsequent washing. The test tube method is an alternative technique that is valuable if the sample is rare or very limited. It uses no catch membrane as is used in the "tea bag" technique. The digestion and the washing steps are completed in the test tube without any internal sieve as the sample never leaves the tube. At the end of the digestion, the test tube is loaded with wash buffer and spun down to remove all cellular debris, leaving only the nuclei at the bottom of the tube. I favor (depending on the tissue type and the tissue availability) the tube technique over the "tea bag" technique. The "tea bag" technique probably has a higher net yield, but the final retrieval of the nuclei from the mesh, while approaching 100%, never reaches this level. Scrapping the mesh is often necessary in order to release the nuclei. The test tube technique is faster as no recovery from a mesh is necessary, and the sample is in the bottom of the tube.

2. Materials

1. Paraffin-embedded tissue or cell block.
2. Xylene.
3. Ethanol, 100%, 95%, and 50%.
4. Hydrochloric acid (concentrated).
5. Dulbecco's Phosphate Buffered Saline (PBS), pH 7.4 without Ca^{2+} and Mg^{2+}: 2.7 mM KCl, 1.2 mM KH_2PO_4, 138 mM NaCl, and 8.1 mM Na_2HPO_4 without Ca^{2+} and Mg^{2+}, pH 7.2.

6. Phosphate Buffered Saline (PBS) pH 1.5, adjust with 1 N HCl.
7. Pepsin: stock solution 10 mg/mL in PBS at pH 1.5.
8. Microfuge tubes.
9. Vortex mixer.
10. HEPES buffer, 10 mM, made in PBS pH 7.0.
11. Syringes, 5 mL and 10 mL.
12. 16, 18, and 25 gauge emulsifying needles.
13. Disposable pipets, plastic.
14. Water bath, 37°C.
15. Propidium iodide (PI), stock 50 mg/mL water (*see* Note 1).
16. RNase, DNase free.
17. "Tea Bags" (*see* Note 2).
18. Microslides, glass.
19. Blades, surgical, no.11.
20. 40 μm nylon mesh.
21. 15 mL conical centrifuge tubes, polycarbonate or polypropylene.
22. 1.5 mL, xylene resistant microfuge tubes.

3. Methods

3.1. Slide Technique

1. Mount one 30-80 μm section on a glass slide (*see* Notes 3 and 4).
2. Clear the sections in two changes of xylene.
3. Hydrate with decreasing per cent alcohols, and then water.
4. Air Dry.
5. If necessary, remove necrotic, inflammatory, and/or nontumorigenic portions of the tissue section by scraping with a sharp blade.
6. Dilute the stock pepsin solution 1:20 in PBS to make 0.5% pepsin solution: 1 mL 10 mg/mL pepsin in PBS, pH 1.5 and 19 mL PBS, pH 1.5.
7. Add 200 μL of 0.5% pepsin in PBS, pH 1.5, covering the tissue section on the glass microslide.
8. Use a no.11 blade to dislodge and disrupt the tissue section.
9. Aspirate the suspension into a pipet, and place it in a microfuge tube.
10. Incubate for 30-60 min at 37°C, vortexing intermittently (*see* Note 5).

11. Draw the contents of the microfuge tube into a syringe.
12. Homogenize the contents by sequentially passing it through smaller gauge emulsifying needles until a smooth texture is obtained.
13. Draw all of the liquid up into the syringe, remove the needle, and place a small square of 40 µm mesh between the needle and the syringe.
14. Push out the contents (nuclei) of the syringe through the mesh into the tube.
15. Add 1 mL PBS 10 mM Hepes buffer in PBS to each tube.
16. Spin the tubes at 500g for 5 min.
17. Decant supernatant and vortex the pellet.
18. Repeat once.
19. After the final wash, add 250 µL PBS.
20. OPTION. If sample is to be stored before staining, while vortexing, add 750 µL cold (-20°C) 100% ETOH dropwise to each tube.
21. Add staining solution: 50°µg/mL propidium iodide and 1,000 units/mL Ribonuclease A per mL of PBS.
22. Incubate 20 min at room temperature before analysis (*see* Note 6).
23. Analyze.

3.2. "Tea Bag" Technique

1. Cut 2-3 sections each 50 µm thick, and place them in properly identified "tea bags" (*see* Note 4).
2. Dewax sections in two changes of xylene for 10 min each.
3. Hydrate section through graded alcohols with changes of 100%, 95%, 50% for 10 min each and then two changes of distilled water.
4. Open "tea bags," remove tissue, and scrape into test tube.
5. Add 1 mL of a prewarmed solution of 0.5% pepsin in 0.9% NaCl, pH 1.5, to each test tube.
6. Incubate 1-2 h at 37°C, vortex intermittently (*see* Note 5).
7. Fill tube with cold PBS without Ca^{2+} and Mg^{2+}.
8. Filter through syringe fitted with 40 µm nylon mesh.
9. Wash cells twice by centrifugation, with PBS without Ca^{2+} and Mg^{2+}. Add 0.5 mL of 50 µg/mL of propidium iodide.

3.3. Test Tube Technique

1. Cut 2-3 sections each 50 µm thick, and place them in properly identified 15 mL centrifuge tubes (*see* Note 4).
2. Dewax sections in two changes of xylene for 10 min each.
3. Hydrate sections through graded alcohols with changes of 100%, 95%, 50% for 10 min each and then two changes of distilled water.

4. Add 1 mL of a prewarmed solution of 0.5% pepsin in 0.9% NaCl, pH 1.5, to each test tube.
5. Incubate 1-2 h at 37°C (*see* Note 5).
6. Draw the contents of the centrifuge tube into a 2 cc syringe. Homogenize the sample by repeatedly passing it through a 23 gauge needle attached to the syringe.
7. Add 2 mL cold PBS w/o Ca^{2+} and Mg^{2+}.
8. Wash twice by centrifugation in PBS w/o Ca^{2+} and Mg^{2+}.
9. Add 1 mL 95% EtOH (-20°C) to cell pellet.
10. Store at 4°C until ready to analyze.

4. Notes

1. Propidium iodide is a possible carcinogen and should be handled with caution. The stock solution should be stored refrigerated in the dark.
2. "Tea Bags" (Shandon Biopsy Bags) are available from the Anatomical Pathology group of Thermo Electron Corporation, 81 Wyman Street, Waltham, MA 02454 USA.
3. Use extra caution when the sections exceed 30 µm as they detach easily.
4. Tissue thickness is dependent upon the type of cell nuclei to be isolated. Endothelial nuclei tend to be long and narrow, while other cell types tend to have a more cuboidal shape.
5. The time for nuclear isolation can be a greatly reduced or increased depending upon tissue type, extent of suboptimally fixed, partially autolysed samples, and thickness of the tissue sections.
6. The 20 min stain time at room temperature for PI is the minimum required for reproducible DNA staining. I prefer to allow the cell suspension to incubate in the refrigerator overnight before analysis on the flow cytometer. The control values are usually better and the control size measurements more univariate.

References

1. Coon JS, Landay AL, Weinstein RS (1986) Flow cytometric analysis of paraffin-embedded tumors: implications for diagnostic pathology. Hum Pathol 17:435–437
2. Hedley DW, Friedlander ML, Taylor IW, Rugg CA, Musgrove EA (1983) Method for analysis of cellular DNA content of paraffin-embedded pathological material using flow cytometry. J Histochem Cytochem 31:1333–1335
3. Hedley DW, Friedlander ML, Taylor IW (1985) Application of DNA flow cytometry to paraffin-embedded archival material for the study of aneuploidy and its clinical significance. Cytometry 4:327–333

Part V

Colloidal Gold Detection Systems for Electron Microscopic Analysis

Chapter 37

Fixation and Embedding

Constance Oliver and Maria Célia Jamur

Abstract

For electron microscopic immunocytochemistry, the fixation procedure is always a compromise between good morphological preservation and retention of antigenicity. The choice of fixative depends on whether the immunogold labeling will be done before or after the samples are embedded and on how resistant the antigen is to fixation. For preembedding staining, it is possible to immunolabel the samples prior to fixation or after only a very mild fixation. Following immunolabeling, the samples can be refixed in a stronger fixative, such as 2% glutaraldehyde, to give good morphological preservation. Since it is not possible to refix the tissue after immunolabeling, for postembedding labeling, the composition of the initial fixative must be such that morphological detail and antigenicity are both preserved. While virtually any embedding resin may be used for immunogold staining, for postembedding methods, the resin can affect the immunostaining. In this chapter, methods are given for conventional fixation and microwave fixation as well as for embedding in various resins.

Key words: Fixation, Immunolabeling, Embedding, Electron microscopy, Microwave, Resin

1. Introduction

For electron microscopic immunocytochemistry, the fixation procedure is always a compromise between good morphological preservation and retention of antigenicity (1–3). If tissue is taken from an animal, it is preferable to fix tissues by perfusion, but if that is not possible, the time between removal of the tissue and fixation should be kept as short as possible. The fixative used will depend on whether the immunogold labeling will be done before or after the samples are embedded and on how resistant the antigen is to the fixative. In order to preserve the ultrastructural detail, it is desirable to include glutaraldehyde in the fixative. However, some antigens are extremely sensitive to crosslinking by glutaraldehyde, and the concentration of glutaraldehyde will have to be reduced

C. Oliver and M.C. Jamur (eds.), *Immunocytochemical Methods and Protocols*, Methods in Molecular Biology, Vol. 588,
DOI 10.1007/978-1-59745-324-0_37, © Humana Press, a part of Springer Science+Business Media, LLC 1995, 1999, 2010

or, in the most extreme cases, omitted entirely. For preembedding staining, it is possible to immunolabel the samples prior to fixation or after only a very mild fixation. Following incubation in the primary antibody or at subsequent steps, the samples can then be refixed in a stronger fixative, such as 2% glutaraldehyde, to give good morphological preservation. For postembedding labeling, it is not possible to refix the tissue after immunolabeling. Therefore, the composition of the initial fixative must be such that morphological detail and antigenicity are both preserved. The composition of the fixative will have to be determined empirically for each antigen. However, a fixative containing 0.5% glutaraldehyde and 2% formaldehyde generally is suitable for a wide variety of antigens. Adding 0.1% picric acid to the fixative can also help preserve morphological detail while retaining antigenicity.

In addition to composition, time and temperature of fixation can also affect the ability to immunolabel a particular antigen. It may be possible to preserve antigenicity by reducing the time of fixation, by altering the temperature of the fixative, or by doing both simultaneously. Many antigens can be preserved quite successfully by fixing at room temperature, but in some instances, fixation and processing at 4°C will help preserve antigenicity. Alternatively, warming (37–50°C) can increase penetration of the fixative into the tissue, and thus, fixation times can be reduced. Recently, microwave fixation has been introduced as an alternative to standard immersion fixation for electron microscopy (4, 5). Samples are immersed in fixative and microwaved for a few seconds. The combination of the chemical fixative and the heating action of the microwave gives good morphological preservation while retaining antigenicity.

Virtually, any embedding resin may be used for immunogold staining. However, for postembedding methods, the resin can affect the immunostaining (2, 4, 6–8). The hydrophilic resins, such as LR Gold, LR White, and Lowicryl, generally give better results than the epoxy-based hydrophobic resins, such as the Epon substitutes or Spurr.

Fixation by rapid freezing followed by either freeze substitution (9) or cryosectioning can also overcome some of the problems of standard immersion fixation and resin embedding. These are more specialized techniques and will not be discussed here. Discussion of the methods can be found in Polak and Varndell (10), Hayat (11), and Verkleij and Leunissen (12).

2. Materials

1. 70% EM-grade glutaraldehyde.
2. 20% EM-grade formaldehyde (*see* Note 1).

3. Dulbecco's phosphate-buffered saline (PBS): 100 mg anhydrous calcium chloride, 200 mg potassium chloride, 200 mg monobasic potassium phosphate, 100 mg magnesium chloride · 6 H_2O, 8 g sodium chloride, and 2.16 g dibasic sodium phosphate ·7 H_2O; bring volume to 1 L with deionized glass-distilled water, pH 7.4.
4. Dulbecco's PBS without calcium and magnesium: 200 mg potassium chloride, 200 mg monobasic potassium phosphate, 8 g sodium chloride, and 2.16 g dibasic sodium phosphate·7 H_2O; bring volume to 1 L with deionized distilled water, pH 7.4.
5. 0.1 M Cacodylate buffer: 21.4 g cacodylic acid·3 H_2O, sodium salt; bring volume to 1 L with deionized glass-distilled water; adjust pH to 7.4 with HCl.
6. 0.5% Glutaraldehyde-2% formaldehyde fixative: 0.5 mL 70% glutaraldehyde, 7 mL 20% formaldehyde, 3 mg calcium chloride, and 62.5 mL PBS or 0.1 M cacodylate buffer, pH 7.4.
7. Saturated picric acid solution: Fill 500 g bottle of picric acid with deionized glass-distilled water (*see* Note 2).
8. 0.1 M glycine: 750 mg glycine; bring volume to 100 mL with PBS, pH 7.4.
9. Osmium tetroxide (4% stock): 1 g osmium tetroxide and 25 mL deionized glass-distilled water (*see* Note 3).
10. Microwave oven (*see* Note 4).
11. Giemsa solution (Sigma-Aldrich).
12. Electrophoresis-grade agar.
13. 35-mm plastic tissue culture dishes.
14. Epon 812 substitute; Epon A: 62 mL Epon 812 substitute and 100 mL dodecenyl succinic anhydride (DDSA); Epon B: 100 mL Epon 812 substitute and 89 mL nadic methyl anhydride (NMA); mix together 10 mL Epon A and 15 mL Epon B; add 0.5 mL 2,4,6-tri (dimethylaminomethyl) phenol (DMP-30), and mix well (*see* Note 5).
15. Araldite 502: 100 g araldite 502 resin and 75 g DDSA; add 2.5–3.5 g 2,4,6-tri (dimethylaminomethyl) phenol (DMP-30) just prior to use (*see* Note 6).
16. Spurr's resin: 26 g nonenyl succinic anhydride (NSA), 10 g vinyl-4-cyclohexene dioxide (ERL 4206), 4 g DER 736, and 0.4 g 2-Dimethylaminothanol (DMAE) (*see* Note 7).
17. Lowicryl K4M: 4.0 g K4M crosslinker, 26.0 g K4M monomer, and 150 mg initiator; mix just prior to use, and degas under vacuum for 15–30 min (*see* Note 8).
18. LR White resin: Store at 4°C; let the bottle come to room temperature before opening; stable for 1 year.

19. LR Gold resin: 25 mL LR Gold resin and 125 mg benzoin methyl ether; mix just prior to use.

3. Methods

3.1. Fixation

1. Rinse samples twice in PBS, and fix for 30 min to 1 h at room temperature in 0.5% glutaraldehyde and 2% formaldehyde in PBS, or fix by perfusion with 0.5% glutaraldehyde and 2% formaldehyde (*see* Note 9).
2. Following fixation, rinse the samples three to five times over a period of 30 min in PBS (*see* Note 10).
3. Quench free aldehyde groups by rinsing the samples for 5 min in 0.1 M glycine in PBS (*see* Note 11).
4. Samples may be fixed in 2% OsO_4 in 0.1 M cacodylate buffer for 1 h at room temperature and then rinsed in 0.1 M cacodylate buffer prior to embedding.

3.2. Microwave Fixation

1. Place a glass beaker containing 100 mL of distilled water in the right rear corner of the microwave oven.
2. Preheat the water load for 2 min to warm up the magnetron.
3. Replace the water load with 100 mL distilled water at 25°C.
4. Using Giemsa/agar blocks (*see* Note 12), map the microwave oven (*see* Note 13).
5. Place the samples in fixative, one at a time, at the location determined during calibration, and irradiate at full power for the appropriate length of time (*see* Note 14).
6. Immediately after irradiation, quench the samples by rinsing them with PBS or 0.1 M cacodylate buffer at 4°C.
7. Rinse the sample in 0.1 M cacodylate buffer.
8. Postfix for 1 h in 2% OsO_4 in 0.1 M cacodylate buffer, and then rinse in 0.1 M cacodylate buffer prior to embedding.

3.3. Embedding

3.3.1. Epon 812 Substitutes

1. Dehydrate the tissue, and infiltrate according to the following schedule:
   (a) 50% Ethanol, 15 min.
   (b) 75% Ethanol, 15 min.
   (c) 95% Ethanol, 15 min.
   (d) 100% Ethanol, 15 min.
   (e) 100% Ethanol, 15 min.
   (f) 100% Propylene oxide, 15 min.
   (g) 100% Propylene oxide, 30 min.

(h) 1:1 Complete resin:propylene oxide, 1–2 h.

(i) 2:1 Complete resin:propylene oxide, 1–2 h.

(j) 100% Complete resin, 3–6 h (*see* Notes 15 and 16).

2. Transfer to polyethylene or gelatin-embedding capsules containing complete resin.
3. Polymerize overnight at 45°C and then for 24 h at 60°C.

3.3.2. Araldite

1. Dehydrate the tissue, and infiltrate according to the following schedule:
   (a) 50% Ethanol, 15 min.
   (b) 75% Ethanol, 15 min.
   (c) 95% Ethanol, 15 min.
   (d) 100% Ethanol, 15 min.
   (e) 100% Ethanol, 15 min.
   (f) 100% Propylene oxide, 15 min.
   (g) 100% Propylene oxide, 30 min.
   (h) 1:1 Complete resin:propylene oxide, 1–2 h.
   (i) 2:1 Complete resin:propylene oxide, 1–2 h.
   (j) 100% Complete resin, 3–6 h.
2. Transfer to polyethylene or gelatin-embedding capsules containing complete resin. Polymerize overnight at 35°C, 24 h at 45°C, and 24 h at 60°C. Alternatively, araldite may be polymerized overnight at 60°C.

3.3.3. Spurr's Resin

1. Dehydrate the tissue, and infiltrate according to the following schedule:
   (a) 50% Ethanol, 15 min.
   (b) 75% Ethanol, 15 min.
   (c) 95% Ethanol, 15 min.
   (d) 100% Ethanol, 15 min.
   (e) 100% Ethanol, 15 min.
   (f) 100% Propylene oxide, 15 min.
   (g) 100% Propylene oxide, 30 min.
   (h) 1:1 Complete resin:propylene oxide, 1–2 h.
   (i) 2:1 Complete resin:propylene oxide, 3–6 h.
   (j) 100% Complete resin, overnight.
2. Transfer to polyethylene or gelatin-embedding capsules containing complete resin. Polymerize overnight at 70°C.

3.3.4. Lowicryl (13)

1. Dehydrate the tissue, and infiltrate with resin according to the following schedule:
   (a) 30% Methanol, 5 min, 4°C.

(b) 50% Methanol, 5 min, 4°C.
(c) 70% Methanol, 5 min, –10°C.
(d) 90% Methanol, 30 min, –20°C.
(e) 1:1 Complete resin:90% methanol, 60 min, –20°C.
(f) 2:1 Complete resin:90% methanol, 60 min, –20°C.
(g) 100% Complete resin, 60 min, –20°C.
(h) 100% Complete resin, overnight, –20°C.

2. Transfer tissue to polyethylene-embedding capsules or gelatin capsules, fill the capsules with complete resin, and cap. Oxygen will inhibit polymerization.
3. Polymerize the plastic with UV light (366 nm, two 15-W Sylvania F15T8/BLB bulbs) placed 10 cm from the capsules. Expose the capsules to the UV light for 24 h at –20°C (*see* Notes 17 and 18).

3.3.5. LR White

1. Dehydrate the tissue, and infiltrate with resin according to the following schedule:
(a) 50% Ethanol, 30 min.
(b) 75% Ethanol, 30 min.
(c) 1:1 LR White:75% ethanol, 1–2 h.
(d) 2:1 LR White:75% ethanol, 1–2 h.
(e) 100% LR White, 1–2 h.
(f) 100% LR White, 3 h to overnight.
2. Transfer tissue to polyethylene-embedding capsules or gelatin capsules, fill the capsules with 100% LR White, and cap. Oxygen will inhibit polymerization.
3. Polymerize 24 h at 50–55°C (*see* Note 19).

3.3.6. LR Gold (14)

1. Dehydrate the tissue, and infiltrate with resin according to the following schedule; samples should be in capped glass vials during dehydration and infiltration:
(a) 50% Acetone, 5 min, 0°C.
(b) 50% Acetone, 45 min, 0°C.
(c) 70% Acetone, 45 min, 0°C.
(d) 90% Acetone, 45 min, 0°C.
(e) 1:1 LR Gold:acetone, 60 min, –20°C.
(f) 7:3 LR Gold:acetone, 60 min, –20°C.
(g) 100% LR Gold, 60 min, –20°C.
(h) 100% LR Gold, 5 h to overnight, –20°C.
(i) 100% LR Gold + initiator (0.5% benzoin methyl ether), 60 min, –20°C.

(j) 100% LR Gold + initiator, 60 min, –20°C.

(k) 100% LR Gold + initiator, 5 h to overnight, –20°C.

2. Transfer tissue to polyethylene-embedding capsules or gelatin capsules, fill the capsules with 100% LR Gold + initiator, and cap. Oxygen will inhibit polymerization.
3. Polymerize the plastic with UV light (366 nm, two 15-W Sylvania F15T8/BLB bulbs) placed 10 cm from the capsules. Expose the capsules to the UV light for 24 h at –20°C.

4. Notes

1. The use of distilled formaldehyde, not formalin, which contains alcohol, is recommended. Freshly prepared paraformaldehyde can also be used, especially if large volumes of fixative are needed for perfusion fixation. To prepare an 8% solution of paraformaldehyde, in a fume hood, add 2 g of paraformaldehyde (trioxymethylene) powder to 25 mL of deionized glass-distilled water. With constant stirring, heat solution to 55–60°C. Once the solution has reached the proper temperature, continue to stir for 15 min. The solution will be milky. Add one to two drops of 1 N NaOH, with stirring, until the solution clears. A slight milkiness may persist. Cool and filter through Whatman No. 1 filter paper. This solution should be used the same day it is prepared.
2. The picric acid will dissolve in the water, resulting in a saturated solution. It will remain indefinitely at room temperature. Do not let picric acid dry, since the powder is explosive.
3. Clean the vial and score it with a diamond scribe. Place it in a clean glass bottle, and add the water. With a glass rod, break the vial. The solution is stable if kept refrigerated and protected from light. The stock solution should be stored away from other chemicals, since osmium vapors may escape from the bottle. Alternatively, aqueous solutions of osmium tetroxide in sealed glass ampules are available commercially. Dilute them to 1–2% with 0.1 M cacodylate buffer for use.
4. A conventional microwave oven, with a maximal power output of 550 W and an operating frequency of 2,450 MHz, or an oven designed specifically for laboratory use can be used. The microwave should have a fixed plate on the bottom, not a turntable.
5. Epon A and B solutions may be stored at 4°C for at least 6 months. Let them come to room temperature before opening.
6. Mix components together in a glass screw-cap bottle. The resin solution may be stored at 4°C for at least 6 months. Let it come to room temperature before opening.

7. Mix components together just before use. Store unused resin under vacuum; it is stable for 2–3 days. Store opened bottles of NSA under vacuum.
8. Avoid contact with the skin, and avoid breathing the vapors. Wear chemically resistant gloves, and use the resin in a fume hood. Mono Step Lowicryl, a premixed form of Lowicryl, is now available from electron microscopy suppliers.
9. The composition of the fixative may vary depending on the sensitivity of the antigen. For some antigens, it may be necessary to omit the glutaraldehyde entirely and fix in 4% formaldehyde in PBS for 1–4 h. Picric acid (0.1%) may also be added to the fixative. For very sensitive antigens, it may be desirable to fix and process tissue at 4°C.
10. Phosphate buffer (0.1 M), pH7.4, may be substituted for PBS.
11. Following fixation in formaldehyde or glutaraldehyde, tissue is generally quenched. The purpose of this step is to block any free aldehyde groups that remain after fixation and washing. This step is especially critical after glutaraldehyde fixation. Glutaraldehyde is a bifunctional aldehyde. During fixation, one end may bind to cellular constituents, leaving the other end free to react. If this end is not blocked, it can bind to the protein in the blocking solution or to the primary antibody. Although any small molecular-weight compound containing an amino group may be used, the most commonly used quenching agents are glycine, ammonium chloride, and sodium borohydride.
12. Giemsa agar blocks are made by preparing a solution of 2% agar in 0.9% saline and then adding Giemsa solution to the liquid agar to a final concentration of 0.5%. The Giemsa agar solution is then poured into flat embedding molds and allowed to solidify. The Giemsa/agar blocks can be trimmed into cubes (0.5 cm^3) or used as they come from the molds.
13. Microwaves are not dispersed evenly over the oven, leaving "hot" and "cold" spots on the oven floor. The radiation pattern inside the oven may be mapped using either an array of neon bulbs or with Giemsa/agar blocks. To map the microwave oven with Giemsa/agar blocks, immerse the blocks in 5 mL of fixative solution in a 35-mm tissue culture dish. Use only one block per dish. Place the dish (one at time, a fresh one for each run) at various locations on the floor of the microwave unit, and expose to microwave radiation at 100% power. The amount of microwave radiation that an area is receives can be determined by the changes in the Giemsa/agar blocks. The correct amount of irradiation is achieved if the Giemsa/agar block turns from blue to violet without showing any signs of melting. If level of radiation is too low,

there will be no change in the block, and if it is too high, the block will begin to melt. Once the ideal position for the sample has been determined, subsequent samples should be placed in the same location. A gridded acetate sheet may be placed in the bottom of the oven to act as a reference guide.

14. To ensure that the sample receives the correct amount of irradiation, place a Giemsa/agar block in the same type of container with the same amount of fixative to be used for the sample at the predetermined location on the floor of the oven and irradiate. 0.05% Glutaraldehyde, 2% formaldehyde, 0.025% $CaCl_2$ in 0.1 M cacodylate buffer, pH 7.4, is a reliable fixative for microwave fixation. The sample receives the correct amount of irradiation if the Giemsa/agar block turns from blue to violet without showing any signs of melting. The irradiation time can be adjusted to achieve optimum sample fixation.
15. Other solvents, such as methanol or acetone, can be used during dehydration, depending on the tissue. However, acetone should not be used with LR White.
16. During infiltration of samples with embedding resin, samples should be placed on a rotator to provide adequate mixing of the sample with the resin. Infiltration schedules for embedding resins will vary with the size of the sample, the viscosity of the resin, and the density of the tissue. Larger samples, more viscous resins, and dense tissue will all require longer times to ensure adequate infiltration of the sample. Certain samples, such as pellets of cultured cells and lung, may trap air or solvents in the samples. More complete infiltration and better polymerization of the resin will be obtained if following infiltration, specimens are transferred to embedding capsules containing just enough resin to cover the samples, and the samples are placed under vacuum overnight. The capsules can then be filled with resin, and samples can be polymerized.
17. For complete polymerization, it may be necessary to continue curing the blocks by UV for up to 2 weeks at either –20°C or room temperature. Temperature for infiltration and polymerization of Lowicryl K4M can be as low as –35°C.
18. Samples that are embedded in resins that are polymerized by UV light (Lowicryl, LR White) should not be osmicated. The osmium may interfere with the polymerization by preventing the light from penetrating the samples.
19. LR White is very hygroscopic and will readily adsorb water. If the 1:1 LR White:75% ethanol is cloudy, increase the concentration of ethanol up to 95%.

References

1. Brandtzaeg P (1982) Tissue preparation methods for immunocytochemistry. In: Bullock GR, Petrusz P (eds) Techniques in immunocytochemistry, vol. 1. Academic, New York, pp 1–76
2. Larsson LI (1988) Fixation and tissue pretreatment. In: Larsson L-I (ed) Immunocytochemistry: theory and practice. CRC, Boca Raton, FL, pp 41–76
3. Skepper JN (2000) Immunocytochemical strategies for electron microscopy: choice or compromise. J Microsc 199:1–36
4. Login GR, Dvorak AM (1988) Microwave fixation provides excellent preservation of tissue, cells and antigens for light and electron microscopy. Histochem J 20:373–387
5. Jamur MC, Faraco CD, Lunardi LO, Siraganian RP, Oliver C (1995) Microwave fixation improves antigenicity of glutaraldehyde-sensitive antigens while preserving ultrastructural detail. J Histochem Cytochem 43:307–311
6. Brorson SH (1998) Antigen detection on resin sections and methods for improving the immunogold labeling by manipulating the resin. Histol Histopathol 13:275–281
7. Newman GR, Hobot JA (1999) Resins for combined light and electron microscopy a half century of development. Histochem J 8: 495–505
8. Causton BE (1984) The choice of resins for electron immunocytochemistry. In: Polak JM, Varndell IM (eds) Immunolabelling for electron microscopy. Elsevier, New York, pp 29–70
9. Shiurba R (2001) Freeze-substitution: origins and applications. Int Rev Cytol 206:45–96
10. Polak JM, Varndell IM (1984) Immunolabelling for electron microscopy. Elsevier, New York
11. Hayat MA (1989) Colloidal gold: principles, methods, and applications, vol 1. Academic, New York
12. Verkleij AJ, Leunissen JLM (1989) Immunogold labeling in cell biology. CRC, Boca Raton, FL
13. Bendayan M (1984) Protein A-gold electron microscopic immunocytochemistry: methods, applications, and limitations. J Electron Microsc Tech 1:243–270
14. Berryman MA, Rodewald RD (1990) An enhanced method for post-embedding immunocytochemical staining which preserves cell membranes. J Histochem Cytochem 38:159–170

Chapter 38

Preparation of Colloidal Gold

Constance Oliver

Abstract

Colloidal gold probes have become widely used for immunocytochemical staining at the electron microscopic level. Gold sols are producing by boiling a solution of tetrachloroauric acid with a reducing agent. The type of reducing agent and the concentration of components determine the final particle size. Gold sols that have a particle size ranging from 2 to 40 nm can be made in the laboratory, depending on the type and concentration of the reducing agent. This chapter details methods for producing various sizes of gold. The methods are relatively simple and very reproducible from batch to batch.

Key words: Colloidal gold, Tetrachloroauric acid, Tannic acid, Trisodium citrate, Thiocyanate

1. Introduction

Since their introduction by Faulk and Taylor (1), colloidal gold probes have become widely used for immunocytochemical staining at the electron microscopic level. Many different methods of producing colloidal gold sols have been published (2–10). Gold sols are producing by boiling a solution of tetrachloroauric acid with a reducing agent. At the beginning of the reduction process, gold atoms are liberated from the chloroauric acid. The gold atoms aggregate forming microcrystals. As more chloroauric acid is reduced, the microcrystals grow in size until all of the chloroauric acid is reduced. The type of reducing agent and the concentration of components determine the ratio between nucleation and growth, and thus determine the final particle size. Gold sols that have a particle size ranging from 2 to 40 nm can be made in the laboratory, depending on the type and concentration of the reducing agent. The methods given below for various sizes of gold are relatively simple and very reproducible from batch to batch.

C. Oliver and M.C. Jamur (eds.), *Immunocytochemical Methods and Protocols*, Methods in Molecular Biology, Vol. 588, DOI 10.1007/978-1-59745-324-0_38,

2. Materials

1. Detergent, such as Haemo Sol, Micro-clean, or 7X. These may be purchased from suppliers of laboratory products such as Fisher Scientific, Hampton, NH; Thomas Scientific, Swedesboro, NJ.
2. Deionized, glass-distilled water.
3. 10% Chloroauric acid: 1 g glass vial chloroauric acid (available from suppliers of laboratory chemicals such as Electron Microscopy Sciences, Hatfield, PA; Polysciences, Warrington, PA, and Fisher Scientific, Hampton, NH) and 10 mL deionized glass-distilled water (*see* Note 1).
4. 1% Trisodium citrate: 100 mg trisodium citrate and 10 mL deionized glass-distilled water; dissolve sodium citrate in water; prepare immediately prior to use.
5. 1% Tannic acid: 100 mg low molecular weight tannic acid and 10 mL deionized glass-distilled water; dissolve tannic acid in water; prepare immediately prior to use (*see* Note 2).
6. 0.025 M Potassium carbonate: 34 mg potassium carbonate; bring the volume to 10 mL with deionized glass-distilled water.
7. 1 M Sodium thiocyanate: 81 mg sodium thiocyanate and 10 mL deionized glass-distilled water; dissolve sodium thiocyanate in water; prepare immediately before use.
8. 0.2 M Potassium carbonate: 276 mg potassium carbonate and 10 mL deionized glass-distilled water.
9. Stirring hot plate and Teflon™ stir bars.
10. Glassware: 250-mL volumetric flask, two 100-mL screw-cap glass bottles, and 50-mL beaker.

3. Methods

3.1. Preparation of Glassware

1. Clean glassware by boiling in detergent, such as Haemasol, Micro, or 7X (*see* Note 3).
2. Rinse free of detergent, and rinse additionally 10–15 times in deionized glass-distilled water (*see* Note 4).

3.2. Sodium Citrate Gold, 15 nm (2, 5)

1. Add 10 μL of 10% chloroauric acid to 100 mL of deionized glass-distilled water (*see* Note 1).
2. Bring the solution to a boil (*see* Note 5).
3. While vigorously stirring the solution using a Teflon™ stir bar and a stirring hot plate, quickly add 4 mL of freshly prepared 1% aqueous trisodium citrate (*see* Note 6).

4. Continue to boil the solution, with stirring. The solution will first turn blue and then red in about 5–7 min. After 2–3 additional min, the solution will reach its end point, a red-orange color.
5. Let it boil an additional 5 min, then cool, and transfer it to a clean screw-cap glass bottle. The gold sol is stable if kept refrigerated and protected from light.

3.3. Tannic Acid–Sodium Citrate Gold, 6 nm (9)

1. Place 79 mL deionized glass-distilled water and 100 µL of 10% chloroauric acid in a clean 250 mL Erlenmyer flask (*see* Note 1).
2. In a 50 mL beaker, mix 4 mL of 1% freshly prepared aqueous trisodium citrate, 0.5 mL 1% tannic acid, and 0.5 mL 0.025 M potassium carbonate (to adjust pH). Add 15 mL of deionized glass-distilled water (*see* Note 7).
3. Heat the gold solution and the reducing solution separately on a stirring hot plate.
4. When the gold solution reaches 60°C, stir vigorously and add quickly the reducing solution.
5. Continue stirring, and maintain temperature at approx 60°C until solution turns red.
6. Heat to boiling after the sol is formed. Solution evaporation can be avoided by using a reflux column or covering the top of the flask with a glass slide. Alternatively, a siliconized 250 mL volumetic flask can be used.
7. Cool the solution, and transfer it to a clean screw-cap bottle. Gold sol is stable if kept refrigerated and protected from light.

3.4. Thiocyanate Gold, 2.8 nm (10)

1. Add 0.3 mL of 1 M sodium thiocyanate, with stirring, to 50 mL of deionized glass-distilled water containing 0.5 mL 10% chloroauric acid and 0.75 mL of 0.2 M potassium carbonate.
2. Continue to stir for 15–30 min. A straw yellow color will develop.
3. Let it stand overnight in the dark at room temperature to complete the reaction (*see* Notes 8 and 9).

4. Notes

1. To prepare 10% chloroauric acid solution, remove the label from the glass vial containing 1 g of chloroauric acid and thoroughly clean the vial. Rinse in deionized glass-distilled water. Score the vial with a diamond scribe, but do not break it. Add 10 mL of deionized glass-distilled water to clean glass bottle. Add the vial of chloroauric acid to the bottle containing the water. Break the vial into the water using a clean glass rod.

The resulting solution is stable for years if kept refrigerated and protected from light. Do not use chloroauric acid that was not sealed in a glass vial. Powdered chloroauric acid is very hygroscopic and adsorbs water readily.

2. The tannic acid should be low molecular weight. This tannic acid is predominately a mixture of tetra and pentagalloyl glucose and should be used for making gold sols. Low molecular weight tannic acid is available from suppliers of electron microscopic supplies.
3. All glassware, stir bars, and so forth, used in preparing gold sols must be free of any contamination, or the sol will not form properly. Glassware may be siliconized if desired.
4. The water used in all solutions and to wash and rinse the glassware should be of the highest purity possible. Sterile deionized glass-distilled water is recommended for all procedures.
5. Care should be taken not to allow the solution to evaporate, thereby changing the concentration of the components. A siliconized 250 mL volumetric flask works well. Alternatively, a reflux apparatus can be used.
6. For 19 nm gold, add 3 mL of 1% trisodium citrate; for 12.5 nm gold, add 6 mL of 1% trisodium citrate.
7. For 15 nm gold, add 20 μL 1% tannic acid and 19.98 mL deionized glass-distilled water; for 10 nm gold, add 100 μL 1% tannic acid and 19.9 mL deionized glass-distilled water; for 3.5 nm gold, add 3 mL 1% tannic acid, 3 mL 0.025 M potassium carbonate, and 14 mL deionized glass-distilled water. Sodium citrate remains constant at 4 mL.
8. Gold colloid will aggregate with age. Use within 3 days of preparation.
9. The size of the gold colloid may be determined in the electron microscope by first wetting a formvar-carbon-coated grid with 0.01% bacitracin. Using a triangle of filter paper, moistened at one end, wick off the bacitracin, and apply a drop of gold colloid to the grid. After 1–2 min, wick off the excess gold colloid. Air-dry, and examine it in the electron microscope.

References

1. Faulk W, Taylor G (1971) An immunocolloid method for the electron microscope. Immunochemistry 8:1081–1083
2. Bendayan M (1984) Protein-A gold electron microscopic immunocytochemistry: methods, applications, and limitations. J Electron Microsc Tech 1:243–270
3. Leunissen JLM, DeMey JR (1989) Preparation of gold probes. In: Verkleij AJ, Leunissen JLM (eds) Immuno-gold Labeling in Cell Biology. CRC, Boca Raton, FL, pp 3–16
4. Handley DA (1989) Methods for synthesis of colloidal gold. In: Hayat MA (ed) Colloidal Gold, vol. 1. Academic Press, New York, NY, pp 13–33
5. Frens G (1973) Controlled nucleation for the regulation of particle size in monodisperse gold suspensions. Nature Phys Sci 241: 20–22

6. Horisberger M, Rosset J (1977) Colloidal gold, a useful marker for transmission and scanning electron microscopy. J Histochem Cytochem 25:295–305
7. Roth J (1982) The preparation of protein A-gold complexes with 3 nm and 15 nm gold particles and their use in labeling multiple antigens on ultra-thin sections. Histochem J 14:791–801
8. Slot JW, Geuze HJ (1985) A new method of preparing gold probes for multiple-labeling cytochemistry. Eur J Cell Biol 38:87–93
9. Muhlpfordt JA (1982) The preparation of colloidal gold particles using tannic acid as an additional reducing agent. Experientia 38: 1127–1128
10. Bashong W, Lucocq JM, Roth J (1985) "Thiocyanate-Gold:" small (2–3 nm) colloidal gold for affinity cytochemical labeling in electron microscopy. Histochem 83: 409–411

Chapter 39

Conjugation of Colloidal Gold to Proteins

Constance Oliver

Abstract

The ability to conjugate proteins to colloidal gold sols provides a wide variety of probes for electron microscopy. Antibodies, protein A, protein G, lectins, enzymes, toxins, and other proteins have all been conjugated to colloidal gold. The nature of the interaction between the colloidal gold and the protein is poorly understood. Proteins are conjugated to gold sols by adjusting the pH of the gold sol to approximately 0.5 pH unit higher than the pI of the protein being conjugated. This chapter gives a general method for conjugating proteins to colloidal gold as well as more specific methods for conjugating antibodies and protein A to colloidal gold.

Key words: Antibody, Protein A, Protein G, Conjugation, Colloidal gold

1. Introduction

The ability to conjugate proteins to colloidal gold sols provides a wide variety of probes for electron microscopy. In addition to antibodies, protein A, protein G, lectins, enzymes, toxins, and other proteins have all been conjugated to colloidal gold (1–7). The nature of the interaction between the colloidal gold and the protein is poorly understood. Colloidal gold is a negatively charged lyophobic sol. The surface of the particle displays not only electrostatic characteristics, but also hydrophobic properties. In conjugating proteins to a gold sol, the electrostatic interactions must be reduced so that the hydrophobic interactions can prevail. This is accomplished by adjusting the pH of the gold sol to approx 0.5 pH unit higher than the pI of the protein being conjugated. Roth (7) gives a table of optimum pH for a number of commonly used proteins. Once the pH is properly adjusted, the net charge of the protein is zero or slightly negative.

C. Oliver and M.C. Jamur (eds.), *Immunocytochemical Methods and Protocols*, Methods in Molecular Biology, Vol. 588, DOI 10.1007/978-1-59745-324-0_39, © Humana Press, a part of Springer Science+Business Media, LLC 1995, 1999, 2010

This prevents the aggregation of the protein owing to electrostatic attraction, while maintaining the hydrophobic interactions, and facilitates the conjugation of the protein to the gold.

2. Materials

1. Cold water fish gelatin (Sigma Aldrich, St. Louis, MO): Warm in 37°C water bath to liquefy; prepare dilute solutions just prior to use; keep stock bottle at 4°C.
2. 0.1 N Hydrochloric acid (HCl): 8.15 mL concentrated HCl and 1 L deionized glass-distilled water.
3. 0.2 M Potassium carbonate (K_2CO_3): 276 mg K_2CO_3; bring volume to 10 mL with deionized glass-distilled water.
4. Dulbecco's phosphate-buffered saline (PBS): 100 mg anhydrous calcium chloride, 200 mg potassium chloride, 200 mg monobasic potassium phosphate, 100 mg magnesium chloride · $6H_2O$, 8 g sodium chloride, and 2.16 g dibasic sodium phosphate · $7H_2O$; bring volume to 1 L with deionized glass-distilled water, pH 7.4.
5. 10% Polyethylene glycol (PEG): 100 mg polyethylene glycol (20,000 mol. wt.) and 10 mL deionized glass-distilled water; dissolve PEG in deionized glass-distilled water; prepare just before use.
6. 10% Sodium chloride: 100 mg NaCl and 10 mL deionized glass-distilled water; dissolve NaCl in deionized glass-distilled water; prepare shortly before using.
7. 0.2 M Borate–NaCl buffer: 76.3 g sodium borate · $10H_2O$ and 9 g sodium chloride; bring volume to 1 L with deionized glass-distilled water, pH 9.0.
8. Tris-buffered saline (TBS): 2.4 g Tris–HCl and 8.76 g sodium chloride; bring vol to 1 L with deionized glass-distilled water, pH 7.4. 10 mM sodium azide (650 mg) may be added as a preservative.

3. Methods

3.1. General Method for Conjugating Proteins to Colloidal Gold

1. Adjust pH to at least 0.5 pH point on the basic side of the pI of the protein to be adsorbed, using either 0.2 M K_2CO_3 or 0.1 N HCl. The pIs for some commonly used proteins can be found in Roth (7).

2. Add two drops of 1% PEG (20,000 mol. wt.) to 5 mL aliquots of the colloidal gold to avoid clogging the pH meter when adjusting the pH. Do not add the PEG to the colloidal gold stock. Discard aliquots after reading pH. Alternatively, narrow-range pH paper can be used.
3. Perform a saturation isotherm to determine the protein:gold ratio for each protein and each size colloidal gold (*see* Note 1).
4. Add 10 mL of colloidal gold to 0.2 mL of protein solution containing the minimal amount of protein needed to stabilize the gold plus 10% (as determined in step 3) (*see* Note 2).
5. Let the solution stand 10 min, and then add 1% PEG to a final concentration of 0.04%.
6. Let the solution stand another 30 min, and then centrifuge it for 45 min at 60,000 × *g*.
7. Remove and discard the clear supernatant.
8. Resuspend the soft gold pellet in 1.5 mL PBS with 0.04% PEG. The hard gold pellet is uncoated gold.
9. For use: dilute the stock solution 1:10–1:20 with PBS containing 0.02% PEG.

3.2. Preparation of Protein A Gold (2)

1. Adjust pH of colloidal gold to 6.0 with either 0.1 N HCl or 0.2 M K_2CO_3 (*see* Note 3).
2. Add 10 mL colloidal gold to 0.3 mg Protein A dissolved in 0.2 mL water for 15 nm gold.
3. Let the solution stand 10 min; add 1% PEG to a final concentration of 0.04%.
4. Let the solution stand 30 min, and then centrifuge for 45 min at 60,000 × *g*.
5. Remove the supernatant, and resuspend the soft pellet in 1.5 mL PBS containing 0.04% PEG. Store at 4°C.
6. For use: dilute 1:10–1:20 in PBS containing 0.02% PEG.

3.3. Preparation of Antibodies Conjugated to Colloidal Gold (8)

1. Use affinity-purified antibodies (*see* Note 4).
2. Dialyze the antibody: For monoclonal antibodies etc., already diluted with 0.2 M borate–NaCl buffer, dialyze against 2 mM borate–NaCl buffer, pH 9.0 for 2 h; for all other antibodies, first dialyze overnight against 0.2 M borate buffer–NaCl, pH 9.0, and then for 2 h against 2 mM borate buffer, pH 9.0. Do not leave the antibodies in the 2 mM borate buffer for extended periods, or the antibodies may aggregate.
3. Determine the optimal amount of antibody needed by running a saturation isotherm (*see* Notes 1 and 5).

4. Add the colloidal gold to the antibody with stirring, and allow to react for 10–30 min. Use 10 mL of colloidal gold and the amount of antibody as determined in step 3.
5. In order to stabilize the probes, add warmed (37°C) cold-water fish gelatin to give a final concentration of 1%.
6. Remove excess antibody by centrifuging the colloidal gold preparation twice on a glycerol step gradient (*see* Note 6).
7. Remove the supernatant, and discard it. Collect the soft pellet (it may be suspended in 1–2 mL of TBS to reduce viscosity), and dialyze for 1 h at room temperature against TBS to remove the glycerol.
8. Repeat the centrifugation. Remove and discard the supernatant, and resuspend the soft pellet in 1–2 mL TBS containing 1% cold-water fish gelatin.
9. Dialyze for 1 h at room temperature against TBS.
10. Dilute the resulting preparation with TBS containing 1% cold-water fish gelatin, and store in the refrigerator.

4. Notes

1. The minimal amount of protein necessary to stabilize the gold is determined by adding 1 mL of the colloidal gold to 0.1 mL of serial aqueous dilutions of the protein. The order of addition of gold to the protein is critical. After 10 min, add 0.1 mL of 10% NaCl to each tube. If there is not enough protein to stabilize the gold, the solution will change from red to blue. For gold sols prepared with tannic acid, it may be necessary to add 0.1% H_2O_2 to the preparations in order to visualize the color change. If the color change cannot be assessed visually, it can be assessed spectrophotometrically (maximum absorbance of 510–550 nm).
2. If you wish to make larger quantities of gold, prepare multiple 10-mL aliquots rather then one large batch.
3. To measure the pH, remove 5 mL aliquots from the stock of colloidal gold, and add two drops of 1% polyethylene glycol. Do not add the PEG to the colloidal gold stock. Discard aliquots after reading pH.
4. IgG conjugated colloidal gold is less stable than Protein A or Protein G gold. A recent study suggests that IgY from chickens may produce a more stable colloidal gold conjugate than IgG (9).
5. If the amount of antibody is limited, the isotherm may be run using 100 µL of colloidal gold and 10 µL each of antibody and NaCl.

6. Prepare the glycerol step gradients by layering 1 mL each 60%, 40%, and 20% glycerol in TBS containing 1% cold-water fish gelatin over a cushion of 0.5 mL 100% glycerol. Keep the gradients on ice once they are made. Layer the colloidal gold over the gradients, and centrifuge at 4°C for 1 h in a swinging bucket rotor at $r_{av} = 200{,}000 \times g$.

References

1. Leunissen JLM, DeMey JR (1989) Preparation of gold probes. In: Verkleij AJ, Leunissen JLM (eds) Immuno-gold Labeling in Cell Biology. CRC, Boca Raton, FL, pp 3–16
2. Bendayan M (1984) Protein A-gold electron microscopic immunocytochemistry: methods, applications, and limitations. J Electron Micros Technol 1:243–270
3. Bendayan M (1989) Protein A-gold and protein G-gold postembedding immunoelectron microscopy. In: Hayat MA (ed) Colloidal Gold, vol. 1. Academic Press, New York, NY, pp 34–96
4. Horisberger M (1981) Colloidal gold: a cytochemical marker for light and fluorescent microscopy and for transmission and scanning electron microscopy. In: Johari O (ed) Scanning Electron Microscopy II. SEM, Inc., AMF O'Hare, Chicago, IL, pp 9–31
5. Horisberger M (1989) Quantitative aspects of labeling colloidal gold with proteins. In: Verkleij AJ, Leunissen JLM (eds) Immuno-gold Labeling in Cell Biology. CRC, Boca Raton, FL, pp 49–60
6. Geoghegan WD, Ackerman GA (1977) Adsorption of horseradish peroxidase, ovomucoid and anti-immunoglobulin to colloidal gold for the indirect detection of concanavalin A, wheat germ agglutinin and goat anti-human immunoglobulin G on cell surfaces at the electron microscopic level: a new method, theory and application. J Histochem Cytochem 25:1187–1200
7. Roth J (1983) The colloidal gold marker system for light and electron microscopic cytochemistry. In: Bullock GR, Petrusz P (eds) Techniques in Immunocytochemistry, vol. 2. Academic Press, New York, NY, pp 217–284
8. Birrell GB, Hedberg KK, Griffith PH (1987) Pitfalls of immunogold labeling: analysis by light microscopy, transmission electron microscopy, and photoelectron microscopy. J Histochem Cytochem 35:843–853
9. Gasparyan VK (2005) Hen egg immunoglobulin Y in colloidal gold agglutination assay: Comparison with rabbit immunoglobulin G. J Clin Lab Anal 19:124–127

Chapter 40

Colloidal Gold/Streptavidin Methods

Constance Oliver

Abstract

Biotin–avidin detection systems are widely used in both immunocytochemistry and molecular biology. They take advantage of the high affinity of biotin, a low-molecular-weight vitamin, for avidin, an egg-white protein. Because of the problem of nonspecific binding of avidin, streptavidin has largely replaced avidin for immunocytochemical procedures. Streptavidin/colloidal gold-biotin detection systems for electron microscopy are most commonly used in postembedding immunocytochemistry. Usually, the primary antibody is unlabeled, the secondary antibody is biotinylated, and the colloidal gold is conjugated to streptavidin. In certain applications, the primary antibody may be biotinylated and no bridging antibody is needed. This chapter details the use of streptavidin-gold for postembedding labeling.

Key words: Colloidal gold, Avidin, Streptavidin, Biotin, Electron microscopy, Postembedding labeling

1. Introduction

Biotin–avidin detection systems are widely used in both immunocytochemistry and molecular biology (1, 2) (*see* Chapters 7, 26, and 27). They take advantage of the high affinity of biotin, a low-molecular-weight vitamin, for avidin, an egg-white protein. The avidin–biotin complex has one of the highest dissociation constants known, 10^{-15} M. This high dissociation constant has made it a convenient system for linking indicators to antibodies. However, egg-white avidin binds nonspecifically to many tissue sites. This nonspecific binding has been attributed both to its high isoelectric point (pI = 10) and to the fact that the protein is glycosylated (3, 4). Because of the problem of nonspecific binding of avidin, streptavidin has largely replaced avidin for immunocytochemical procedures. Streptavidin, produced by Streptomyces avidinni, has properties that are very similar to avidin, but it is not glycosylated (5). Streptavidin generally gives little or no

C. Oliver and M.C. Jamur (eds.), *Immunocytochemical Methods and Protocols*, Methods in Molecular Biology, Vol. 588, DOI 10.1007/978-1-59745-324-0_40, © Humana Press, a part of Springer Science+Business Media, LLC 1995, 1999, 2010

background staining, and is superior to avidin for immunocytochemical uses.

Streptavidin/colloidal gold-biotin detection systems for electron microscopy are most commonly used in postembedding immunocytochemistry. A bridging technique is generally used. In this method, the primary antibody is unlabeled, the secondary antibody is biotinylated, and the colloidal gold is conjugated to streptavidin. In certain applications, the primary antibody may be biotinylated and no bridging antibody is needed. It is also possible to use streptavidin–biotin complexes during detection. These complexes contain multiple gold particles and can enhance a weak signal.

High-quality reagents needed for biotin–avidin immunostaining are all available commercially. Kits are also available commercially for biotinylating antibodies (*see* Chapter 7). The major consideration in biotinylating antibodies is the use of biotin with a carbon spacer arm at least 1 nm long, since the binding site of biotin on avidin and probably streptavidin is in a deep depression (4).

2. Materials

1. Dulbecco's phosphate-buffered saline (PBS): 100 mg anhydrous calcium chloride, 200 mg potassium chloride, 200 mg monobasic potassium phosphate, 100 mg magnesium chloride · $6H_2O$; 8 g sodium chloride, and 2.16 g dibasic sodium phosphate · $7H_2O$; bring volume to 1 L with deionized glass-distilled water, pH 7.4.
2. Fixative: 2% EM-grade formaldehyde in PBS and 0.5% EM-grade glutaraldehyde in PBS.
3. 0.1 M Cacodylate buffer: 21.4 g cacodylic acid, sodium salt · $3H_2O$; bring volume to 1 L with deionized glass-distilled water; adjust pH to 7.4 with HCl.
4. 0.1 M Glycine: 750 mg glycine; bring volume to 100 mL with PBS, pH 7.4.
5. Osmium tetroxide (4% stock): 1 g glass vial osmium tetroxide, and 25 mL deionized glass-distilled water (*see* Note 1).
6. Nickel grids: Clean in acetone or alcohol before use.
7. Saturated solution of sodium *meta*-periodate prepared daily in deionized glass-distilled water.
8. Tris-buffered saline (TBS): 2.4 g Tris–HCl and 8.76 g NaCl; bring volume to 1 L with deionized glass-distilled water, pH 7.4.
9. High-salt Tween-20 buffer: 2.4 g Tris–HCl, 29.2 g sodium chloride, and 1 mL Tween-20; bring volume to 1 L with deionized glass-distilled water, pH 7.4.

10. 1% Bovine serum albumin (BSA): 1 g BSA and 100 mL TBS or high-salt Tween-20 buffer; add BSA to buffer with stirring.
11. Dulbecco's PBS without calcium and magnesium: 200 mg potassium chloride, 200 mg monobasic potassium phosphate, 8 g sodium chloride, and 2.16 g dibasic sodium phosphate · $7H_2O$; bring volume to 1 L with deionized glass-distilled water, pH 7.4.
12. Primary antibody diluted in PBS without calcium and magnesium, and 1% BSA or TBS with 1% BSA (*see* Note 2).
13. Biotinylated secondary antibody (*see* Chapter 7) diluted in PBS without calcium or magnesium with 1% BSA or TBS with 1% BSA.
14. Colloidal gold conjugated with streptavidin (*see* Note 3).
15. 0.1 M Maleate buffer: 1.16 g maleic acid and 3.5 g sucrose; add deionized glass-distilled water to make 100 mL, and adjust to pH 6.5.
16. 2% Uranyl acetate: 2 g uranyl acetate and 100 mL maleate buffer; add uranyl acetate to the buffer, and adjust to pH 6.0.
17. Reynolds' lead citrate (6): 1.33 g lead nitrate, 1.76 g trisodium citrate · $2H_2O$; 30 mL deionized glass-distilled water, and 8.0 mL 1 N NaOH (*see* Note 4).
18. 0.05 M Borate buffer: 1.9 g sodium borate · $10H_2O$; bring volume to 100 mL with deionized glass-distilled water, pH 8.6.

3. Method

3.1. Postembedding Labeling with Streptavidin-Gold

1. Rinse the samples twice in PBS, and fix for 30 min to 1 h at room temperature in 0.5% glutaraldehyde and 2% formaldehyde in PBS (*see* Note 5).
2. Following fixation, rinse the samples three to five times over a period of 30 min in PBS (*see* Note 6).
3. Rinse the samples for 5 min in 0.1 M glycine in PBS to quench the free aldehyde groups (*see* Note 7).
4. Then, rinse the samples in buffer, and postfix in 1–2% osmium tetroxide for 1 h at room temperature (*see* Note 8).
5. Dehydrate the samples, and embed (*see* Note 9).
6. Cut the resulting blocks with a diamond knife, and mount sections on nickel grids (*see* Note 10).
7. Etch the plastic in the sections slightly in order to allow for penetration of reagents into the samples. Float the grids section

side down on drops of a freshly prepared saturated solution of sodium *meta*-periodate (*see* Note 11).

8. Rinse the grids three to five times in deionized glass-distilled water.
9. Block nonspecific binding by incubating the sections in 1% BSA or normal serum in PBS without calcium and magnesium, or in TBS for 15 min.
10. Rinse the grids five times in PBS without calcium and magnesium or in TBS.
11. Incubate for 1–2 h at room temperature in primary antibody diluted in PBS without calcium and magnesium containing 1% BSA or in TBS containing 1% BSA.
12. Rinse as in step 10.
13. Incubate the grids in biotinylated secondary antibody diluted in PBS without calcium and magnesium containing 1% BSA or in TBS plus 1% BSA for 30 min at room temperature.
14. Rinse as in step 10.
15. Incubate grids for 30 min at room temperature in colloidal gold conjugated with streptavidin.
16. Rinse as in step 10.
17. Rinse the grids in a stream of deionized glass-distilled water from a squirt bottle and dry.
18. At this point, the grids may be examined in the electron microscope to evaluate the staining.
19. Stain the grids with uranyl acetate for 5–10 min, rinse in water, and stain with lead citrate for 1–2 min. They are now ready for final examination in the electron microscope (*see* Note 12).

4. Notes

1. Clean the vial, and score it with a diamond scribe. Place it in a clean glass bottle, and add the water. With a glass rod, break vial. The solution is stable if kept refrigerated and protected from light. The stock solution should be stored away from other chemicals since osmium vapors may escape from the bottle. Alternatively, aqueous solutions of osmium tetroxide in sealed glass ampules are available commercially. Dilute to 1–2% with cacodylate buffer for use.
2. The concentration of the primary antibody can range from 1–20 μg/mL with 5 μg/mL being average. If background staining is high, the antibody may be diluted in high-salt Tween-20 buffer.

3. The colloidal gold should be diluted in PBS without calcium and magnesium containing 1% BSA or 0.01% polyethylene glycol (mol. wt. 20,000), or in TBS plus 1% BSA or 0.01% polyethylene glycol (mol. wt. 20,000).
4. Add the lead nitrate and sodium citrate to the water in a 50 mL volumetric flask. Shake vigorously for 1 min, and allow to stand with intermittent shaking for 30 min. Add 8.0 mL 1 N NaOH. Dilute the suspension to 50 mL with deionized glass-distilled water, and mix by inversion. The solution is stable up to 6 months. Turbidity can be removed by centrifugation.
5. The composition of the fixative may vary depending on the sensitivity of the antigen. For some antigens, it may be necessary to reduce the glutaraldehyde concentration or omit it entirely, and fix in 4% formaldehyde in PBS for 1–4 h.
6. 0.1 M Phosphate or cacodylate buffer, pH 7.4, may be substituted for PBS.
7. The amino group on the glycine will bind to any free aldehyde groups left on the cells after fixation and prevent them from binding to the antibody or blocking solution, thus reducing the nonspecific background.
8. If embedding in a resin that is polymerized by UV light, such as Lowicryl and LR Gold, do not osmicate the samples. Any effect of the osmium on antigenicity can usually be eliminated by using sodium *meta*-periodate during etching to oxidize the unbound osmium (*see* Subheading 3.1, step 7).
9. The choice of embedding resin can affect the degree of immunostaining. Although all embedding resins may be used, the epoxy resins, such as Epon substitutes and Spurr, may reduce the intensity of staining. The acrylic resins (LR White, LR Gold, and Lowicryl) are more hydrophilic and usually result in better immunolabeling (see Chapter 37).
10. It is often advisable to cut the sections slightly thicker than normal (light gold). The sections will adhere to the grids better during the staining process if, after the sections are picked up, the grids are placed in a 50°C oven for an hour. The nickel grids can become magnetized and should be handled with nonmagnetic forceps. They may also need to be degaussed before viewing in the electron microscope, and the astigmatism may need to be adjusted for each grid.
11. If the primary antibody is directed against a carbohydrate-containing epitope, keep the exposure to the *meta*-periodate as brief as possible, since the *meta*-periodate may remove the carbohydrate. If this is a problem, it may be necessary to etch in hydrogen peroxide or sodium ethoxide. The incubation can be done in Petri dishes lined with parafilm or in spot plates. The time required for etching depends on the embedding resin,

and can vary from 30 min for Epon substitutes to <5 min for LR White and LR Gold. From this step until the staining is completed, the grids should not be allowed to dry.

12. If the nonspecific background is high, it may be because of the streptavidin binding to endogenous biotin. In that instance, it is necessary to block the endogenous biotin with streptavidin. After etching, grids are floated on drops of unconjugated streptavidin (5 μg/mL) in TBS for 15 min. Rinse five times in TBS. The streptavidin must then be reacted with unconjugated biotin, or it will react with the biotinylated antibody. Float grids on biotin (5 μg/mL) in TBS for 15 min. Rinse five times in TBS. At this point, the sections may be blocked again with BSA or incubated with the primary antibody.

References

1. Bonnard C, Papermaster DS, Kraehenbuhl J-P (1984) The streptavidin–biotin bridge technique: application in light and electron microscope immunocytochemistry. In: Polak JM, Varndell IM (eds) Immunolabelling for Electron Microscopy. Elsevier, New York, NY, pp 95–111
2. Larsson L-I (1988) Immunocytochemical detection systems. In: Larsson L-I (ed) Immunocytochemistry: Theory and Practice. CRC, Boca Raton, FL, pp 77–146
3. Wooley DW, Longsworth LG (1942) Isolation of an antibiotin factor from egg white. J. Biol. Chem. 142:285–290
4. Green NM (1975) Avidin. Adv. Prot. Res. 29:85–133
5. Chaiet L, Wolf FJ (1964) The properties of streptavidin, a biotin-binding protein produced by Streptomycetes. Arch. Biochem. Biophys. 106:1–5
6. Reynolds ES (1963) The use of lead citrate at high pH as an electron opaque stain in electron microscopy. J. Cell Biol. 17:208–212

Chapter 41

Pre-embedding Labeling Methods

Constance Oliver

Abstract

Colloidal gold conjugates generally do not readily penetrate cells, even after permeabilization. Therefore, their use in pre-embedding immunostaining has been largely restricted to labeling cell-surface antigens for scanning or transmission electron microscopy or for tracing endocytic pathways in living cells. One nanometer gold conjugates that do penetrate cells and tissues much more readily have also been used successfully to immunolabel intracellular structures. For pre-embedding labeling, all of the immunostaining is done prior to embedding the tissue in resin or preparing the samples for scanning electron microscopy. This chapter provides methods for pre-embedding staining with unconjugated primary antibody or with primary antibody conjugated to colloidal gold. The use of colloidal gold for tracing endocytic pathways is also given.

Key words: Colloidal gold, Pre-embedding labeling, Electron microscopy, Endocytic pathways, Immunostaining

1. Introduction

Colloidal gold conjugates generally do not readily penetrate cells, even after permeabilization. Therefore, their use in pre-embedding immunostaining has been restricted to labeling cell-surface antigens for scanning (1) or transmission electron microscopy (Fig. 1a) or for tracing endocytic pathways in living cells (2) (Fig. 1b). One nanometer gold conjugates that do penetrate cells and tissues much more readily have also been used successfully to immunolabel intracellular structures (3, 4). A variety of 1 nm gold conjugates are now commercially available (*see* Note 1). For pre-embedding labeling, all of the immunostaining is done prior to embedding the tissue in resin or preparing the samples for scanning electron microscopy. This method is especially useful if the antigen to be detected is sensitive to fixation. The immunostaining may be done on unfixed or lightly (4% formaldehyde)

C. Oliver and M.C. Jamur (eds.), *Immunocytochemical Methods and Protocols*, Methods in Molecular Biology, Vol. 588, DOI 10.1007/978-1-59745-324-0_41, © Humana Press, a part of Springer Science+Business Media, LLC 1995, 1999, 2010

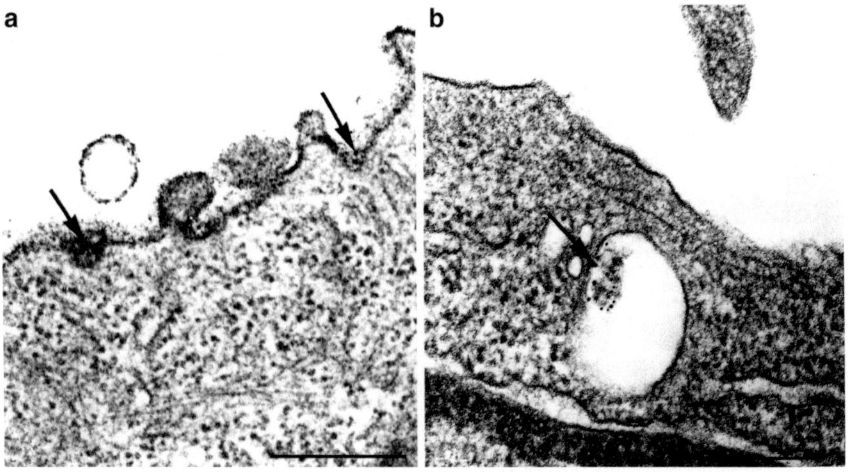

Fig. 1. Transmission electron micrograph of RBL-2H3 cells with colloidal gold conjugated to a monoclonal antibody against the IgE receptor. (**a**) Gold conjugate is localized primarily in coated pits. (**b**) Five minutes after exposing cells to antibody-coated gold, gold particles are localized in early endosomes. Bar = 0.5 μm.

fixed samples. Following the immunolabeling, the samples may then be refixed in 2% glutaraldehyde–2% formaldehyde to improve ultrastructural preservation.

When immunolabeling cell-surface components, it is important to be aware that redistribution of membrane components may be induced by the immunolabeling. Crosslinking of membrane components in unfixed or lightly fixed cells by antibodies may result in aggregation, capping, or intemalization of the molecule of interest. Usually, brief fixation in a fixative containing low concentrations of glutaraldehyde is sufficient to prevent redistribution. Fixation in formaldehyde alone or performing the immunostaining at 4°C may not be sufficient to prevent lateral diffusion of molecules in the plasma membrane.

2. Materials

1. Dulbecco's phosphate-buffered saline (PBS): 100 mg anhydrous calcium chloride, 200 mg potassium chloride, 200 mg monobasic potassium phosphate, 100 mg magnesium chloride. $6H_2O$; 8 g sodium chloride, and 2.16 g dibasic sodium phosphate. $7H_2O$; bring volume to 1 L with deionized glass-distilled water, pH 7.4.
2. 0.5% Glutaraldehyde–2% formaldehyde fixative: 0.5 mL 70% EM-grade glutaraldehyde, 7 mL 20% EM-grade formaldehyde, 3 mg calcium chloride, and 62.5 mL 0.1 M cacodylate buffer or PBS, pH 7.4 (*see* Note 2).
3. 0.1 M Glycine: 75 mg glycine, bring the volume to 100 mL with PBS.

4. Dulbecco's PBS without calcium and magnesium: 200 mg potassium chloride, 200 mg monobasic potassium phosphate, 8 g sodium chloride, and 2.16 g dibasic sodium phosphate. $7H_2O$; bring volume to 1 L with deionized glass-distilled water, pH 7.4.
5. 1% Bovine serum albumin (BSA): 1 g BSA and 100 mL PBS without calcium and magnesium; add BSA to PBS with stirring. Make fresh daily or aliquote and store at −20°C. Centrifuge if a precipatate appears after freezing.
6. Primary antibody (*see* Note 3).
7. Colloidal gold conjugate (*see* Note 4).
8. 0.1 M Cacodylate buffer: 21.4 g cacodylic acid $3H_2O$, sodium salt; bring volume to 1 L with deionized glass-distilled water; adjust pH to 7.4 with HCl.

3. Methods

3.1. Cell-Surface Labeling

3.1.1. Unlabeled Primary Antibody

1. Rinse cells twice in PBS, and fix for 30 min to 1 h at room temperature in 0.5% glutaraldehyde and 2% formaldehyde in PBS (*see* Note 5).
2. Following fixation, rinse the cells 3 to 5 times over a period of 30 min in PBS (*see* Note 6).
3. Rinse the cells for 5 min in 0.1 M glycine in PBS to quench free aldehyde groups (*see* Note 7).
4. Rinse the cells for 15 min in a solution of 1% BSA in PBS without calcium and magnesium to block nonspecific binding of the primary antibody (*see* Note 8).
5. Expose the cells to the primary antibody. Incubation times usually range from 1–2 h at room temperature.
6. Rinse cells five times in PBS without calcium and magnesium over a period of 30 min to remove unbound primary antibody (*see* Note 9).
7. Incubate the cells in colloidal gold conjugate for 30 min at room temperature (*see* Note 4).
8. Rinse cells in PBS without calcium and magnesium five times over a period of 30 min.
9. For better morphological preservation, refix the cells in 2% glutaraldehyde–2% formaldehyde in 0.1 M cacodylate buffer, pH 7.4 for 1 h at room temperature.
10. Rinse in cacodylate buffer, postfix in 1–2% osmium tetroxide, and embed as usual (*see* Note 10 and Chapter 37).

3.1.2. Primary Antibody Conjugated to Colloidal Gold

1. Perform steps 1–4 as outlined in Subheading 3.1.1.
2. Incubate the cells in primary antibody conjugated to colloidal gold diluted in PBS without calcium and magnesium containing 1% BSA for 1 h at room temperature (*see* Note 3).
3. Continue with step 8 in Subheading 3.1.1.

3.1.3. Tracing Endocytic Pathways

1. Rinse cells in sterile medium containing 1–2% BSA.
2. Add ligand conjugated to the colloidal gold, i.e., colloidal gold conjugated with antibody to a specific receptor.
3. Allow to bind at 4°C for 30–60 min, or return to incubator immediately.
4. At various time intervals, stop endocytosis with cold (4°C) PBS or balanced salt solution.
5. Rinse twice in cold PBS.
6. Fix and embed as usual (*see* Note 10 and Chapter 37).

4. Notes

1. Nanoprobes (www.nanobrobes.com) supplies 1 nm gold particles conjugated to a wide variety of compounds including antibodies, fluorochromes and lipids. Conjugates are available that may be applied not only to electron microscopy, but also light microscopy, and fluorescence microscopy.
2. The purity of the reagents is critical. Always use the highest quality available, i.e., affinity-purified antibodies, EM-grade glutaraldehyde, distilled formaldehyde, or freshly prepared paraformaldehyde. The use of distilled formaldehyde, not formalin which contains alcohol, is recommended. Freshly prepared paraformaldehyde can also be used, especially if large volumes of fixative are needed. To prepare an 8% solution of paraformaldehyde, in a fume hood add 2 g of paraformaldehyde (trioxymethylene) powder to 25 mL of double distilled water. With constant stirring, heat solution to 60–70°C. Once the solution has reached the proper temperature, continue to stir for 15 min. The solution will be milky. Add one to two drops of 1 N NaOH, with stirring, until the solution clears. A slight milkiness may persist. Cool and filter through Whatman no. 1 filter paper. This solution should be used the same day that it is prepared.
3. Primary antibody is usually at a concentration of 1–5 μg/mL, in PBS without calcium and magnesium, containing 1% BSA.

4. The colloidal gold conjugate should be an IgG directed against IgGs of the same species as the primary antibody, i.e., if your primary antibody was produced in rabbits, your secondary antibody should be an anti-rabbit IgG. The secondary antibody may be from any species other than that of the primary antibody. In the above example, the secondary antibody could be donkey, goat, sheep, mouse, etc. anti-rabbit IgG. The secondary antibody may diluted to 1–5 μg/mL in PBS without calcium and magnesium plus 1% BSA.
5. The composition of the fixative may vary depending on the sensitivity of the antigen. For some antigens, it may be necessary to omit the glutaraldehyde entirely and fix in 4% formaldehyde in PBS for 1–4 h (*see* Chapter 37).
6. 0.1 M Phosphate buffer, pH 7.4, may be substituted for PBS.
7. Following fixation in formaldehyde or glutaraldehyde, tissue is generally quenched. The purpose of this step is to block any free aldehyde groups that remain after fixation and washing. This step is especially critical after glutaraldehyde fixation. Glutaraldehyde is a bifunctional aldehyde. During fixation, one end may bind to cellular constituents, leaving the other end free to react. If this end is not blocked, it can bind to the protein in the blocking solution or to the primary antibody, increasing the nonspecific background. Although any small molecular-weight compound containing an amino group may be used, the most commonly used quenching agents are glycine, ammonium chloride, and sodium borohydride.
8. Following queching, the samples are blocked to reduce nonspecific binding of the primary antibody and to reduce the background. The proteins in the blocking solution are chosen so as not to react with the secondary antibody or the detection system. They bind to sites in the samples that bind proteins through nonspecific interactions, such as charge. Although 2–10% BSA is most commonly used, other proteins, such as ova albumin, normal serum, or IgG fractions, can also be used. The exact composition of the blocking solution may have to be determined empirically if background staining is high.
9. If the nonspecific staining is high, 0.1 M EDTA can also be added to the rinse solutions.
10. Appropriate controls should always be run with any immunocytochemical procedure. Controls may include omitting the primary antibody, substituting preimmune serum, normal serum, or normal IgG for the primary antibody, adsorbing the primary antibody against the antigen, or immunostaining with an unrelated antibody.

References

1. Becker RP, Johari O (eds) (1979) Cell Surface Labeling. SEM, Inc., AMF O'Hare, Chicago, IL
2. Oliver C, Fujimura A, Silveirae Souza AM, Orlandini de Castro R, Siraganian RP, Jamur MC (2007) Mast cell-specific gangliosides and FcepsilonRI follow the same endocytic pathway from lipid rafts in RBL-2H3 cells. J Histochem Cytochem 55:315–325
3. Vandre DD, Burry RW (1992) Immunoelectron microscopic localization of phosphoproteins associated with the mitotic spindle. J Histochem Cytochem 40:1837–1847
4. Burry RW, Vandre DD, Hayes DM (1992) Silver enhancement of gold antibody probes in pre-embedding electron microscopic immunocytochemistry. J Histochem Cytochem 40: 1849–1856

Chapter 42

Postembedding Labeling Methods

Constance Oliver

Abstract

Since it was first introduced, postembedding immunogold labeling has become the most widely used method of immunolabeling for electron microscopy. For postembedding labeling, samples are first fixed, embedded, and sectioned. All immunostaining is performed on sections mounted on grids. The immunostaining may be done with a direct labeling technique with the primary antibody conjugated to colloidal gold, or by an indirect method where the primary antibody is unlabeled and the gold is conjugated to a secondary or tertiary antibody, protein A, protein G, etc. Colloidal gold-antibody conjugates are also widely used, especially in indirect immunocytochemical methods. This chapter gives the standard method for post embedding labeling as well as one in which the cell membranes are enhanced.

Key words: Colloidal gold, Postembedding, Membrane enhancement, Antibody conjugates, Protein A, Protein G

1. Introduction

Since it was first introduced (1), postembedding immunogold labeling has become the most widely used method of immunolabeling for electron microscopy (2–8). For postembedding labeling, samples are first fixed, embedded, and sectioned. All immunostaining is performed on sections mounted on grids. The immunostaining may be done with a direct labeling technique with the primary antibody conjugated to colloidal gold, or by an indirect method where the primary antibody is unlabeled and the gold is conjugated to a secondary or tertiary antibody, protein A, protein G, etc. Colloidal gold has several advantages as a marker for electron microscopy. The gold particles are distinct and readily visualized, they are easily quantifiable, and they do not diffuse on the sections. The most popular reagents for postembedding colloidal gold immunocytochemistry are the protein A and pro-

C. Oliver and M.C. Jamur (eds.), *Immunocytochemical Methods and Protocols*, Methods in Molecular Biology, Vol. 588, DOI 10.1007/978-1-59745-324-0_42, © Humana Press, a part of Springer Science+Business Media, LLC 1995, 1999, 2010

tein G conjugates. Protein A, a cell-wall component of *Staphylococcus aureus*, has a high affinity toward the Fc region of IgG molecules from a number of species, including rabbit and human (9). However, protein A has a low affinity for most classes of mouse IgG molecules. Protein G, an immunoglobulin-binding molecule present in the cell wall of the group G *Streptococcal* strain (G 148), has a high affinity for immunoglobulins from a wider range of species, including mouse (10). Thus, protein G has been used with mouse monoclonal antibodies. Colloidal gold-antibody conjugates are also widely used, especially in indirect immunocytochemical methods. However, the stability of these gold conjugates is less than that for protein A, and depending on the antibody, the affinity may be less. However, a recent study suggests that IgY from chickens may produce a more stable colloidal gold conjugate than IgG (11). Colloidal gold conjugated to avidin (*see* Chapter 40), lectins (12), and enzymes (13), has also been used for postembedding staining.

2. Materials

1. Dulbecco's phosphate-buffered saline (PBS): 100 mg anhydrous calcium chloride, 200 mg potassium chloride, 200 mg monobasic potassium phosphate, 100 mg magnesium chloride·6 H_2O, 8 g sodium chloride, and 2.16 g dibasic sodium phosphate·7 H_2O; bring volume to 1 L with deionized glass-distilled water, pH 7.4.
2. 0.5% Glutaraldehyde–2% formaldehyde fixative: 0.5 mL 70% EM-grade glutaraldehyde, 7 mL 20% EM-grade formaldehyde, 3 mg calcium chloride, and 61 mL 0.1 M cacodylate buffer or PBS, pH 7.4 (*see* Note 1).
3. 0.1 M Glycine: 750 mg glycine; bring volume to 100 mL with PBS, pH 7.4.
4. Osmium tetroxide (4% stock): 1 g glass vial osmium tetroxide and 25 mL deionized glass-distilled water (*see* Note 2).
5. Embedding medium, e.g., LR Gold and initiator (*see* Chapter 37).
6. Nickel grids: Clean in acetone or alcohol just prior to use.
7. Saturated aqueous solution of sodium *meta*-periodate; prepare daily.
8. Tris-buffered saline (TBS): 2.4 g Tris–HCl and 8.76 g NaCl; bring volume to 1 L with deionized glass-distilled water, pH 7.4.
9. 1% Bovine serum albumin (BSA): 1 g BSA and 100 mL TBS (*see* Note 3).

10. High-salt Tween-20 buffer: 2.4 g Tris–HCl, 29.2 g sodium chloride and 1 mL Tween-20; bring volume to 1 L with deionized glass-distilled water, pH 7.4.
11. Dulbecco's PBS without calcium and magnesium: 200 mg potassium chloride, 200 mg monobasic potassium phosphate, 8 g sodium chloride, and 2.16 g dibasic sodium phosphate·7 H_2O; bring volume to 1 L with deionized glass-distilled water, pH 7.4.
12. Primary antibody (*see* Note 4).
13. Secondary antibody (*see* Note 5).
14. Colloidal gold conjugate (*see* Note 6).
15. 0.1 M Cacodylate buffer: 21.4 g cacodylic acid·3 H_2O, sodium salt; bring volume to 1 L with deionized glass-distilled water; adjust pH to 7.4 with HCI.
16. Saturated picric acid solution: Fill 500 g bottle of picric acid with deionized glassdistilled water (*see* Note 7).
17. Membrane enhancement fixative: 1 mL 70% glutaraldehyde, 14 mL 20% formaldehyde, 3 mg calcium chloride, 150 μL saturated picric acid, and 55 mL 0.1 M cacodylate buffer, pH 7.4.
18. Acetone.
19. Polyethylene embedding capsules or gelatin capsules.
20. UV light source, e.g., 366 nm, two 15-W Sylvania FI5t8/BLB bulbs.
21. 0.1 M Maleate buffer: 1.16 g maleic acid and 3.5 g sucrose; add deionized glass distilled water to make 100 mL; adjust pH to 6.5.
22. 2% Uranyl acetate: 2 g uranyl acetate and 100 mL maleate buffer; add uranyl acetate to buffer; adjust pH to 6.0.
23. Reynolds' lead citrate (14): 1.33 g lead nitrate, 1.76 g trisodium citrate·2 H_2O, 30 mL deionized glass-distilled water, and 8.0 mL 1 N NaOH (*see* Note 8).

3. Methods

3.1. Standard Method

1. Rinse samples twice in PBS, and fix for 30 min to 1 h at room temperature in 0.5% glutaraldehyde and 2% formaldehyde in PBS (*see* Note 9).
2. Following fixation, rinse the samples 3–5 times over a period of 30 min in PBS (*see* Note 10).
3. Quench free aldehyde groups by rinsing the samples for 5 min in 0.1 M glycine in PBS (*see* Note 11).

4. Rinse the samples in cacodylate buffer or PBS, and postfix in 1–2% osmium tetroxide for 1 h at room temperature (*see* Note 12).
5. Following postfixation, dehydrate the samples and embed (*see* Note 13).
6. Cut the resulting blocks with a diamond knife, and mount sections on nickel grids. It is often advisable to cut the sections slightly thicker than normal such that the interference color of the sections is light gold (*see* Note 14).
7. Etch the plastic in the sections slightly in order to allow for penetration of reagents into the samples (*see* Note 15).
8. Rinse 3–5 times in deionized glass-distilled water.
9. Block nonspecific binding by incubating sections in 1% BSA or 5% normal serum in PBS without calcium and magnesium, or in TBS for 15 min (*see* Note 16)
10. Rinse five times in PBS without calcium and magnesium, or in TBS.
11. Incubate the sections for 1–2 h at room temperature in primary antibody diluted in PBS without calcium and magnesium containing 1% BSA or in TBS containing 1% BSA (*see* Note 4).
12. Rinse as in step 10.
13. If an unlabeled secondary antibody is necessary as a bridging antibody, incubate the grids in the secondary antibody diluted in PBS without calcium and magnesium containing 1% BSA or in TBS plus 1% BSA for 30 min at room temperature, and then rinse as in step 10 (*see* Note 5).
14. Incubate grids for 30 min at room temperature in colloidal gold conjugated with protein A, protein G, immunoglobulin, or if a biotinylated secondary antibody was used, streptavidin (*see* Note 6).
15. Rinse as in step 10.
16. Rinse the grids in a stream of deionized glass-distilled water from a squirt bottle and dry.
17. At this point, the grids may be examined in the electron microscope to evaluate the staining.
18. Stain the grids with uranyl acetate and lead citrate for final examination in the electron microscope (*see* Notes 16 and 17).

3.2. Membrane Enhancement Method (15)

1. Fix samples in membrane enhancement fixative (see 2. Materials 17.) for 2–3 h at room temperature.
2. Rinse tissue five times with cold (4°C) PBS or cacodylate buffer over a period of 1–2 h (*see* Note 18).

3. Rinse samples with 0.1 M glycine in phosphate or cacodylate buffer for 1 h at 4°C to quench free aldehyde groups.
4. If phosphate buffer has been used, rinse tissue five times over a period of 1 h in 0.1 M maleate buffer containing 3.5% sucrose, pH 6.5, to remove phosphate ions.
5. Stain the tissue *en bloc* with 2% uranyl acetate in maleate-sucrose buffer, pH 6.0, for 2 h at 4°C in the dark.
6. Dehydrate the tissue and infiltrate with resin according to the following schedule:

   50% Acetone, 5 min, 0°C.

   50% Acetone, 45 min, 0°C.

   70% Acetone, 45 min, 0°C.

   90% Acetone, 45 min, 0°C.

   1:1 LR Gold:acetone, 60 min, –20°C.

   7:3 LR Gold:acetone, 60 min, –20°C.

   100% LR Gold, 60 min, –20°C.

   100% LR Gold, 5 h to overnight, –20°C.

   100% LR Gold + initiator (0.5% benzoin methyl ether), 60 min, –20°C.

   100% LR Gold + initiator, 60 min, –20°C.

   100% LR Gold + initiator, 5 h to overnight, –20°C (*see* Note 19).
7. Transfer tissue to polyethylene embedding capsules or gelatin capsules, till the capsules 100% LR Gold + initiator and cap (*see* Note 20).
8. Polymerize the plastic with UV light placed 10 cm from the capsules. Expose the capsules to the UV light for 24 h at –20°C (*see* Note 21).
9. Cut gold sections with a diamond knife, and mount on nickel grids. To increase the adherence of the sections to the grids, after sectioning, the grids may be placed in a 60°C oven for 1 h.
10. Hydrate sections for 5 min in TBS (*see* Note 22).
11. Rinse in distilled water.
12. Block sections with 1% BSA or 5% normal goat serum in TBS.
13. Incubate grids for 60 min with primary antibody diluted with TBS containing 1% BSA or 5% normal goat serum (*see* Note 4).
14. Rinse grids five times in TBS.
15. If a secondary antibody is necessary as a bridging antibody, incubate the grids in the secondary antibody diluted in TBS plus 1% BSA for 30 min at room temperature and then rinse five times in TBS.

16. Incubate grids for 30 min at room temperature in colloidal gold conjugated with protein A, protein G, immunoglobulin, or if a biotinylated secondary antibody was used, streptavidin (*see* Note 6).
17. Rinse grids five times in TBS.
18. Rinse in deionized glass-distilled water.
19. Fix with 2% aqueous glutaraldehyde for 5 min.
20. Rinse grids three times in deionized glass-distilled water.
21. In order to enhance membrane contrast, stain for 15 min in 2% aqueous osmium tetroxide.
22. Rinse five times in deionized glass-distilled water.
23. Stain in Reynolds' (13) lead citrate for 1–2 min.
24. Rinse grids five times in deionized glass-distilled water and in a stream of deionized glass-distilled water from a squirt bottle.
25. Dry grids by placing on fine filter paper, i.e., Whatman no. 50.
26. Examine with the electron microscope (*see* Notes 17 and 18).

4. Notes

1. The use of distilled formaldehyde, not formalin, which contains alcohol, is recommended. Freshly prepared paraformaldehyde can also be used, especially if large volumes of fixative are needed. To prepare an 8% solution of paraformaldehyde, ***in a fume hood***, add 2 g of paraformaldehyde (trioxymethylene) powder to 25 mL of double-distilled water. With constant stirring, heat solution to 55–60°C. Once the solution has reached the proper temperature, continue to stir for 15 min. The solution will be milky. Add one to two drops of 1 N NaOH, with stirring, until the solution clears. A slight milkiness may persist. Cool and filter through Whatman no. 1 filter paper. This solution should be used the same day that it is prepared.
2. Clean the vial, and score with a diamond scribe. Place in a clean glass bottle, and add water. With a glass rod, break the vial. The solution is stable if kept refrigerated and protected from light. Stock solution should be stored away from other chemicals since osmium vapors may escape from bottle. Alternatively, aqueous solutions of osmium tetroxide in sealed glass ampules are available commercially. Dilute to 1–2% with cacodylate buffer for use.

3. Add the BSA to the buffer with stirring. High-salt Tween-20 buffer or PBS without calcium and magnesium may be substituted for TBS.
4. The concentration of the primary antibody can range from 1 to 20 μg/mL with 5 μg/mL being the average. If nonspecific staining is a problem, the antibody may be diluted in high-salt Tween-20 buffer.
5. The bridging antibody is directed against IgG of the same species as the primary antibody. For example, if the primary antibody is a mouse monoclonal, then the bridging antibody would be an anti-mouse IgG.
6. The colloidal gold should be diluted in PBS without calcium and magnesium containing 1% BSA or 0.01% polyethylene glycol (mol wt 20,000), or in TBS plus 1% BSA or 0.01% polyethylene glycol (mol wt 20,000).
7. Let the picric acid/water stand; it will keep indefinitely at room temperature.
8. Do not let the picric acid dry since the powder is explosive.
9. Add 1.33 g lead nitrate and 1.76 g sodium citrate to 30 mL glass-distilled water in a 50-mL volumetric flask. Shake vigorously for 1 min and allow to stand with intermittent shaking for 30 min. Add 8.0 mL 1 N NaOH. Dilute the suspension to 50 mL with deionized glass-distilled water and mix by inversion. The solution is stable up to 6 months. Turbidity can be removed by centrifugation.
10. The composition of the fixative may vary depending on the sensitivity of the antigen. For some antigens, it may be necessary to reduce the glutaraldehyde concentration, or omit it entirely and fix in 4% formaldehyde in PBS for 1–4 h (*see* Chapter 37).
11. 0.1 M Phosphate buffer, pH 7.4, may be substituted for PBS.
12. The amino group on the glycine will bind to any free aldehyde groups left on the cells after fixation, and prevent them from binding to the antibody or blocking solution and increasing the nonspecific background. Following fixation in formaldehyde or glutaraldehyde, tissue is generally quenched. The purpose of this step is to block any free aldehyde groups that remain after fixation and washing. This step is especially critical after glutaraldehyde fixation. Glutaraldehyde is a bifunctional aldehyde. During fixation, one end may bind to cellular constituents, leaving the other end free to react. If this end is not blocked, it can bind to the protein in the blocking solution or to the primary antibody. Although any small molecular-weight compound containing an amino group may

be used, the most commonly used quenching agents are glycine, ammonium chloride, and sodium borohydride.

13. If the samples are to be embedded in a resin that is polymerized by UV, such as Lowicryl or LR Gold, do not postfix in osmium tetroxide. Any effect of the osmium on antigenicity can usually be eliminated by using sodium *meta*-periodate during etching (*see* step 7).
14. The choice of embedding resin can affect the degree of immunostaining. Although all embedding resins may be used, the epoxy resins, such as Epon substitutes and Spurr, can reduce the intensity of staining. The acrylic resins (LR White, LR Gold, and Lowicryl) are more hydrophilic and usually result in better immunolabeling (*see* Chapter 37).
15. Sections will adhere to the grids better during the staining process if after the sections are picked up, the grids are placed in a 60°C oven for an hour. The nickel grids can become magnetized and should be handled with nonmagnetic forceps. They may also need to be degaussed before viewing in the electron microscope, and the astigmatism may need to be adjusted for each grid.
16. Grids are floated, section side down, on drops of a freshly prepared saturated solution of sodium *meta*-periodate. If the primary antibody is directed against a carbohydrate-containing epitope, keep the exposure to the *meta*-periodate as brief as possible, because the *meta*-periodate may remove the carbohydrate. If this is a problem, it may be necessary to etch in hydrogen peroxide or sodium ethoxide. The incubation can be done in Petri dishes lined with parafilm or in spot plates. The time required for etching depends on the embedding resin and can vary from 30 min for Epon substitutes to <5 min for LR White and LR Gold. From this step until the staining is completed, the grids should not be allowed to dry.
17. Following quenching, the samples are blocked to reduce nonspecific binding of the primary antibody and to reduce the background. The proteins in the blocking solution are chosen so as not to react with the secondary antibody or detection system. They bind to sites in the samples that bind proteins through nonspecific interactions such as charge. Although 2–10% BSA is most commonly used, other proteins (e.g., ova albumin, normal serum, or IgG fractions) can also be used. The exact composition of the blocking solution may have to be determined empirically if background staining is high.
18. If the nonspecific staining is high, 0.1 M EDTA can also be added to the rinse solution.
19. Appropriate controls should always be run with any immunocytochemical procedure. Controls may include omitting the

primary antibody, substituting preimmune serum, normal serum, or normal IgG for the primary antibody, adsorbing the primary antibody against the antigen, or immunostaining with an unrelated antibody.

20. To enhance preservation, 3–5% purified sucrose and 0.5 mM calcium chloride may be added to the buffer.
21. Samples should be in capped glass vials during dehydration and infiltration.
22. Oxygen will inhibit polymerization.
23. Instead of hydrating the sections, they may be etched for 1 or 2 min with a freshly prepared saturated solution of sodium *meta*-periodate.

References

1. Romano EL, Romano M (1984) Historical aspects. In: Polak JM, Varndell LM (eds) Immunolabelling for electron microscopy. Elsevier, New York, NY, pp 3–16
2. Roth J (1982) The protein A-gold (pAg) technique-a qualitative and quantitative approach for antigen localization on thin sections. In: Bullock GR, Petrusz P (eds) Techniques in immunocytochemistry, vol 1. Academic Press, New York, NY, pp 107–154
3. Roth J (1984) The protein A-gold technique for antigen localization in tissue sections by light and electron microscopy. In: Polak JM, Varndell LM (eds) Immunolabelling for electron microscopy. Elsevier, New York, NY, pp 113–122
4. Slot JW, Geuze HJ (1984) Gold markers for single and double immunolabeling of ultrathin cryosections. In: Polak JM, Varndell LM (eds) Immunolabelling for electron microscopy. Elsevier, New York, NY, pp 129–142
5. Bendayan M (1989) Protein A-gold electron microscopic immunocytochemistry: methods, applications, and limitations. J Electron Microsc Tech 1:243–270
6. Bendayan M (1989) Protein A-gold and protein G-gold postembedding immunoelectron microscopy. In: Hayat MA (ed) Colloidal gold, vol 1. Academic Press, New York, NY, pp 34–95
7. Bendayan M, Stephens H (1984) Double immunostaining procedures: techniques and applications. In: Polak JM, Varndell LM (eds) Immunolabelling for electron microscopy. Elsevier, New York, NY, pp 143–154
8. Merighi A (1992) Postembedding electron microscopic immunocytochemistry. In: Polak JM, Priestley JV (eds) Electron microscopic immunocytochemistry. Oxford University Press, Oxford, UK, pp 51–88
9. Forsgren A, Sjöquist J (1966) 'Protein A' from *S. aureus*. 1. Pseudoimmune reaction with human γ-globulin. J Immunol 97:8 22–827
10. Björck L, Kronvall G (1984) Purification and some properties of streptococcal protein G, a novel IgG-binding reagent. J Immunol 133:969–974
11. Gasparyan VK (2005) Hen egg immunoglobulin Y in colloidal gold agglutination assay: comparison with rabbit immunoglobulin G. J Clin Lab Anal 19:124–127
12. Benhamou N (1989) Preparation and application of lectin-gold complexes. In: Hayat MA (ed) Colloidal gold, vol 1. Academic Press, New York, NY, pp 96–145
13. Bendayan M (1984) Enzyme-gold electron microscopic cytochemistry: a new affinity approach for the ultrastructural localization of macromolecules. J Electron Micros Tech 1:349–372
14. Reynolds ES (1963) The use of lead citrate at high pH as an electron opaque stain in electron microscopy. J Cell Biol 17:208–210
15. Berryman MA, Rodewald RR (1990) An enhanced method for postembedding immunocytochemical staining which preserves cell membranes. J Histochem Cytochem 38:16

Part VI

The Clinical Laboratory

Chapter 43

The Clinical Immunohistochemistry Laboratory: Regulations and Troubleshooting Guidelines

Patricia A. Fetsch and Andrea Abati

Abstract

The Clinical Laboratory Improvement Amendments (CLIA) set standards designed to improve the quality of all laboratory testing. In the first portion of this chapter, we discuss the CLIA requirements that apply to most Immunohistochemistry laboratories, and explain topics such as certification, test complexity, patient test management, proficiency testing, personnel, quality control, quality assurance, and compliance.

The second portion of this chapter addresses the most common problems encountered in immunohistochemical procedures and the appropriate solutions to correct them.

Key words: CLIA-88, Immunohistochemistry regulations, College of American Pathologists

1. Introduction

Immunohistochemical procedures have become an integral part of the clinical laboratory routine, evolving from a research tool to a diagnostic necessity in pathology. In some instances, immunohistochemical tests provide valuable information on prognosis as well as predictive response to anticancer therapies. As a specifically defined laboratory section, the Immunohistochemistry Laboratory must meet federally mandated standards of operation as defined in the Clinical Laboratory Improvement Amendments of 1988 (CLIA-88) (*see* Note 1)(1). These regulations set forth uniform quality standards for laboratories and apply to all entities that perform tests for health purposes on human specimens. All laboratories must register with the United States Department of Health and Human Services to obtain a CLIA certificate and pay a certificate fee. The published guidelines for the practice of pathology do not include regulations devoted exclusively to

C. Oliver and M.C. Jamur (eds.), *Immunocytochemical Methods and Protocols*, Methods in Molecular Biology, Vol. 588,
DOI 10.1007/978-1-59745-324-0_43, © Humana Press, a part of Springer Science+Business Media, LLC 1995, 1999, 2010

immunohistochemistry; however, within the Federal Register are CLIA regulations governing the use of "special histologic stains" in the practice of pathology which can be applied to the immunostaining procedures.

Discussed herein are the general requirements of the immunohistochemistry laboratory for compliance with CLIA-88. In addition, a troubleshooting guide for immunohistochemical procedures is included at the end.

2. Clinical Laboratory Regulations (CLIA-88)

Congress passed the Clinical Laboratory Improvement Amendments of 1988 to set criteria to improve the quality of clinical laboratory services. The goal of this law was to standardize laboratory testing across the United States in all sites conducting testing on human specimens for health assessment or for the diagnosis, prevention, or treatment of disease. Failure to comply with these requirements may result in sanctions by the Health Care Financing Administration (HCFA), whose task is that of implementing CLIA-88 (*see* Note 2). These sanctions may include changes in specific aspects of the laboratory operation, the suspension of part or all of Medicare payment for services, or even a complete shutdown of a facility. The regulations as printed in the Federal Register of Feb. 28, 1992 (Vol. 57, pp. 7001–7288) can be found in many regional, university, law, and reference libraries. In addition, the College of American Pathologists (CAP) provides a highly regarded laboratory accreditation program that may be of benefit prior to federal inspection (2). The guidelines discussed in this chapter provide a general reference for CLIA-88.

2.1. Procedure Manual

Procedure manuals should be well organized and contain a table of contents, all applicable procedures, and associated forms. The procedure manual must address all methods and antibodies currently in use. Procedures must be written in compliance with the Clinical and Laboratory Standards Institute (CLSI) GP2-A5 (3). Manufacturer's package inserts may be used to supplement a procedure but may not replace it. Technical procedures designed for the use at the bench should be complete, easy to follow, and readily available for testing personnel. These procedures must contain the following information for each assay performed:

1. *Title.* Concise and descriptive, clearly stating the intent of the document.
2. *Principle.* Open the document with a section that states its purpose, which may include information regarding the theory and clinical implications of the test.

3. *Specimen requirements.* Information regarding specimen type, collection, processing, storage, preservation, and the criteria for specimen rejection.
4. *Reagents, standards, and controls.* Instructions on preparation, labeling requirements, storage, and shelf life, and any special safety requirements (e.g., general category or class of hazard).
5. *Equipment/supplies.* Examples: staining racks, dishes, disposable pipettes, microscope slides, and other applicable supplies.
6. *Instrumentation/calibration.* Instructions for calibration and maintenance of automated equipment only for those activities that are performed each time the procedure is done. Instrument operators' manuals may be used to describe what the operator needs to do and how to do it.
7. *Step-by-step directions.* A detailed set of instructions for all methods, sample types (frozen tissue, formalin-fixed tissue, air dried imprints, cytologic preparations), and antibodies currently in use, including fixatives used and any pretreatment protocols required.
8. *Calculations.* Applies to quantitative procedures.
9. *Quality control.* Frequency and tolerance of controls, instructions for the documentation of quality control (QC) data and the corrective action to be taken if controls fail to meet the laboratory criteria for acceptability.
10. *Interpretation.* Reporting of results and expected values.
11. *Procedure notes.* Description of the course of action to be taken in the event that a test system becomes inoperable.
12. *Limitations.* Test sensitivity/specificity, interfering substances, etc.
13. *Safety precautions.* Instructions for collection and processing of biohazardous samples, chemical safety, and the use of chemical hoods and personal protective equipment (gloves, face shields).
14. *References.* Information such as the manufacturer's product literature, text books, and publications.
15. Author.
16. *Distribution.* Documentation that the procedure has been reviewed by all testing personnel.
17. *Effective date and schedule for review.* The laboratory director or designee reviews and signs all procedures; procedures must be re-signed and redated if there is a change in the laboratory director.

Technical approaches must be scientifically valid and clinically relevant, and documentation that the laboratory director or designee has reviewed all procedures on an annual basis is required. All changes are reviewed and approved before being placed in service, and the signed approvals of new and changed documents must be dated. A copy of discontinued procedures must be maintained for 2 years thereafter, recording initial date of use and retirement date.

2.2. Reagents

All reagents must be properly labeled and dated as to content and quality (i.e., titer, concentration), date prepared or received, when placed in service, expiration date, and storage requirements. If necessary, this information may be recorded on a log as long as reagent containers are identified so as to be traceable to the appropriate data in the log. Reagents must be stored as recommended by the manufacturer. If ambient temperature is indicated, there must be documentation that the defined temperature range is maintained, and corrective action is taken when tolerance limits are exceeded. The laboratory must routinely monitor the pH of buffers.

Reagent performance and adequacy are verified before placing the material in service. This can be accomplished through direct analysis of the new reagent or by parallel testing with reagents currently in use.

Antibody titration records are required for new antibody lots or when new antibodies are introduced into the laboratory. For newly introduced antibodies, this is accomplished by running the assay at various antibody dilutions using a known positive and negative control to determine the appropriate concentration for maximum sensitivity and specificity. Since incubation times, buffers, specimen processing, pretreatment conditions, fixation, and other processing reagents will affect the dilution used, optimal dilutions must be determined by each laboratory under its own special conditions. Parallel testing for new lots of established antibodies to verify optimum antibody titer and controls is usually sufficient.

Antibodies and other reagents for immunostaining are to be disposed off after the manufacturer's expiration date.

2.3. Equipment Maintenance

The daily monitoring of temperatures on various types of laboratory equipment is critical. Tissue processing temperatures (water baths, ovens) may affect the quality of immunohistochemical staining, and thus need to be verified each day. In addition, refrigerators and freezers require daily temperature checks, as the storage conditions of immunoreagents must be optimal for maintaining expected shelf life. If a "frost-free" freezer is in use, there must be assurance that the specimens, tissues, and reagents that are stored in that freezer are not damaged due to the cycle of freezing, thawing, and refreezing.

In accordance with Environmental Protection Agency guidelines, mercury thermometers should be eliminated and replaced with alcohol-based types. All thermometers are to be calibrated with an appropriate National Institute of Standards and Technology (NIST) thermometer when put in service and every 6 months thereafter. Large volume refrigerators/freezers can be monitored with an upper and lower limit alarm system or a recording thermometer.

Scheduled preventive maintenance is performed to prevent breakdowns or malfunctions, prolong the life of an instrument, and maintain optimum operating characteristics. For automated immunostainers, the performance and documentation of maintenance/function checks should be done as defined by the manufacturer with at least the frequency as specified. In general, common laboratory equipment such as pipettes, centrifuges, and balances need to be serviced or calibrated twice yearly.

All instrument maintenance, service, and repair records should be available to, and usable by, the technical staff operating the equipment. These records are to be retained for the life of the instrument. This information can be invaluable for troubleshooting purposes.

Specific guidelines for laboratory information systems include regulations for computer configuration, procedure manuals, system security, data entry/reports/retrieval, hardware and software, and system maintenance.

2.4. Quality Control

Controls are used to ensure proper technique and specificity of the stain. The use of similarly processed positive and negative staining controls is essential for the interpretation of immunohistochemical reactions and must be done for each antibody. These controls may be commercially prepared, previously tested patient samples, or proficiency testing specimens for which results have been confirmed.

The use of separate positive control tissues known to contain the antigen being evaluated must be included for each antigen in a run. It is most cost effective to use large in-house tissues that have been fixed with the regular workday's surgical cases for this type of control. Autopsy tissues may also be used as control material. For cytology, cell culture material, effusions, and fine needle aspiration material can be prepared in the form of cytospins and stored (unfixed, desiccated) at –20°C for 6–12 months for use as controls on similarly processed material. All controls should be fixed and prepared with the same protocol as the patient's slide material.

Internal or built-in controls are present when the specimen contains the target marker not only in the tumor to be identified, but also in adjacent normal tissue. The evaluation of internal controls (when present) can be used as an indication of appropriate immunoreactivity. For ubiquitous antigens, internal controls are acceptable for use as a positive control, but the laboratory manual must clearly state the manner in which internal positive controls are used on a case-by-case basis for quality assurance (QA).

A negative reagent control is used to assess nonspecific background staining of the specimen. In lieu of primary antibody, the use of nonimmune IgG from the same species as the primary antibody on one slide of each particular specimen is tested along with the rest of the case slides. Isotype-matched immunoglobulin negative controls, while optimal, are not always feasible and therefore not essential. If numerous pretreatment steps are performed (i.e., heat induced epitope retrieval (HIER), enzyme digestion), the negative reagent control is done using the most aggressive retrieval procedure in the particular antibody panel.

A negative tissue control is also assessed to verify that there is no staining of tissues known to lack the antigen. A separate negative tissue control for each antibody can be used, or the patient test slide itself may be used for this purpose if it contains appropriate tissue components known to lack the target antigens.

The quality control program must clearly define goals for monitoring performance, procedures, policies, tolerance limits, corrective action, and related information. Records must be maintained regarding the reactivity of positive and negative controls on a daily basis, along with an ongoing mechanism to evaluate the corrective actions taken when a control is unacceptable. These quality control records must be maintained for 2 years.

2.5. Storage of Slides

The immunostained slides are filed with the remainder of slides from the case. Slides (and reports) are kept for a minimum of 10 years.

2.6. Quality Assurance

An active program of surveillance of the quality of the immunostains produced must be defined. The primary elements of such a QA program include procedures and policies for patient test management, quality control, proficiency testing, comparison of test results, relationship of clinical information to patient test results, personnel assessment, communications, complaint investigations, quality assurance review with staff, and quality assurance records. The documentation and review by the laboratory director of all QA procedures are imperative and cannot be overstressed. A brief explanation of each of the QA elements is as follows:

1. A patient test management system must assure optimum specimen integrity and identification from the pretesting to posttesting process. Criteria must be established for patient preparation, specimen collection, labeling, preservation, and transportation. An appropriate specimen identification and accessioning system is in place to minimize sample mixups. A turnaround time (i.e., the interval between specimen receipt by laboratory personnel and results reporting) for each test is defined and adhered to. Accuracy and reliability of test

reporting systems, appropriate storage of records, and prompt retrieval of test results should be included. Note: On all reports for tests using analyte specific reagents (ASR), a U.S. Food and Drug Administration (FDA)-required disclaimer is included which states that the FDA has not cleared these tests through the 510 (k) process. The mandatory language is as follows:

"These tests were developed and their performance characteristics determined by the *name of institution,* Pathology Laboratory. They have not been cleared or approved by the FDA. However, the FDA has determined that such clearance or approval is not necessary. These tests are used for clinical purposes. They should not be regarded as investigational or for research. This laboratory is certified under the Clinical Laboratory Improvement Amendments of 1988 (CLIA) as qualified to perform high complexity clinical laboratory testing." This disclaimer does not apply to immunohistochemistry reagents labeled by the manufacturer with directions for use and performance claims. For example, the HercepTest (DakoCytomation, Carpinteria, CA) is an FDA-approved test kit and is not classified as an ASR.

For immunohistochemical studies used to provide diagnostic predictive/prognostic information independent of other histologic findings (e.g., hormone receptors in breast cancer, HER-2/*neu,* EGFR), the laboratory should include in the patient report the type of specimen fixation and processing, antibody clone and detection system used, and the criteria used to determine a positive versus negative result and/or scoring system.

2. The laboratory must have an ongoing mechanism to evaluate corrective actions and review their effectiveness when quality control is unacceptable.
3. Successful participation in a CLIA-88 approved proficiency testing program is mandated. Proficiency testing determines how well a laboratory's results compare with those of other laboratories that use the same methodologies and can identify performance problems not recognized by internal mechanisms. Proficiency testing samples are tested along with the laboratory's regular workload by staff who usually perform the testing using routine methods. An example of this type of external audit system is the CAP, MK series, which provides two sets of challenges per year. Additional surveys are available for CD20, CD117, Her2/neu, Estrogen Receptor, and Epidermal Growth Factor Receptor. Written procedures of the proper handling, analysis, review, and reporting of proficiency testing materials are required. There must be evidence of the identification and review of problems discovered through the use of this program and the documentation of

corrective actions taken. If external proficiency testing is not available, blind testing of specimens with known results, exchange of specimens with other laboratories, or an equivalent system can be used to assess the reliability of test procedures on a semiannual basis. Under CLIA-88 regulations, interlaboratory communication about proficiency testing samples before the submission of data to the proficiency testing provider is strictly prohibited as is the referral of proficiency testing specimens to another laboratory. The documented review of proficiency testing reports are retained for 2 years.

4. When the laboratory uses different methodologies or instruments, or performs testing at multiple testing sites, a system has to be in place that evaluates and verifies the comparability between these test results. For example, correlation studies must ensure that manual and automated methods of immunostaining within a laboratory are in agreement. This must be documented biannually. In addition, any reference laboratories utilized must be CLIA-88 certified, and the lab director must monitor the quality of test results received from these outside sources.
5. A mechanism must be in place to evaluate immunohistochemical results that are inconsistent with clinicopathologic studies. This evaluation should be performed and recorded by a laboratory physician.
6. Personnel qualifications for high complexity testing are stated in the CLIA-88 regulations. The director of the laboratory must be a qualified physician or a doctoral level clinical scientist. Detailed job descriptions as well as a system of documenting that all analysts are knowledgeable about the contents of procedure manuals relevant to the scope of their testing activities are required. The competency of each person to perform the duties assigned must be assessed annually. Continuing education programs are an essential part of the laboratory quality improvement plan.
7. Documentation of problems due to breakdowns in communication, complaints reported to the laboratory, and records of the corrective action taken should be available. Quality assurance meetings with the staff are necessary to discuss problems identified and corrective actions taken to prevent reoccurrences.
8. Laboratory inspection programs assure that the laboratory maintains up-to-date documentation, procedure manuals, qualified personnel, and properly maintained laboratory equipment. Successful laboratory inspections are required to maintain accreditation by the Joint Commission on Health Care Organizations and the HCFA.

2.7. Safety/Environment

The work area should be well-lighted with sufficient space, and have the necessary water, air, gas, and electrical outlets.

Water quality (reagent grade II is appropriate for immunohistochemical procedures) must be regularly monitored as to bacterial contamination, resistivity, and silica content. If glassware is washed in the laboratory, a specific procedure is followed which requires rinsing with deionized or distilled water prior to drying, as well as a determination that glassware is free of cleaning agents prior to use.

Temperature and humidity are controlled to minimize evaporation of reagents and to keep performance of electronic equipment optimal. Ventilation is adequate for the removal of noxious fumes and odors. Formaldehyde and xylene vapor concentrations must be below the maximum permissible levels. For formaldehyde, this level is 0.75 ppm for an 8 h time weighted average, or 2.0 ppm for a 15 min short-term exposure. For xylene, the level is 100 for an 8 h time weighted average, and 200 for a 15 min short-term exposure. The monitoring of the work area and employees can be performed on a yearly basis. Chemical and biological safety cabinets are checked for proper airflow on a yearly basis.

Waste disposal of infectious specimens, contaminated materials, and chemicals must be in compliance with local, state, and federal regulations. Flammable safety cabinets are required for storage of alcohols, xylenes, and other combustible materials.

Safety policies and procedures are documented, and Material Safety Data Sheets are provided for all chemicals used in the laboratory. In addition, a chemical hygiene plan that defines the safety procedures for all hazardous chemicals is written in detail. All laboratory personnel must review these policies on an annual basis.

A documented ergonomics program should be in place to prevent musculoskeletal disorders in the workplace through prevention and engineering controls. Universal precautions training that complies with the Occupational Safety and Health Administration's standard on occupational exposure to blood borne pathogens as well as a fire training program should be provided on an annual basis for all laboratory employees. Personnel are required to use proper personal protective devices when handling corrosive, flammable, biohazard, or carcinogenic substances. Eye wash stations should be readily available and tested regularly.

3. Troubleshooting of Imunoperoxidase Assays (*See* Note 3 and Chapters 24 and 25)

When analyzing an immunostained specimen, deposits of the colored chromogen indicate the presence of the antigen and represent specific positive staining. The pattern of staining in the cells can be cytoplasmic, nuclear, membranous, or surface; focal or diffuse.

This section addresses some of the most common problems encountered in immunoperoxidase procedures and the appropriate solutions to correct them. Note that we address manual immunohistochemical staining methods only; see appropriate operator's manual for troubleshooting of automated immunostainers.

3.1. Absence of Staining

1. *Procedure not followed:* Perform staining steps in the correct order. Follow appropriate pretreatment protocols such as enzymatic digestion or HIER. Verify that reagents were prepared according to procedural requirements. Review manufacturer's package inserts.
2. *Sodium azide present in buffers:* The presence of sodium azide will prevent the development of the peroxidase color reaction.
3. *Improper fixation and processing:* Review manufacturer's package inserts for appropriate fixation techniques, as overfixation/wrong fixative can destroy antigens (4). Paraffin embedded tissue should never be exposed to temperatures >60°C as this can destroy some antigens. Do not store unstained slides (both cytologic smears and tissue sections) for long periods of time as this can diminish immunoreactivity of certain antigens. Follow appropriate pretreatment protocols (i.e., digestion, HIER).
4. *Drying out of specimens during staining:* Samples must be kept moist by applying sufficient reagent to prevent evaporation and by using a humidity chamber. When wiping off excess liquid, process only a few slides at a time. Repeated drying of specimens will result in poor morphology and staining. Slides must not be allowed to dry out at any time during or following the HIER procedure.
5. *Decolorization of stained slide:* Avoid decolorization procedures. Remove coverslip and rehydrate only prior to the start of the immunocytochemical procedure.
6. *Improper counterstain:* If alcohol soluble chromogens such as 3-amino-9-ethylcarbazole (AEC) are used, avoid counterstains containing alcohol, dehydration steps, and xylene/toluene based mounting media as they will dissolve soluble colored precipitates.

3.2. Weak Staining

1. *Too much buffer left on slides:* After rinsing, as much liquid as possible should be wiped from around the specimen to avoid the dilution of antibody.
2. *Use of old substrate:* Prepare chromogen immediately before use, or according to manufacturer's specifications.
3. *Incubation times too short:* Refer to laboratory procedure and manufacturer's antibody specifications.

4. *Antibody too dilute:* Verify appropriate titer.
5. *Improper storage/expired reagents:* Refer to manufacturer's antibody specifications for proper storage of reagents. Avoid the use of outdated reagents.

3.3. Excess Background Staining

Positive staining that is not a result of antigen–antibody binding is termed nonspecific background stain. The most common cause of this is the attachment of protein to highly charged collagen and connective tissue elements of the specimen. Therefore, it is imperative to consistently include a negative reagent control slide on all test samples for background staining assessment. There are a number of conditions which may contribute to excess background:

1. *Endogenous peroxidase activity not removed:* Perform peroxidase blocking step.
2. *Nonspecific binding of protein to the specimen:* Perform a protein block using nonimmune serum from same animal species as the secondary antibody to reduce nonspecific binding (3–5% solution for 20 min incubation). Use a higher concentration of salt in the buffer solutions, such as use of a 1:10 Tris:saline solution. Do not use albumin when preparing cytospin slides or use gelatin in histologic water baths; charged or silanated slides are optimal.
3. *Improper antibody dilutions:* Verify titer. The use of concentrated antibody solutions can cause high background. This is especially common when changes are made in the incubation times of a procedure: for example, 2 h incubation at room temperature is lengthened to 18 h at 4°C. It may also be observed when different specimen types (paraffin versus frozen tissue) are being tested.
4. *Improper fixation:* Verify appropriate fixative and time of fixation. Check that specimen is not too thick so that fixative can penetrate completely.
5. *Paraffin incompletely removed:* Follow appropriate deparaffinization procedures. Use fresh xylene baths.
6. *Improper rinsing of slides:* Slides should be rinsed thoroughly after each incubation in three buffer baths. The only exception to not rinsing is after incubation with the blocking serum. Use fresh solutions in buffer baths.
7. *Overdevelopment of substrate reaction:* Check for excess chromogen in the solution, a high concentration of antigen in the specimen, or increased temperatures that can cause an accelerated reaction. Polyclonal antibodies, in particular, should be monitored carefully during the substrate reaction.
8. *Excessive application of tissue adhesive:* Use charged or silanated microscope slides when mounting the specimen. Avoid the use of gelatin in histology water baths.

9. *Increased thickness of specimen:* Tissue sections should be cut 4–5 μm thick, cell smears should be spread as thinly as possible, and cytospins should only be a monolayer in thickness.
10. *Endogenous biotin:* Endogenous biotin is usually found in high concentrations in kidney, liver, brain, and adipose tissue. Samples from these tissues and their metastases can show a false-positive staining artifact and a high level of background staining in procedures that employ avidin or steptavidin-conjugated detection systems. Endogenous biotin can be blocked by preincubation of the sample with a dilute avidin solution, followed by incubation with a dilute biotin solution before the application of the primary antibody.
11. *Microwave heating:* Perform biotin block step following microwave antigen retrieval (5).
12. *Necrotic tissue:* Autopsy tissues may be suboptimal for immunocytochemical studies due to compromised antigen preservation.
13. *Effusion samples:* Immunocytochemical stains should be performed on formalin-fixed, paraffin embedded cell block sections.

3.4. Positive Control Acceptable/Specimen Stains Weakly

1. *Improper fixation and processing of specimen:* Process controls and patient samples in an identical manner.
2. Antigen present in low concentration.
3. *Excess buffer or nonimmune serum allowed to remain on specimen:* Remove excess buffer before application of antibodies.
4. *Antigen partly destroyed or masked by fixation:* If the antigen was masked due to overfixation in formalin, the use of enzyme digestion or HIER prior to the application of the primary antibody may increase the staining intensity (*see* Chapter 8).

3.5. Artifacts

1. *Undissolved granules of chromogen or counterstain:* Precipitates are not confined to cells but spread randomly across the specimen. This can be corrected by filtering the chromogen or counterstain.
2. *Mercury deposits:* This is observed as a black precipitate which is spread randomly across the specimen. It can be corrected by removing the mercury through dezenkerization of B5-fixed material prior to immunostaining.
3. *Bacterial or yeast contamination:* Practice sanitary laboratory techniques.
4. *Pigments such a melanin and hemosiderin:* These differ in texture and color from the chromogen, but may be difficult for interpretation. However, the negative control will demonstrate their true character, and by using a chromogen of a contrasting

color (for example, AEC stains positive cells a red color) this problem can be minimized.

4. Notes

1. To order a copy of the Clinical Laboratory Improvement Amendments of 1988, mail request to: New Orders, Superintendent of Documents, P.O. Box 371954, Pittsburgh, PA 15250-7954. Telephone 202-512-1800; FAX 202-512-2250.
2. Additional resources for assistance in meeting CLIA-88 regulations can be obtained from:
   (a) Clinical and Laboratory Standards Institute (CLSI), 940 West Valley Road, Suite 1400, Wayne, PA 19087-1898, USA. Telephone: 610-688-0100; FAX: 610-688-0700; E-mail: standard@clsi.org; Website: wwwclsi.org
   (b) College of American Pathologists (CAP), 325 Waukegan Road, Northfield, IL 60093-2750. 800-323-4040. FAX 800-289-1815.
   (c) Health Care Financing Administration (HCFA), P.O. Box 26687, Baltimore, MD 21207-0487. 410-290-5850.
   (d) Occupational Safety and Health Administration (OSHA), Dept. of Labor, 200 Constitution Ave NW, N3647, Washington, DC. 202-219-8151.
   (e) O'Leary TJ (2001) Standardization in immunohistochemistry. Appl Immunohistochem Mol Morphol 9:3–8
3. Additional resources for troubleshooting assistance can be found in:
   (a) Bourne J. (1983) Handbook of immunoperoxidase staining methods. DAKO Corp.: Carpinteria, CA.
   (b) Wordinger R., Miller G., and Nicodemus D. (1987) Manual of immunoperoxidase techniques, 2nd ed. ASCP (Chicago, IL).
   (c) Fetsch P., Abati A. (2003) Ancillary Techniques, in *Atlas of Difficult Diagnosis in Cytopathology* (Atkinson, B.F. and Silverman, J.F., eds.) 2nd ed., pp. 747–806. W.B. Saunders (Philadelphia, PA).
   (d) Taylor C.R., Shi S-R., Barr N.J., and Wu N. (2002) Techniques of Immunohistochemistry: Principles, Pitfalls, and Standardization, in *Diagnostic Immunohistochemistry* (Dabbs, D.J., ed.), pp. 3–43. Churchill Livingstone (Philadelphia, PA).

References

1. Department of Health and Human Services, Health Care Financing Administration (2003) Clinical Laboratory Improvement Amendments of 1988: final rule. Fed Regist 68:3640–3714
2. College of American Pathologists Laboratory Accreditation Program (2007) Standards for laboratory accreditation, Commission on Laboratory Accreditation inspection checklist, Laboratory general and anatomic pathology checklists. College of American Pathologists, Northfield, IL
3. Clinical and Laboratory Standards Institute (2007) The CLSI Procedure Manual Toolkit: improving procedure writing in the clinical laboratory, CLSI document GP02–A5-C. CLSI, Wayne, PA
4. Battifora H (1990) Assessment of antigen damage in immunohistochemistry: the vimentin internal control. Anat Pathol 96:669–671
5. Rodriguez-Soto J, Warnke R, Rouse R (1997) Endogenous avidin-binding activity in paraffin-embedded tissue revealed after microwave treatment. Appl Immunohistochem 5:59–62

INDEX

MIX
Papier aus verantwortungsvollen Quellen
Paper from responsible sources
FSC® C105338

If you have any concerns about our products,
you can contact us on
ProductSafety@springernature.com

In case Publisher is established outside the EU,
the EU authorized representative is:
Springer Nature Customer Service Center GmbH
Europaplatz 3, 69115 Heidelberg, Germany

Printed by Libri Plureos GmbH
in Hamburg, Germany